THE PSYCHOLOGY OF SEX ROLES

THE PSYCHOLOGY OF SEX ROLES

Edited by David J. Hargreaves and Ann M. Colley

University of Leicester

⭘ **HEMISPHERE PUBLISHING CORPORATION**
A subsidiary of Harper & Row, Publishers, Inc.

Cambridge   New York   Philadelphia   San Francisco   London
Mexico City   São Paulo   Singapore   Sydney   Washington

THE PSYCHOLOGY OF SEX ROLES

1 2 3 4 5 6 7 8 9 0   H R U K   8 9 8 7

Library of Congress Cataloging in Publication Data

The Psychology of sex roles.

 Includes bibliographies and indexes.
  1. Sex role—Psychological aspects. 2. Identification
(Psychology) I. Hargreaves, David, 1948–
II. Colley, Ann M. [DNLM: 1. Identification (Psychology)
BF 692.2 P9745]
BF692.2.P77   1987   155.3′3   87-17708
ISBN 0-89116-776-5

CONTENTS

EDITORS' INTRODUCTION

This book is a review of psychological research on sex roles. The growth of interest in sex roles has been extremely rapid over the last decade or so, and their explanation has become a central concern in disciplines including sociology, anthropology and education as well as in psychology. These different perspectives all contribute towards the new interdisciplinary fields of Women's Studies and Men's Studies. Any surveys in such broad and socially important fields will inevitably have their own biases and selective emphases: it is almost certainly better to acknowledge these and to make them explicit than to deny that they exist. Like ourselves, the majority of our contributors are psychologists who are actively engaged in empirical research: the book reflects this bias, and could perhaps be regarded as an attempt to provide the objective empirical background to the pressing social issues.

It may be useful to distinguish between what is commonly thought of as research on *sex differences* and that on *sex roles*. The former has largely been concerned with the identification and measurement of discrepancies between the *levels* of male and female performance on a wide range of psychological variables — measures of thinking, personality, attitudes, skills and so on. Until relatively recently, such research was likely to have been carried out as subsidiary to some more substantive line of investigation: but the publication of Maccoby and Jacklin's (1974) comprehensive handbook on sex differences clearly established that the field now has its own intrinsic interest. Research on *sex roles*, whilst overlapping to a considerable extent with that on sex differences, is more concerned with explaining the ways in which psychological differences between the sexes are structured and maintained by the process of *socialization*. It is concerned, in other words, with the way in which (biological) males and females become (psychologically) masculine and feminine: with people's progression along what Archer (1984) calls the *developmental pathways* of sex roles.

The book is in three main parts: the four chapters in Part I provide the theoretical background for what is to follow. In Chapter 1, Chris Singleton surveys sex roles from a variety of disciplinary perspectives, adopting a transactional approach to biological and social influences upon them. One useful strategy is to look at abnormal cases in trying to unravel these influences, and Singleton contrasts the phenomena of transsexualism, homosexuality and transvestism in doing so. In Chapter 2, David Hargreaves reviews and evaluates the psychological theories that have been developed to explain sex-role stereotyping. He surveys three traditional theories, namely psychoanalytic theory, social learning theory and cognitive-developmental theory, and then looks at the distinctions between masculinity, femininity and 'psychological androgyny' in the light of recent developments such as gender schema theory. In Chapters 3 and 4, Sarah Hampson and Chris Singleton consider the ways in which sex roles manifest themselves in the general areas of personality and thinking respectively. Hampson emphasizes that sex roles in personality are socially constructed, discussing them in terms of the cognitive basis of the individual's self-concept: and Singleton looks at the cognitive aspects of sex roles from the point of view of differential patterns of ability.

Part II of the book covers the developmental aspects of the sex role system from infancy through to adolescence. In Chapter 5 Charlie Lewis reviews the rapidly growing empirical literature on sex roles in infants and toddlers. A good deal of this work has investigated the influence of mothers and fathers, and Lewis argues for an 'ecological' understanding of early sex-role development. Peter Smith follows this through into the preschool and school years in Chapter 6, emphasizing the importance of the child's own understanding of gender roles in the process of their formation. In Chapter 7, 'Family and sex roles in middle childhood', John and Elizabeth Newson present some original data from their own well-known longitudinal research on social patterns of child-rearing: this work fills a significant and sizeable lacuna in developmental research. The immense influence of the school system upon sex-role behaviour is evaluated by Colin Rogers in Chapter 8: and Clive Hollin undertakes a thorough and systematic review of theories and research on sex roles in adolescence, in Chapter 9.

Sex roles exert their ubiquitous influence in just about every sphere of adult life: six of these are documented in Part III. Kevin Durkin considers the pervasive influence of the mass media in Chapter 10, suggesting that research on *counterstereotyping* has important future implications for theory as well as for practice. In Chapter 11, Oonagh Hartnett and Jenny Bradley discuss how sex roles structure the working lives of men and women. They apply a psychological perspective to account for the different employment patterns of the two sexes, and point out that most of the research to date has emphasized problems associated with female employment patterns. They suggest that, particularly at a time when unemployment is high, there are problems in male employment patterns which should be given more attention. In Chapter 12 Ann Colley reviews empirical literature in the complementary area of leisure and sport participation. Constraints on leisure participation which result from the division of labour and responsibility within the home are discussed, and the effects of sex-stereotyping on sport participation are examined.

In Chapter 13 Suzanne Skevington critically evaluates findings which suggest that the mental disorders suffered by men and women differ in frequency and type. Social and psychological factors which influence the occurrence and reporting of symptoms are examined, and some emphasis is placed on the concept of 'control'. Kevin Howells discusses sexual maladjustment, homosexual behaviour, and sexual aggression in Chapter 14, exploring the implications of recent empirical and theoretical work on sex roles for the explanation of these three types of behaviour. Finally, in Chapter 15, Ann Taylor examines the theoretical and empirical evidence for diminished sex-role stereotyping of behaviour in old age.

We should like to thank Naomi Roth for her help and support in the planning stages of the book, and also Rita-Jean Benford and Margaret Frape for secretarial assistance.

References

Archer, J. (1984) Gender roles as developmental pathways. *British Journal of Social Psychology*, *23*, 245–256.
Maccoby, E. E. & Jacklin, C. N. (1974) *The psychology of sex differences*. Stanford, California: Stanford University Press.

LIST OF CONTRIBUTORS

Ann Colley: Department of Psychology, University of Leicester, Leicester LE1 7RH.

Kevin Durkin: Social Psychology Research Unit, University of Kent at Canterbury, Beverley Farm, Canterbury, Kent CT2 7LZ.

Sarah Hampson: Department of Psychology, Birkbeck College, University of London, Malet St., London WC1E 7HX.

David Hargreaves: Department of Psychology, University of Leicester, Leicester LE1 7RH.

Oonagh Hartnett and Jenny Bradley: Department of Applied Psychology, University of Wales Institute of Science and Technology, Llwyn-y-Grant, Penylan, Cardiff CF3 7UX.

Clive Hollin: Department of Psychology, University of Leicester, Leicester LE1 7RH.

Kevin Howells: Department of Psychology. University of Birmingham, Birmingham B15 2TT.

Charlie Lewis: Department of Psychology, University of Reading, Building 3, Earley Gate, Whiteknights, Reading RG6 2AL.

John and Elizabeth Newson: Child Development Research Unit, University of Nottingham, University Park, Nottingham NG7 2RD.

Colin Rogers: Department of Educational Research, University of Lancaster, Cartmel College, Bailrigg, Lancaster LA1 4YL.

Chris Singleton: Department of Psychology, University of Hull, Hull HU6 7RX.

Suzanne Skevington: School of Humanities and Social Sciences, University of Bath, Claverton Down, Bath BA2 7AY.

Peter K. Smith: Department of Psychology, University of Sheffield, Sheffield S10 2TN.

Ann Taylor: Department of Psychology, University of Leicester, Leicester LE1 7RH.

PART I

THEORETICAL BACKGROUND

CHAPTER ONE **Biological and Social Explanations of Sex-Role Stereotyping**
C. H. Singleton

Introduction

The development of the child integrates and reintegrates biological and environmental influences in a complex transactional process. Both the individual and the environment are continuously changing over time, and the reciprocal interaction between them, which moulds and directs psychological growth, is fluid and dynamic. But while researchers may appear to endorse a transactional model of development in general terms, such endorsement rarely finds expression in more specific theorizing. It is not just that transactionality is conceptually difficult: in fact, the main problem lies in translating it into testable theory.

This gulf between the complexity of general models and the relative simplicity of specific theories is still very apparent in research on sex-role stereotyping. The merits of the transactional approach and the similar but somewhat more static interactional approach have been proclaimed (e.g. Archer & Lloyd 1974, 1982; Lewis 1975, 1982; Parsons 1980, Petersen 1980; Singleton 1978; Sameroff 1977) but when one looks for theories which manifest real integration of biological and environmental factors in the explanation of some aspect of sex-role stereotyping the transactional ethos is found to have evaporated and the residue which remains has either a strongly biological or a strongly environmental taint to it. Petersen (1980) has argued that a comprehensive transactional view – which she refers to as the 'biopsychosocial model' – cannot be formulated into a proper model at all since it is overidentified – i.e. it contains too much information relative to the number of parameters to be estimated. But it can be useful in structuring our concepts.

The ubiquitous term 'sex role' has rarely been defined with clarity. Angrist (1969) observed that its usage differed across disciplines, in anthropology referring to social positions, in sociology more to social relationships, and in psychology to differences in behaviour, personality and ability. The predominant view in psychology at the present time is that the term 'sex role' refers to the set of behaviours and characteristics that are typical of men and women, and that 'sex-role stereotype' refers to consensual beliefs about those characteristics. There is some debate as to how this distinction relates to that between descriptive and prescriptive beliefs (see Archer 1984). The term 'sex-typing' is usually taken to mean the process whereby males and females come to have role characteristics different from the other sex and different in degree to other members of their own sex (Archer 1980; Pleck 1981; Spence & Helmreich 1978).

Sex roles are shaped by common social assumptions and expectations about masculinity and femininity – that boys should be tough and girls should be tender, for example. Such assumptions readily become stereotyped, for it is easy for people to use their notions of the 'typical male' and the 'typical female' in assigning attributes to a person or in responding to them. Furthermore, the categories 'male' and 'female' are dichotomous, so there is an inevitable tendency for this dichotomy to be reflected in sex-role stereotypes, with the result that traits are regarded as *either* masculine *or* feminine. With the ascription of distinct traits comes the assignment of distinct life-styles and role options. As children grow up they become increasingly aware that to step outside the conventional stereotyped boundaries is to be regarded as abnormal, or even psychologically unhealthy. The mentally healthy man, for example, is typically portrayed by clinicians as aggressive, independent, objective and autonomous, while the mentally healthy woman is seen as submissive, dependent, subjective and suggestible (Broverman *et al.* 1970).

The perplexing questions the psychologist must face here are: why does 'society' expect male and female roles to conform to these stereotypes, and from where comes the psychological force which generally constrains our behaviour into these stereotyped or normative patterns? A naive answer might be that we have all been socialized to behave in this manner, but this fails to resolve the question of why socialization pressures have created these particular stereotypes rather than any others. An alternative, but equally naive retort might be that our social roles accord with our biological functions – for example that women are nurturant because their biology destines them to become mothers, and men are aggressive because their biology preordains them to become fathers. Among other things, this answer assumes that the biological basis of psychological differences between the sexes is a straightforward matter, which is a very long way from the truth (Maccoby & Jacklin 1975; Singleton 1978).

To attempt serious answers to these issues clearly requires consideration not only of social and biological factors but also of the complex and dynamic interaction between the two. Environment works upon the biological base, but at the same time biology is continuously being modified by the environment, so that biological differences between the sexes can become amplified or attenuated in the processes of child-rearing and socialization. We need to decide how we are to establish the existence of a biological basis for sex-role stereotyping: and if such a basis does exist, what its nature might be.

The search for a biological basis

In what ways might biological influences on sex roles be established? Two ways spring readily to mind. The first is to look for similarities in sex-role behaviour between animals and humans. The second is to look for evidence of sex role-related differences in young infants. Neither are very satisfactory. Comparisons of humans and animals are notoriously problematic because although we may formulate general conceptual similarities between the two, when it comes to testing specific hypotheses we have to compare overt behaviour, and here we run into difficulties. For example, if we wanted to make comparisons between humans and animals in terms of aggression, in animals our measures would refer to threat displays, latency of attack, duration and outcome of fights, etc., whereas in humans our measures would probably refer to verbal hostility, teachers' ratings of assertiveness, self-report inventories, etc. How are we to assess valid correspondence here?

Investigation of sex differences in early infancy is motivated by the conviction that the effects of the culture are at a minimum at this time, and therefore that any biological factors should reveal themselves in relatively 'pure' form. Accurate assessment of infant behaviours is methodologically difficult because of the fluctuating state of the baby and the general inconsistency of response. Moreover, since female infants develop more rapidly than male infants in some respects, early sex differences may merely be reflections of developmental differences. Actually, it turns out that there are few behavioural gender differences detectable during the early years of life which cannot be attributed to maturational sex differences (Maccoby & Jacklin 1975). Baby boys tend to be larger, stronger in some respects, and sometimes more irritable than baby girls, who are by contrast generally more responsive to tactile and oral stimulation. The importance of these seemingly minor differences is that they may provide a foundation upon which several important aspects of sex-role stereotypes can be built by the amplifying effect of parental responses and child-rearing practices generally

(Singleton 1978). Subtle differences between boys and girls at birth can initiate differential parental treatment that amplifies differences in the offspring, which in turn can bring about further modification of parental behaviour, and so on. Sex-role stereotypes are therefore created within the reciprocal processes of child-rearing (see Chapter 5).

Studies of sex-related differences in animals and in human infants are therefore not as helpful in teasing out biological influences as might have been imagined. This leaves us with two further principal areas of research which may shed light on the problem, and these are: studies of hormonal variation in animals and humans; and studies within a broad anthropological or cross-cultural framework. The rationale behind the former is that hormonal sex differences, particularly in the prenatal period, influence brain differentiation which in turn predisposes differential role behaviours. In the latter category, the identification of sex-role stereotypes which are universal across all cultures would arguably provide support for a biological basis for such stereotypes.

It is the purpose of this chapter to examine these two important areas of research in some detail in order to discover what explanations of the processes of sex-role stereotyping they have generated. Although some evaluation of these explanations will be made as we progress through the research work, I will conclude with an attempted synthesis and overall evaluation from the transactional point of view.

The process of sexual differentiation

One of the first things which happens after a baby is born is the assignment of gender on the basis of external genital appearance. This raises the question of whether gender identity – our personal feelings of being a male or a female – is normally dependent upon being labelled a boy or a girl, and on the social consequences of gender labelling. Although most children are able to appreciate gender by about three years of age (Thompson 1975) the awareness that gender is an unvarying state does not stabilize until about seven (Slaby & Frey 1975; Wehren & Di Lisi 1983), and attitudes towards the meaning of one's own gender are subject to modification throughout the lifespan (Livson 1983). Adolescence, the early years of marriage, and late adulthood are periods of particular vulnerability in this respect (Katz 1979) and special problems may also arise in cases of infertility (Karahasanoglu, Barglow & Growe 1972). Hence, in its fullest sense, gender identity is not a straightforward matter, but its foundation is normally established in mid-childhood. In most cases this identity is congruent with the sex role adopted by the individual, although incongruities do arise occasionally: for example, in cases of transvestism and transsexuality, and sometimes when there are anomalies in sexual differentiation.

Before we consider these issue, however, we must first have some understanding of the main factors involved in the process of prenatal sexual differentiation. At conception the sex chromosome of the father's sperm (X or Y) determines the child's genetic sex (XX for a female and XY for a male). The presence of a Y chromosome in the embryo stimulates the gonadal buds to develop into testes. In the absence of a Y chromosome the buds normally begin to differentiate into ovaries. Thereafter the sex chromosomes appear to have no influence in the process. The embryo also possesses potential internal female (Mullerian) and male (Wolffian) structures. The testes secrete androgenic (male) sex hormones which cause the Wolffian structures to develop into the internal male reproductive organs and inhibit the development of the Mullerian ducts. Without this hormonal inhibition the Mullerian ducts develop without the necessity of further stimulation into the internal female genitalia. It should be emphasized here that the commonly used terms 'male sex hormones' and 'female sex hormones' are misleading, for both 'male' (androgenic) and 'female' (estrogenic) hormones are produced by males and females. The mature male usually produces more androgens than estrogens and the mature female usually produces more estrogens than androgens, but both types have a pervasive influence on bodily functions (Petersen 1979). The prenatal hormonal mix also determines how the external genitalia will develop: if androgenic then the pattern will be male, otherwise female. Androgenic hormones also act upon the developing brain of the fetus causing the hypothalamus and pituitary gland to adopt an acyclical (male) rather than a cyclical (female) pattern of hormonal activity from puberty onwards (Wilson 1978).

Thus at each stage of the process, if male differentiation does not occur, female differentiation will result automatically and does not depend upon the prior presence of ovaries. This is illustrated in the clinical condition known as Turner's syndrome, in which the individual has a missing sex chromosome so that the pattern is not XX or XY but XO. In such individuals there are no ovaries yet both internal and external genitalia are clearly female, although somewhat immature in form owing to the absence of gonadal hormones. By contrast, in Klinefelter's syndrome, which is characterized by an XXY pattern, the presence of the additional X chromosome, while not preventing the differentiation of male genitals, does result in the expression of some female features at puberty, such as breast development and lack of facial hair. Mental retardation is common in these individuals which makes assessment of gender identity and sex role somewhat inconclusive (Scott & Thomas 1973). However, girls with Turner's syndrome are reported to exhibit conventionally feminine behaviour and interest patterns (Ehrhardt, Greenberg & Money 1970).

At one time it was believed that the presence of additional Y chromosomes (XYY, XYYY, etc.) causes hyperaggressiveness, and for this reason individuals with this type of chromosome pattern have been described as 'supermales'. It is now clear however, that this conclusion may have resulted from the fact that early studies were carried out on prison populations in which XYY males appear to be over-represented. An associated finding, that XYY males are likely to be mentally retarded remains controversial, but it seems fairly clear that even if not hyperaggressive they nevertheless exhibit typically masculine patterns of behaviour (Owen 1972).

Hormonal studies in animals

It has been well known for some time that in the rat, modification of the hormonal environment at birth can result in alterations in adult sexual behaviour. Levine (1966) suggested that there is a critical period during which the presence or absence of the male sex hormone testosterone has a permanent effect on the sex hormone receptivity of the brain. If the androgenic hormone testosterone is present during this critical period it is argued that it permanently desensitizes the animal, whether male or female, to female hormones. Thus injection of testosterone into newborn female rats eradicates the normal female sexual response and this is not restored by subsequent injections of female hormones. If subsequently injected with testosterone, however, she does tend to exhibit male sexual behaviour patterns. By contrast, male rats castrated at birth and given female sex hormones tend to adopt typically female sexual behaviour.

In other species similar organizational effects of androgens have been postulated. In the female guinea pig the prenatal administration of androgens results in genital, physiological and psychosexual masculinization (Goy 1970). In rhesus monkeys, the organizing action of testosterone appears to be completed at or shortly after birth so that castration has little effect on normal male behaviour patterns, whereas female offspring of pregnant mothers treated with testosterone tend to exhibit characteristically male patterns of behaviour (Phoenix 1974).

These studies lend some support to the idea that testosterone organizes the brain and nervous system during a critical period so that the behavioural repertoire of males and females is differentially primed (Reinisch 1974; Timiras 1982). There are, however, factors which prevent us from being sure about this. Linton (1971) has pointed out that the observed behavioural differences in the experimentally treated animals may in some respects be due to differential responses by their peers triggered by pheromones or by perceived differences in physical appearance. Furthermore, in these research studies attention has usually been confined to sexual behaviour, rough-and-tumble play, and threat behaviour. Many other sex-related behaviours, including maternalism, were not evaluated. However, Quadagno, Briscoe and Quadagno (1977) claim that androgenized female rats do not exhibit reduced maternal behaviour. Nor should it be forgotten that the behaviours assessed in these studies are subject to considerable environmental influence. For example, play and sexual behaviour are seriously disrupted in rhesus monkeys reared in isolation or socially reared in the laboratory (Phoenix 1978).

While perinatal androgens influence the display of aggression in several species, there are considerable differences both within and across species, such that one cannot conclude simply that hormone exposure induces changes in the brain which increase aggression (Quadagno, Briscoe & Quadagno 1977). Perhaps this is not surprising in view of the finding that in older animals, experiences of aggressive encounters generally play an important role in determining reactions to androgen treatment, and hormone levels tend to vary as a function of social experience and environmental conditions (Rogers 1976). Finally, although we might wish to accept that these experimental studies with animals demonstrate a relationship between hormones and various behaviours, the implications of such findings for sex-role development and gender identity in humans are not at all clear. Even across different rodent species, and in some cases within species, we find considerable variation which makes generalization very difficult. As we progress further up the evolutionary scale we find a weakening of the effects of hormones on behaviour as the roles of learning and experience increase in importance. Furthermore, the generalization of findings from animal studies such as these to humans is highly questionable.

Sex hormone anomalies

Experimental fetal androgenization in animals has its clinical counter-part in the adrenogenital syndrome in human beings. In this syndrome the fetus is exposed to excess androgenic hormones due to a genetic defect, the effect of which is a masculinization of the external genitalia of the female proportional to the amount of androgen excess. In extreme cases this may result in a male gender assignment at birth, but partial masculinization is usually corrected by surgery. Similar effects can be caused by synthetic hormones administered for medical reasons to pregnant women (progestin-induced hermaphroditism). Studies of surgically corrected females with adrenogenital syndrome suggest that they are usually more active, independent and energetic than matched controls, and researchers have generally portrayed them as tomboys who are not dissatisfied to be girls (Ehrhardt & Baker 1974). Although these findings might indicate that gender identity and sex-role behaviour are both hormonally determined, there are other factors which should be taken into account in considering these cases. The energetic, tomboyish behaviour of girls with adrenogenital syndrome may be a side-effect of drug therapy, for the drug commonly used to counter the effects of the syndrome is cortisone, which itself increases activity level (Quadagno, Briscoe & Quadagno 1977). Nor can socialization effects be ruled out, for the parents may have consciously or unconsciously treated these children as 'boyish' (Huston 1983).

The adrenogenital syndrome may be compared with cases in which boys have been prenatally exposed to large doses of estrogens which have been administered to their diabetic mothers to prevent miscarriage. These boys appear to be less assertive, less athletic, and less interested in typically male activities than matched controls (Ehrhardt & Meyer-Bahlburg 1981; Yalom, Green & Fisk 1973).

Animal studies in which the testes have been removed during the critical period for brain differentiation are paralleled by the androgen insensitivity syndrome in human beings. In this rare condition, also known as testicular feminization, genetic males with testes are insensitive to androgens. Their bodies respond to naturally circulating estrogens and consequently female external genitalia are formed, and female secondary sexual characteristics develop at puberty. These individuals are raised as females and their sex-role behaviour and gender identity appear to be no different from normal women (Masica, Money & Ehrhardt 1971). In cases of partial androgen insensitivity which occur in either sex, Money and Ogunro (1974) report that sexual orientation, role and identity all follow the sex of rearing almost invariably.

It should be noted that many methodological problems are associated with the studies of human sex hormone anomalies. In particular, the small size of the samples in some of the studies, and the heavy reliance on interview data rather than direct impartial observation, is of concern. These difficulties lead us to draw conclusions of only a tentative nature until more rigorous studies have been conducted. Even the reliable observation of clear behavioural differences would not rule out non-biological mechanisms of influence in many of these cases, for the awareness of genital abnormality may well affect the child's self-perception and the family's perception of the child. For example, in the adrenogenital syndrome it is possible that the masculinizing effect on the genitals changes the family's attitudes towards the girl and her behaviour as well as the girl's feelings about herself. This would amply a cognitive mediational process rather than a direct physiological influence on behaviour.

Psychosexual neutrality?

In their review of studies of sex hormone anomalies Money and Ehrhardt (1972) concluded that the most important factor in the development of sex-role and gender identity is the assigned sex of rearing. Provided the parents have no ambivalence or uncertainty about the child's sexual identity and the child has been raised consistently in his or her assigned sex, Money predicts that the socially imposed identity will normally be accepted. This view, which had been described as psychosexual neutrality, was supported by Hampson (1965) and Lev-Ran (1974), but strongly criticized by Hutt (1972, 1978) and Zuger (1970). Hutt argued that any incongruity between the sex of assignment, on the one hand, and the chromosomal gonadal or reproductive features on the other may be irrelevant to gender identity. Since the chromosomal constitution determines gonadal development in the normal process of sexual differentiation and the gonadal hormones in turn determine the nature of the genitalia, where there has been some aberration in some part of the sequence the elements antecedent to that point are no longer relevant in the same manner. Hence Hutt maintained that given an interruption of the normal sequence of events, the critical factor becomes the exposure, or not, to androgenic influences. The more masculinized the genital features, then correspondingly the more likely is the sex assignment to be male, but also the more likely is the brain to have been organized in a masculine pattern as a result of androgenic influence.

Hutt's critique loses some of its force in the face of one of Money's most dramatic cases, which illustrates the flexibility of gender identity during infancy (Money & Tucker 1975). As a result of a surgical accident during circumcision the penis of one of a pair of seven-month-old twin boys was destroyed. The parents decided to reassign the child as a girl and from then on treated the child in every way as a female. External female genitalia were subsequently constructed by means of plastic surgery, and hormone replacement therapy was provided. Money reported that this child grew up consistently thinking of herself as a girl, pursuing feminine activities, and anticipating a future as an adult woman. As the twins grew, their play interests diverged in stereotyped fashion, although the girl displayed an unusually high activity level.

The difficulties in changing gender identity once it is established, however, are demonstrated in some of the cases described by Money and Ehrhardt (1972) and by Stoller (1974). One such case reported by Stoller involved a genetic female with masculinized genitals who was raised as a boy until the age of six, when she commenced precocious puberty (which is not untypical in some of these conditions). On medical advice her parents reassigned her as a girl, but the outcome was disastrous. She was utterly miserable in her new gender, presenting a clumsy and grotesque appearance in girls' clothes, had very few friends and developed behaviour problems and other manifestations of psychological disturbance. This case suggests that the age of six is apparently much too late to alter gender identity successfully.

However, the qualification 'apparently' is important, for more recently Imperato-McGinley *et al.* (1979) have documented cases of a rare genetic disorder which can result in an incredible but relatively harmonious change in gender at puberty. These authors examined thirty-seven boys from the City of Santa Domingo in the Dominican Republic, who all manifested this particular dysfunction which disrupts testosterone metabolism so that male genitals are not properly formed during prenatal development. Of these thirty-seven boys, seventeen had been thought to be girls and had been raised as such. At puberty the activation of male hormones in these children caused masculinization of the genitals and the development of male secondary sexual characteristics — the 'girls' turned into boys. Despite normal female socialization, these boys are reported to make a fairly smooth transition from female to male role congruent with masculine gender identity and patterns of sexual interest and activity. The apparent ease of this gender transition is probably due in large part to the fact that this disorder is relatively common in that locality, and the sex change is accepted with equanimity by the parents and the community.

Imperato-McGinley *et al*. also investigated eight children in the United States who have this genetic disorder, but these children were all raised as girls after corrective surgery. At present in their teens, five of this group are reported to be experiencing serious difficulties in coping with their condition, which requires hormone injections to maintain female appearance and presents considerable obstacles to sexual and marital fulfilment. The comparison of the two samples not only implicates hormonal factors in gender identity but also points to the environment as a critical influence on the success of gender assignment or reassignment. It therefore seems appropriate to consider whether there are biological factors in other cases where the gender of assignment appears to be 'wrong': in particular, cases of transsexuality, transvestism and homosexuality. The discussion here will be largely restricted to biological influences as these conditions are discussed in wider context in Chapter 14.

Transsexualism

Transsexualism if often confused with transvestism and homosexuality, and it is important to clarify the distinction between these conditions. Both transvestites and homosexuals generally maintain their own gender identity concordant with gender assignment and socialization. They differ from the norm, however, in that homosexuals manifest sexual orientation towards members of their own sex, while transvestites exhibit a predilection for dressing as a member of the opposite sex. Apart from their choice of sexual partner, many homosexuals, both male and female, show no abnormalities of sex role; others adopt an opposite-sex role (Bell 1973). Transvestism, on the other hand, is by definition unconventional sex-role behaviour.

The characteristic feature of transsexualism is a fundamental feeling by the individual that he or she was born into the wrong sex and should rightly belong to the other sex. This conviction may be pursued as far as genital surgery. Although transsexuals may exhibit aspects of both homosexuality and transvestism, when seen from the individual's point of view these are consistent with what is felt to be the correct gender identity and sex role for him or her. Thus the underlying factor is development of a gender identity of the opposite sex (Green 1974a).

One of the most profound insights into the life and feelings of a transsexual was provided by Jan Morris (1974), who lived a conventional male life as James Morris while yearning to be female. Eventually, at the age of forty-six, Morris underwent a transsexual operation and assumed the female role she had always felt was congruent with her gender identity. Morris's revelations, however, still leave the origins of trans-sexuality a mystery. There are no obvious anomalies of sexual differentiation in these individuals, so it would be inaccurate to describe them as hermaphroditic. Bardwick (1971) suggested that the prenatal sexual differentiation of the brain in transsexuals may have proceeded in the wrong direction, resulting in an incongruity between gender identity and anatomical sex. If this were the case then one would expect to find some indications of physiological difference between transsexuals and normal individuals, and so far none has been satisfactorily demonstrated. Furthermore, in circumstances in which an explanation of abnormal brain differentiation is plausible, for example the adrenogenital syndrome, gender identity is commonly found to correspond to sex of assignment and upbringing.

On the basis of his studies of clinic cases of transsexualism, Stoller (1969) proposed a model for the aetiology of the condition which encompassed the following features: a mother who is depressed, unfeminine, possible bisexual; a father who is distant and passive, possibly absent from home much of the time; an empty and resentful marriage between the parents, but not usually overt marital breakdown; a male child who is exceptionally attractive; and an exaggeratedly close symbiotic relationship between the mother and the son which hinders the child's development of individual identity. Person and Ovesey (1974) conclude that transsexualism can take several forms, some of which do not altogether conform to Stoller's aetiological model, but all forms tend to manifest extreme separation anxiety regarding the mother and can probably be traced back to early family relationships.

The proportion of males seeking transsexual surgery is much greater than females (Benjamin & Ihlenfeld 1973), which, in view of the more prestigious position of males in our society, may seem odd. However, the greater social desirability of masculinity makes it more acceptable as a role option for females without the necessity for complete sex-change. There is far less social tolerance of femininity in males (Green 1979). Moreover, the required therapeutic and surgical procedures are much more complicated in cases of female-to-male transsexualism (Pauly 1974).

The therapeutic value of sex-change operations for transsexualism has been questioned in recent years, and the alternative of counselling to assist in the management of the identity conflict has been advocated by some writers (e.g. Lothstein 1979; Meyer & Reter 1979; Raymond 1977). The evaluation of treatment approaches is difficult in the light of the relatively poor understanding we have of the causation of the condition. It may be the case that there is a combination of prenatal predisposing factors, such as androgen deficiency in a critical phase in neural development, which are amplified by early experiences in the child-rearing situation (Green 1974b; Money & Primrose 1969).

Homosexuality

We saw earlier that prenatal or perinatal hormonal manipulations in animals can result in sexual behaviours characteristic of the opposite sex. It is tempting to extrapolate from these findings to cases of apparent sex-role inversion in humans. The principal advocate of this view is Dörner (1976), who has concluded that in genetic males, androgen deficiency during the hypothalamic differentiation phase of brain development results in a more female brain type and neuroendocrine pattern, with consequent predisposition to homosexuality. Similarly, in genetic females Dörner argues that overdoses of androgen lead to a more male differentiation of the brain and a predisposition to female homosexuality. Such effects cannot be treated by hormone administration in adulthood since the critical changes have taken place prenatally, but Dörner's theory has provided the underpinings for neurosurgical treatment involving operations on the hypothalamus, the results of which have generally claimed to be favourable, but this approach remains highly controversial. Meyer-Bahlburg (1977, 1980) argues that since Dörner's theory of the homology of animal sexual inversion and human homosexuality has yet to be established, the psychosurgical approach seems premature.

Although sexual activity and potency of homosexuals is affected by reduction of androgen levels, sexual orientation remains unaffected. In this respect homosexuality is no different to heterosexuality (Money 1970). A proliferation of sex-hormone investigations of homosexuals has resulted in a heterogeneity of findings from which it is difficult to conclude other than that levels and production of hormones in adulthood are highly unlikely to be responsible for either male or female homo-sexuality (Meyer-Bahlburg 1980). However, more recent studies of hormonal response patterns in homosexuals have revealed differences which suggest that a biological factor in homosexuality may exist. The hormonal response patterns which have been the subject of scrutiny are the positive estrogen feedback effect on luteinizing hormone (LH). In animals and humans increasing levels of estrogen in the female trigger an LH surge; this effect is much smaller and less consistent in males. Dörner and his co-workers (Dörner *et al.* 1975, 1976) have reported deviations in the positive feedback phenomenon in several cases of homosexuality and transsexuality, which imply hormonal disturbances in these conditions, but methodological weaknesses dictate caution in interpreting these studies. A more rigorous investigation of this phenomenon in which the responses of male homosexuals were compared with those of male heterosexuals and female heterosexuals has been reported by Gladue, Green & Hellman (1984). In this study baseline hormone levels were assessed and then LH and testosterone changes in response to an injection of an estrogen preparation were measured over a 96-hour period. The LH surge pattern for homosexual men was significantly different from that of the heterosexual men and the heterosexual women: in fact it was intermediate between the two heterosexual groups. The women did not show any significant alterations in testosterone concentrations across the test period, whereas both male groups showed a significant decrease in testosterone immediately after estrogen treatment. Testosterone levels gradually returned to baseline but the homosexual group showed a significant lag in return compared to the heterosexual group. These results suggest that homosexual men have a pattern of neuroendocrine responsiveness intermediate between that of heterosexual men and women, which invites the idea that there may be physiological developmental components in the sexual orientation and sex-role expression of at least some homosexual men.

Anthropological and cross-cultural studies

Anthropologists have developed an alternative approach to the issue of whether sex-role stereotypes have a biological basis – the search for cultural universals. If sex-related differences in behaviour are consistently expressed across most cultures, then it may be argued that this consistency has a biological underpinning (Goldberg 1973). Although the categories 'man' and 'woman' are universal, the behavioural content of those categories varies from culture to culture. In some cultures, for example, men weave and women make pots, whereas in others these roles are reversed; in some parts of the world women are the major agricultural producers, and in others they are prohibited from agricultural activity. Of course, all cultures must adapt to the ecological conditions of their environment, and so it is difficult to determine whether any given division of roles has arisen because of evolutionary factors or whether it reflects a common solution to a common survival problem (Archer 1976).

All cultures use gender as a major criterion for assigning roles and have gender distinctions built into their language, and all expect that certain temperamental differences will inevitably be associated with males and females which suit them for their roles (Rosenblatt & Cunningham 1976). The most extreme sex-role differentiation is encountered in societies based on hunting and fishing, while less marked differentiation is found in societies based on animal husbandry and food storage. Societies where the extended family is the norm and in which social co-operation is important tend to have strong sex-role differentiation, while societies in which small, relatively independent nuclear family groupings are the norm show less strong differentiation (Barry, Bacon & Child 1957).

The only roles which appear to be universally or almost universally linked to one sex or the other are those concerned with child-rearing, hunting and making war. Now it is quite possible that the second two follow as a direct result of the first. Since women were necessary to breast-feed their infants and since they generally had infants to breast feed, the activities of hunting and making war could have become part of the male role by default. This 'female child-raiser' and 'male-warrior-hunter' dichotomy is a pervasive pattern which, some writers have maintained, has evolutionary origins (e.g. Tiger & Fox 1971). If this does have a biological basis it should arguably be observable in our closest evolutionary relatives, the primates. But this division of labour, with males providing economic support and protection for the rest of the group, is not found in non-human primates. With the exception of nursing infants, all individuals gather their own food, and although the females have primary care of infants in most primate species, in some this function is fulfilled by the males (Burton 1977; Redican 1976). The idea that the primate male performs the role of group protector also appears to be anthropomorphic. Of course, in some species the males are substantially larger and heavier than the females, but there is little evidence of these potential defence attributes being put to effective use. The norm seems to be for many animals of both sexes to participate in defence of the group and protection of the young, and in cases of major threat the whole troop tends to flee together. Thus the notion of 'women and children first' has no apparent non-human equivalent (Fedigan 1982)!

It is generally acknowledged that learning and experience are highly significant components of the social behaviours of primates, and thus in order to determine the relative importance of biological factors in sex-role development the social learning component should ideally be eliminated. Attempts to do this were pioneered over twenty years ago by Harlow, who reared rhesus monkeys in isolation with surrogate, dummy mothers, and with only brief periods of social contact each day (Harlow 1965). Limited contact with peers was incorporated because complete isolation rearing of primates has been found to result in such gross disturbances of behaviour that any studies of social roles would thereby be invalidated (McKinney 1974). Harlow reported that monkeys raised in conditions of isolation with limited peer access still developed sex-typical behaviours, so that by two-and-a-half months of age the males were more active and aggressive while the females were more passive. Harlow concluded that these sex differences in the rhesus monkey must be innate, but this conclusion has been strongly criticized on many grounds, including the overall abnormality of the cage environment compared to free-ranging group-living situations; the definition of 'passivity'; and the failure to eliminate or properly control for socialization factors (Fedigan 1982).

Perhaps the single most salient piece of research in this area remains the classic study of three tribes of New Guinea by Mead (1935). Amongst the Arapesh tribe, both men and women were taught to help others and to care about others' needs and feelings and to avoid aggression. In the Mundugamor tribe, however, both men and women were ruthless and aggressive and apparently devoid of maternal feelings. By contrast, in the Tchambuli tribe women were dominant and the men were passive. While the women fished and made articles to trade, the men painted, danced, made music and played games. The men were emotional, easily embarrassed and they deferred to the women who were nevertheless tolerant of this male dependency and quite appreciated the fact that their menfolk were decorative and entertaining. Mead's findings are not unique, for there are several other cultures in which, for example, women do the heavy work because men are believed to be too weak. In these cultures the women generally are stronger because of years of heavy work, but it is considered unmasculine for men to attempt to build up their muscular strength. Mead's study indicates that 'masculinity' or 'femininity' can be the norm for all members of a cultural group, or that the sex-role stereotypes found in typical Western society can be reversed, with the females being 'masculine' and the males being 'feminine'.

One of the most detailed cross-cultural studies of relevance to the present enquiry was the 'Six Cultures Project' (Whiting & Whiting 1975). Child-rearing practices in six different cultures from different parts of the world were studied intensively, and the authors were impressed by the consistency of the sex differences which emerged in the findings. In early childhood rough-and-tumble play and dependency were found to be sexually differentiated in all six cultures, and as the children grew older further differences in sex-role behaviour emerged, with girls increasing in nurturant behaviour and boys increasing in aggressiveness. The growth of nurturance in girls is seen by these authors as a direct consequence of the assignment of infant care and household chores to them, and hence is regarded as culturally rather than biologically determined. Regarding the development of aggression, Maccoby and Jacklin (1975) and Tieger (1980) agree that the data from the Six Cultures project are insufficient to draw firm conclusions.

Unfortunately, cross-cultural, anthropological, and ethnological studies have not furnished many unequivocal answers. Although both child-rearing and aggressive behaviour do appear to be almost universally and consistently sex-differentiated, the striking finding is their malleability, suggesting powerful cultural influences. Moreover, other important factors need to be taken into account in the analysis of these studies. For example, the influence of the ratio of males to females can affect the sexual divisions of labour in a society as well as the relative value placed upon males and females and upon the roles they fulfil (Guttentag & Secord 1983). In some societies female roles are circumscribed because of the nature of the patriarchal kin system and associated systems of male dominance. Analysis of such cultures suggests that sex-role stereotypes are largely a function of power in the society (Rosaldo 1974; Rosenblatt & Cunningham 1976). Broadly speaking, one may sensibly conclude that socialization for sex roles can be predicted from the sex differences in work requirements for males and females in any given society.

Conclusions

Beach (1976, 1978), Diamond (1976) and Fedigan (1982) have argued that the contrast of 'male' with 'female' behaviour which pervades the literature is a false dichotomy born of the fact that genital sex is obviously discrete except in rare cases. The separation and opposition of female and male biology and behaviour is not well supported by the current available evidence. Hormonal sex differences, as we have seen, are a matter of ratios not absolutes as both males and females produce a range of 'male' and 'female' sex hormones. Furthermore, estrogen is not the chemical or behavioural antithesis of androgen; both types of hormone can have the effect of disturbing the developmental process such that the female type of differentiation is abolished. The theory that androgen 'causes' sex-related differentiation in the brain and therefore underlies many of the behavioural differences between the sexes, although plausible, has yet to be articulated with sufficient precision to permit satisfactory evaluation. Hence it may be contended that, at the present time, all the prenatal and perinatal hormone studies demonstrate is that the delicate balance of the developing neuroendocrine system is easily disturbed. It is accepted that prenatal androgens do affect the development of the hypothalamus, which in turn affects behaviour, but this process is much more complex than the androgen causational model would suggest.

If it is inappropriate to conceive of behaviour on a single male-to-female continuum, then how should it be conceptualized? Beach and Diamond argue that both 'male' and 'female' behavioural systems can co-exist in one individual. The development of mechanisms which mediate the former does not necessitate the suppression of the latter. On this basis we are not born psychosexually male or female, nor strictly neutral, but with varying potentials for acquiring given behaviours. These potentials are in all probability related to the prenatal environment, but after birth social forces begin to mould these possibilities into more distinct patterns of behaviour. In fact, from the very moment of birth parents treat boys and girls differently (Will, Self & Datan 1976) and will interact differently with the same infant as a function of the gender label used (Seavey, Katz & Zalk 1975). If no gender information is available sex attributions tend to be made on the basis of stereotypical cues, which suggests that gender labels and associated expectations are deeply ingrained in most, if not all of us. The divergence into male and female sex roles and gender identities is therefore a self-fulfilling process based on the belief that maleness and femaleness are discontinuous, mutually exclusive, and opposing categories. Furthermore, the accomplishment of this divergence reinforces our faith in the sanctity of the dichotomy (Fedigan 1982). Kaplan (1980) suggests that our understanding of this complex process could be greatly enhanced by considering not two but three psychosexual categories: masculine, feminine and androgynous, the latter including those individuals showing evidence of a balance of positively valued masculine and feminine characteristics and for whom this distribution of traits results in adaptive functioning.

This attempt to integrate the biological and social evidence into a broad transactional perspective has many elements missing. In particular, this chapter has not examined the cognitive processes involved in sex-typing (Kohlberg 1966) although it is contended that cognitive-developmental theory is consonant with the arguments presented here. Nor has there been any detailed consideration of the mass of research on socialization processes and general cultural determinants of sex-role stereotypes. These omissions have been quite deliberate, for they comprise the principal focus of the remainder of this volume. The analysis presented here has merely set the transactional stage for the exposition which is to come.

References

Angrist, S. A. (1969) The study of sex-roles. *Journal of Social Issues, 15,* 215–232.

Archer, J. (1976) Biological explanations of psychological sex differences. *In* Lloyd, B. and Archer, J. (eds) *Exploring sex differences.* London: Academic Press, pp. 241–266.

Archer, J. (1980) The distinction between gender stereotypes and sex-role concepts. *British Journal of Social and Clinical Psychology, 19,* 51.

Archer, J. (1984) Gender stereotype and sex-role concepts: a reply to Stoppard and Kalin. *British Journal of Social Psychology, 23,* 89-91.

Archer, J. & Lloyd, B. (1974) Sex roles: biological and social interactions. *New Scientist, 64,* 582–584.

Archer, J. & Lloyd, B. (1982) *Sex and gender.* Harmondsworth: Penguin.

Bardwick, J. (1971) *The psychology of women: a study of bio-cultural conflicts.* New York: Harper & Row.

Barry, H., Bacon, M. K. & Child, I. L. (1957) A cross-cultural survey of some sex differences in socialization. *Journal of Abnormal and Social Psychology, 55,* 327–332.

Beach, F. A. (1976) Cross-species comparisons and the human heritage. *Archives of Sexual Behaviour, 5,* 469–485.

Beach, F. A. (1978) Human sexuality and evolution. *In* Washburn, S. L. & McCown, E. R. (eds) *Human evolution: biosocial perspectives.* Menlo Park: Benjamin/Cummings Publishing, pp. 123–153.

Bell, A. P. (1973) Homosexualities: their range and character. *In* Cole, J. K. &

Dienstbier, R. (eds) *Nebraska symposium on motivation*, vol. 21. Lincoln: University of Nebraska Press, pp. 1–26.

Benjamin, H. & Ihlenfeld, C. L. (1973) Transsexualism. *American Journal of Nursing*, *73*, 457–461.

Broverman, I. K., Broverman, D. M., Clarkson, F. E., Rosenkratz, P. S. & Vogel, S. R. (1970) Sex-role stereotypes and clinical judgments of mental health. *Journal of Consulting and Clinical Psychology*, *34*, 1–7.

Burton, F. D. (1977) Ethology and the development of sex and gender identity in nonhuman primates. *Acta Biotheoretica*, *26*, 1–18.

Diamond, M. (1976) Human sexual development: biological foundations for social development. *In* Beach, F. A. (ed.) *Human sexuality in four perspectives*. Baltimore: Johns Hopkins University Press, pp. 22–61.

Dörner, G. (1976) *Hormones and brain differentiation*. Amsterdam: Elsevier.

Dörner, G., Rohde, W., Seidel, K., Hass, W. & Schott, G. (1976) On the evocability of a positive estrogen feedback action on LH-secretion in transsexual men and women. *Endrocrinology*, *67*, 20–25.

Dörner, G., Rohde, W., Stahl, F., Krell, L. & Masius, W. G. (1975) A neuroendocrine predisposition for homosexuality in man. *Archives of Sexual Behaviour*, *4*, 1–18.

Ehrhardt, A. A. & Baker, S. W. (1974) Fetal androgens, human central nervous system differentiation, and behaviour sex differences. *In* Friedman, R. C., Richart, R. M. & Vande Wiele, R. L. (eds) *Sex differences in behaviour*. New York: John Wiley, pp. 33–52.

Ehrhardt, A. A., Greenberg, N. & Money, J. (1970) Female gender identity and absence of fetal gonadal hormones: Turner's syndrome. *Johns Hopkins Medical Journal*, *126*, 237–248.

Ehrhardt, A. A. & Meyer-Bahlburg, H. F. L. (1981) Effects of prenatal sex hormones on gender-related behaviour. *Science*, *211*, 1312–1318.

Fedigan, L. M. (1982) *Primate paradigms: sex roles and social bonds*. Montreal: Eden Press.

Gladue, B. A., Green, R. & Hellman, R. E. (1984) Neuroendocrine response to estrogen and sexual orientation. *Science*, *225*, 1496–1499.

Goldberg, S. (1973) *The inevitability of patriarchy*. New York: Morrow.

Goy, R. W. (1970) Early hormonal influence on the development of sexual and sex-related behaviour. *In* Quarton, G. C., Melanchuk, T. & Schmitt, F. O. (eds) *Neurosciences: a study program*. New York: Rockefeller University Press.

Green, R. (1974a) *Sexual identity conflict in children and adults*. New York: Basic Books.

Green, R. (1974b) The behaviourally feminine male child: Pretranssexual? Pretransvestic? Prehomosexual? Preheterosexual? *In* Friedman, R. C., Richart, R. M. & Vande Wiele, R. L. (eds) *Sex differences in behaviour*. New York: John Wiley.

Green, R. (1979) Childhood cross-gender behaviour and subsequent sexual preferences. *American Journal of Psychiatry*, *136*, 106–108.

Guttentag, M. & Secord, P. F. (1983) *Too many women? The sex ratio question*. London: Sage.

Hampson, J. L. (1965) Determinants of psychosexual orientation. *In* Beach, F. A. (ed.) *Sex and behaviour*. New York: John Wiley.

Harlow, H. F. (1965) Sexual behaviour in rhesus monkeys. *In* Beach, F. A. (ed.) *Sex and behaviour*. New York: John Wiley.

Huston. A. C. (1983) Sex-typing. *In* Mussen, P. H. (ed.) *Handbook of child psychology*, 4th edn, vol. 4. New York: John Wiley, pp. 388–464.

Hutt, C. (1972) *Males and females*. Harmondsworth: Penguin.

Hutt, C. (1978) Sex-role differentiation in social development. *In* McGurk, H. (ed.) *Issues in childhood social development*. London: Methuen, pp. 171–202.

Imperato-McGinley, J., Petersen, R. E., Gautier, T. & Sturla, E. (1979) Androgens and the evolution of male-gender identity among male pseudoher-maphrodites with 5-reductase deficiency. *New England Journal of Medicine*, *300*, 1233–1237.

Kaplan, A. G. (1980) Human sex-hormone abnormalities viewed from an androgynous perspective: a reconsideration of the work of John Money. *In* Parsons, J. E. (ed.) *The psychobiology of sex differences and sex roles*. New York: McGraw-Hill, pp. 81–91.

Karahasanoglu, A., Barglow, P. & Growe, G. (1972) Psychological aspects of infertility. *Journal of Reproductive Medicine*, *9*, 241–247.

Katz, P. A. (1979) The development of female identity. *Sex Roles*, *5*, 155–178.

Kohlberg. L. (1966) A cognitive-developmental analysis of children's sex-role concepts and attitudes. In Maccoby, E. E. (ed.) *The development of sex differences*. Stanford: Stanford University Press.

Lev-Ran, A. (1974) Gender role differentiation in hermaphrodites. *Archives of Sexual Behaviour*, *3*, 391–424.

Levine, S. (1966) Sex differences in the brain. *Scientific American*, *214 (April)*, 84–90.

Lewis, M. (1975) Early sex differences in the human: studies of socio-emotional development. *Archives of Sexual Behaviour*, *4*, 329–335.

Lewis, M. (1982) The social network systems model: towards a theory of social development. In Field, T. M. (ed.) *Review of human development*. New York: John Wiley, pp. 180–214.

Linton. S. (1971) Primate studies and sex differences. *In* Skolnick, A. S. & Skolnick, J. H. (eds) *Family in transition*. Boston: Little, Brown & Co., pp. 194–197.

Livson, F. B. (1983) Gender identity: a life-span view of sex-role development. In Weg, R. B. (ed.) *Sexuality in the later years: roles and behaviour*. New York: Academic Press, pp. 105–127.

Lothstein, L. M. (1979) Psychodynamics and sociodynamics of gender-dysphoric states. *American Journal of Psychotherapy*, *33*, 214–238.

McKinney, W. T. Jr. (1974) Primate social isolation. *Archives of General Psychiatry*, *31*, 422–426.

Maccoby, E. E. & Jacklin, C. N. (1975) *The psychology of sex differences*. London: Oxford University Press.

Masica, D. N., Money, J. & Ehrhardt, A. A. (1971) Fetal feminisation and gender identity in the testicular feminising syndrome of androgen insensitivity. *Archives of Sexual Behaviour*, *1*, 131–141.

Mead, M. (1935) *Sex and temperament in three primitive societies*. New York: Morrow.

Meyer, J. K. & Reter, D. J. (1979) Sex re-assignment follow-up. *Archives of General Psychiatry, 36*, 1010–1015.

Meyer-Bahlburg, H. F. L. (1977) *Archives of Sexual Behaviour, 6*, 297–325.

Meyer-Bahlburg, H. F. L. (1980) Homosexual orientation in women and men: a hormonal basis? In Parsons, J. E. (ed.) *The psychobiology of sex differences and sex roles*. New York: McGraw-Hill, pp. 105–130.

Money, J. (1970) Sexual dimorphism and homosexual gender identity. *Psychological Bulletin, 74*, 425–440.

Money, J. & Ehrhardt, A. A. (1972) *Man and woman, boy and girl*. Baltimore: Johns Hopkins University Press.

Money, J. & Ogunro, C. (1974) Behavioural sexology: ten cases of genetic male intersexuality with impaired prenatal and pubertal androgenisation. *Archives of Sexual Behaviour, 3*, 181–205.

Money, J. & Primrose, C. (1969) Sexual dimorphism and dissociation in the psychology of male transsexuals. *In* Green, R. & Money, J. (eds) *Transsexualism and sex re-assignment*. Baltimore: Johns Hopkins University Press, pp. 115–131.

Money, J. & Tucker, P. (1975) *Sexual signatures: on being a man or woman*. Boston: Little, Brown & Co.

Morris, J. (1974) *Conundrum*. London: Faber & Faber.

Owen, D. (1972) The 47XYY male: a review. *Psychological Bulletin, 78*, 209–233.

Parsons, J. E. (1980) Psychosexual neutrality: is anatomy destiny? In Parsons, J. E. (ed.) *The psychobiology of sex differences and sex roles*. New York: McGraw-Hill, pp. 3–29.

Pauly, I. B. (1974) Female transsexualism. *Archives of Sexual Behaviour, 3*, 509–526.

Person, E. S. & Ovesey, L. (1974) The transsexual syndrome in males. *American Journal of Psychotherapy, 28*, 4–20, 174–193.

Petersen, A. C. (1979) Female pubertal development. *In* Sugar, M. (ed.) *Female adolescent development*. New York: Brunner/Mazel.

Petersen, A. C. (1980) Biopsychosocial processes in the development of sex-related differences. *In* Parsons, J. E. (ed.) *The psychobiology of sex differences and sex roles*. New York: McGraw-Hill, pp. 31–35.

Phoenix, C. H. (1974) Prenatal testosterone in the nonhuman primate and its consequences for behaviour. In Friedman, R. C., Richart, R. M. & Vande Wiele, R. L. (eds) *Sex differences in behaviour*. New York: John Wiley, pp. 19–32.

Phoenix, C. H. (1978) Sexual behaviour of laboratory and wild-born rhesus monkeys. *Hormones and Behaviour, 10*, 178–192.

Pleck, J. H. (1981) *The myth of masculinity*. Cambridge, Mass.: MIT Press.

Quadagno, D. M., Briscoe, R. & Quadagno, J. S. (1977) Effect of perinatal gonadal hormones on selected nonsexual behaviour patterns: a critical assessment of the nonhuman and human literature. *Psychological Bulletin, 84*, 62–80.

Raymond, J. (1977) Transsexualism: the ultimate homage to sex-role power. *Chrysalis*, *3*, 11–23.

Redican, W. K. (1976) Adult male-infant interactions in non-human primates. *In* Lamb, M. E. (ed.) *The role of the father in child development*. New York: John Wiley, pp. 345–385.

Reinisch, J. (1974) Fetal hormones, the brain and human sex differences. *Archives of Sexual Behaviour*, *3*, 51–90.

Rogers, L. (1976) Male hormones and behaviour. *In* Lloyd, B. & Archer, J. (eds) *Exploring sex differences*. London: Academic Press, pp. 157–184.

Rosaldo, M. Z. (1974) Woman, culture and society: a theoretical overview. *In* Rosaldo, M. Z. & Lamphere, L. (eds) *Woman, culture and society*. Stanford: Stanford University Press.

Rosenblatt, P. C. & Cunningham, M. R. (1976) Sex differences in cross-cultural perspectives. *In* Lloyd, B. & Archer, J. (eds) *Exploring sex differences*. London: Academic Press, pp. 71–94.

Sameroff, A. J. (1977) Early influences on development: fact or fantasy? *In* Chess, S. & Thomas A. (eds) *Annual Progress in Child Psychiatry and Child Development*. New York: Brunner/Mazel, pp. 3–33.

Scott, C. I. & Thomas, G. H. (1973) Genetic disorders associated with mental retardation: clinical aspects. *Pediatric Clinics of North America*, *20*, 121–140.

Seavey, C. A., Katz, P. A. & Zalk, S. R. (1975) Baby X: the effect of gender labels on adult responses to infants. *Sex Roles*, *1*, 103–109.

Singleton, C. H. (1978) Sex differences. *In* Foss, B. M. (ed.) *Psychology survey 1*. London: Allen & Unwin, pp. 116–130.

Slaby, R. & Frey, K. S. (1975) Development of gender constancy and selective attention to same-sex models. *Child Development*, *46*, 849–856.

Spence, J. T. & Helmreich, R. L. (1978) *Masculinity and femininity: their psychological dimensions, correlates and antecedents*. Austin, Texas: University of Texas Press.

Stoller, R. J. (1969) Parental influence in male transsexualism. *In* Green, R. & Money, J. (eds) *Transsexualism and sex re-assignment*. Baltimore: Johns Hopkins University Press.

Stoller, R. J. (1974) Facts and fancies: an examination of Freud's concepts of bisexuality. In Strouse, J. (ed.) *Women and analysis: dialogues on psychoanalytic views of femininity*. New York: Grossman.

Thompson, S. K. (1975) Gender labels and early sex role development. *Child Development*, *46*, 339–347.

Tieger, T. (1980) On the biological basis of sex differences in aggression. *Child Development*, *51*, 943–963.

Tiger, L. & Fox R. (1971) *The imperial animal*. New York: Holt, Rinehart & Winston.

Timiras, P. S. (1982) The timing of hormone signals in the orchestration of brain development. In Emde, R. N. & Harmon, R. J. (eds) *The development of attachment and affiliative systems*. New York: Plenum, pp. 47–63.

Wehren, A. & Di Lisi, R. (1983) The development of gender understanding: judgments and explanations. *Child Development*, *54*, 1568–1578.

Whiting, B. B. & Whiting, J. W. M. (1975) *Children of six cultures: a psychocultural analysis*. Cambridge, Mass.: Harvard University Press.

Will, J. A., Self, P. A. & Datan, N. (1976) Maternal behaviour and perceived sex of infant. *American Journal of Orthopsychiatry*, *46*, 135–139.
Wilson, J. D. (1978) Sexual differentiation. *Annual Review of Physiology*, *40*, 279–306.
Yalom, I. D., Green, R. & Fisk, N. (1973) Prenatal exposure to female hormones: effect on psychosexual development in boys. *Archives of General Psychiatry*, *28*, 554–561.
Zuger, B. (1970) Gender role determinism: a critical review of the evidence from hermaphroditism. *Psychosomatic Medicine*, *32*, 449–467.

CHAPTER TWO   Psychological Theories of Sex-Role Stereotyping
David J. Hargreaves

Introduction

Sex roles are the behaviour patterns which are differentialy displayed by the sexes, and sex-role stereotypes are the beliefs that people hold about these patterns. Since the stereotypes are all-pervasive in Western society, as the contents of this book make clear, it seems very likely that they will shape sex roles. Beliefs about the behaviour of males and females may themselves in part determine that behaviour, and vice versa. Psychological theories of sex-role stereotyping aim to explain this process.

There are three 'traditional' theories of sex-role stereotyping, which are based on the three major theoretical perspectives in developmental psychology, namely psychoanalytic theory, reinforcement or learning theory, and cognitive-developmental theory. These have been comprehensively reviewed elsewhere (e.g. in Maccoby 1966), and I shall make no attempt to duplicate those efforts here. My review will restrict itself to outlining and comparing the main features of the traditional theories. The main emphasis will be upon some recent theoretical developments which focus on the nature of, and relationship between, masculinity and femininity. In particular, I shall discuss the concept of 'psychological androgyny', and the recent formulation of 'gender schema' theories (e.g. Bem 1981a).

Sex-role stereotyping is an integral and fundamental part of the process of *socialization*: this could be thought of as 'the process whereby the individual is converted into the person', and its study has changed dramatically over the last few decades. It could indeed be argued that this change of approach has transformed child development from a quiet backwater of psychology into one of its most vigorous, active areas. The old view of socialization is represented by a body of research on what became known as 'child-rearing practices' (see e.g. Danziger 1971), which was rooted in the learning theory approach. Implicit in this research was the view that socialization is a one-way process in which parents 'shape' the behaviour of their children, without any appreciable influence being exerted in the opposite direction. According to this view, sex roles are seen as patterns of behaviour that parents and teachers 'condition' into children, differentially rewarding masculinity in boys, and femininity in girls. It soon became apparent that this 'one-way' view of socialization had severe limitations; and the shift towards a 'two-way', interactive view of the process is best exemplified by the cognitive-developmental approach. This approach has gained considerable impetus from the revival of interest in Piaget's theory, and forms the basis for most of the recent theoretical developments.

Freud's original psychoanalytic theories of sex-role stereotyping (e.g. Freud 1925) have been the subject of a good deal of controversy. Because Freud's account of child development is primarily from the point of view of psychosexual motivation, his account of the process of sex-role stereotyping is fairly elaborate. It is probably this degree of elaboration which has made the theory difficult to subject to empirical testing.

There is a further theoretical approach which does not *explain* the development of sex-role stereotyping in the same sense as those above, but which is nevertheless worth mentioning here. The *role theory* approach represents the intersection between psychological and sociological explanations of individual behaviour, which have a common focus upon the *self* and its development. I shall draw on the role theory approach in outlining the three traditional theories of sex-role stereotyping, in the first half of this chapter. Recent theoretical and methodological developments in the study of masculinity, femininity and androgyny will then be traced, and this will lead to a consideration of gender schema theory. Finally, I shall attempt in the Conclusion to put all these theories into perspective.

Three traditional theories of sex-role stereotyping

Psychoanalytic theory

Freud's theory of sex-role stereotyping is part of his psychosexual stage theory of development. This is based on the notion that the libidinal energy which provides the motive force for most behaviour shifts its focus to different bodily *erogenous zones* at different stages of development. The lips and mouth form the oral erogenous zone, which is the first focus of the libido in infancy, for example: the first stage of psychosexual development is thus known as the oral stage. This is then followed by the anal, the phallic-urethral, and the genital stages. The theory holds that the degree to which libidinal desires can be gratified at each of these stages will determine the extent to which they influence later adult personality characteristics; different sets of characteristics are associated with each of the stages. Freud's account of sex-role stereotyping centres on developments within the third, phallic-urethral stage, which lasts roughly from the age of three until six years. A central concept of the theory is the *Oedipus complex*, which Freud considered to be one of his most important discoveries. In the Greek myth from which this is derived, Oedipus unwittingly kills his father and then marries his mother, unaware of the incestuous relationship.

In boys, the Oedipus complex takes the form of an initial desire to sexually possess the mother. The result of this desire is that the father is seen as a rival; in particular, the boy fears the possible loss of his penis at the hands of his father. This is what Freud called 'castration anxiety'; and it is accompanied by the boy's assumption that girls have already been castrated as a punishment for inappropriate behaviour. The boy eventually realizes that he will never realistically be able to possess his mother, and represses this desire. He does this by identifying with and taking on the characteristics of his father; 'identification with the aggressor' is one of the ways in which Freud proposed that the threat posed by an aggressor can be neutralized. Identification with the father involves not only the acquisition of masculine behaviour and characteristics, but also the development of the superego, or conscience. Thus the resolution of the Oedipus complex in boys results in the ultimate internalization of social and moral norms, as well as the development of sex-role identity.

Freud's parallel account of the development of sex-role identity in girls is much less coherent, as many critics have pointed out. The girl's equivalent of 'castration anxiety' is 'penis envy'; she assumes that she has already been castrated as a punishment for some misdemeanour, and regards her clitoris as an inferior substitute for the penis. As in the case of the boy, she initially identifies with the mother as a primary love object; but she renounces this identification and initially attempts to transfer it to the father when she discovers that her mother lacks a penis. Eventually she discovers that this desire to share the possession of a penis with her father is unattainable, and she transfers her identification back to her mother. Freud explains that the girl 'gives up her wish for a penis and puts in place of it a wish for a child: and *with that purpose in view* she takes her father as a love-object' (Freud 1925, p. 256). The resolution of the Oedipus complex in girls is thus ultimately accomplished by taking on the feminine characteristics of the mother.

Freud considered that the boy's Oedipus complex is not simply repressed, but 'literally smashed to pieces by the shock of threatened castration' (1925, p. 257): the superego takes over completely as its natural heir. In girls, however, the Oedipus complex is never fully resolved because the threat of castration was never present in such an intense form; castration is in fact regarded as having been carried out already. Freud concluded from this that the superego was never fully developed in females:

> That they show less sense of justice than men, that they are less ready to submit to the great necessities of life, that they are more often influenced in their judgements by feelings of affection or hostility . . . would be amply accounted for by the modification in the formation of their superego. (Freud 1925, pp. 257–258)

It is hardly surprising that Freud's theory of sex-role stereotyping has received a good deal of criticism and hostility from within the psychoanalytic movement (e.g. Horney 1924), as well as from feminists (see e.g. Mitchell 1974); and Freud himself was aware of many shortcomings in various aspects of his theory of infantile sexuality. It nevertheless remains a profound, detailed and influential account of those unconscious aspects of emotional development which are beyond the province of other developmental theories.

Social learning theory

Social learning theory uses the principles of conditioning and reinforcement as its starting point in the explanation of the complexities of human development: but it becomes necessary to complement these with constructs, such as 'identification', which are essentially cognitive in character. Miller (1983) has explained very clearly how modern social learning theory, as propounded for example by Bandura (1977), contrasts with traditional forms of learning theory in its incorporation of some of the concepts of cognitive-developmental theory, as well as of psychoanalysis.

Mischel (1966, 1970) has provided what is probably the most comprehensive and thorough account of the social-learning view of sex-role stereotyping. He starts from the premise that:

> the acquisition and performance of sex-typed behaviours can be described

by the same learning principles used to analyse any other aspect of an individual's behavior. In addition to discrimination, generalization, and observational learning, these principles include the patterning of reward, nonreward and punishment under specific contingencies, and the principles of direct and vicarious conditioning. (Mischel 1966, pp. 55–57)

Now the most powerful reinforcing agents in the young child's life are likely to be the parents: parents use a wide variety of different rewards and punishments such as praise, encouragement, disapproval and anger, in controlling children's behaviour. There is a considerable amount of empirical evidence (e.g. Fling & Manosevitz 1972) which shows that parents tend to reward sex-appropriate behaviour and play activities, and to disapprove of those which are sex-inappropriate. It has also been empirically demonstrated that nursery school teachers engage in this kind of 'shaping' (e.g. Fagot 1977; Serbin *et al.* 1973).

The social learning theory explanation of masculine sex-typing is essentially that the father is the most powerful provider of rewards and punishments, and that the son becomes initially attached to him as a result. From this follows the development of identification with and imitation of the father; and finally a generalized masculine sex-role identity emerges which is independent of the characteristics of the individual father. This process is presumably similar for girls and their mothers although empirical studies of imitation and identification have shown that the question of the symmetry of the process of sex-typing between boys and girls is by no means straightforward.

A classic series of experiments was conducted by Albert Bandura and his associates at Stanford University (e.g. Bandura & Walters 1963; Bandura, Ross & Ross 1961, 1963). In these experiments preschool children were exposed to aggressive and non-aggressive models in a series of carefully controlled experimental designs, and given the opportunity to imitate them under different experimental conditions. The aggressive models were adults and children who punched, kicked and were verbally aggressive towards a life-size inflatable 'Bobo doll'; and they were matched in other experimental conditions by non-aggressive models and controls. The experimental subjects, after observing the models, were frustrated by being forbidden to play with a range of attractive toys. They were then allowed to play freely in a room containing a Bobo doll as well as various toys, such as guns, that were potentially aggressive in their use. Bandura and his associates were primarily interested in the *imitation learning* that might be observed in the subjects' behaviour. They hypothesized that subjects exposed to aggressive models should imitate aggression more than those exposed to non-aggressive models, or than those with no model at all (i.e. the controls).

The general hypothesis that aggressive models would be imitated by the children in the absence of direct reinforcement was supported by the results; but most interesting for the theme of this chapter was the way in which this effect turned out to be mediated by the sex of the model, and by the sex of the subject. Although it was generally true that children were most strongly influenced by same-sex models, there were some circumstances in which this could apparently be overlaid by more powerful effects of sex-role identity. In one study, for example, Bandura, Ross and Ross (1963) compared children's tendency to imitate the behaviour of adult models who either dispensed or received toys and other desirable objects. Models who dispensed rewards were generally imitated more than those who received them, and male models in the 'dispensing' role were more generally imitated than equivalent females. However, boys who watched a female model dispense desirable objects in a situation where an adult male was ignored (that is who did not receive any of these objects) tended to imitate the ignored male rather than the female dispenser.

These results have important implications for the learning theory explanation of sex-role stereotyping. We have seen that a straightforward reinforcement explanation based on the power of the model is insufficient on its own, and needs to be supplemented by further theoretical constructs. It seems clear from the Bandura experiments that aggressive behaviour was being learnt *observationally* – that is in the absence of any direct reinforcement. It is also clear that novel patterns of aggression were being created in the subjects: children were aggressive towards the doll in ways that they had not observed in the model. This suggests that the cognitive components of imitation and identification are of considerable significance, and they are indeed integral to Bandura's (1977) later statement of social learning theory. This draws on some of the concepts of cognitive-developmental theory, but also has some marked contrasts with it, as we shall see next.

Cognitive-developmental theory

Cognitive-developmental theory centres on the child's conception of the world; on how children perceive and categorize the things and people around them. The dominant influence is undoubtedly Piaget's theory;

and the main exponent of this approach in the area of sex-role stereo-typing is Lawrence Kohlberg (Kohlberg 1966). Like Piaget, Kohlberg sees the child as an active agent, striving to make sense of the environment; and he proposes that the categorization of oneself as 'boy' or 'girl' is a fundamental part of this. Now this viewpoint contrasts markedly with that of social learning theory. Social learning theory takes the view that the internalization of sex-role standards (e.g. in the form of identifications) follows on from the rewards and punishments associated with different sex-typed behaviours. Cognitive-developmental theory takes the opposite causal view, that imitation and reinforcement of sex-typed behaviour is actually *guided* by some form of internalized sex-role identity. Kohlberg (1966) summarizes this difference by contrasting the social-learning syllogism 'I want rewards, I am rewarded for doing boy things, therefore I want to be a boy' with the cognitive-developmental equivalent 'I am a boy, therefore I want to do boy things, therefore the opportunity to do boy things (and to gain approval for doing them) is rewarding' (p. 89). Another implication of this difference is that social learning theory views the level of a boy's sex-typing as a *result* of the degree of identification with the father, whereas cognitive-developmental theory regards it as a *cause*.

A central concept in the cognitive-developmental view is that of 'gender identity', which is the categorization of oneself as 'boy' or 'girl'. Once this is established, through the normal mechanisms of concept formation, it determines the ways in which objects and acts are evaluated, that is in terms of the degree of consistency with the individual's gender identity. Gender identity may emerge in some children as early as at 18–24 months of age (Lewis 1975); it manifests itself first in the child's verbal distinctions between 'boy' and 'girl', or 'mummy' and 'daddy'. At this stage it is very unlikely that sex-role concepts exist in any logically ordered way; the verbal labels are likely to be applied in the same way as any name (e.g. 'Tom') might be.

Numerous empirical studies of different aspects of early gender identity have been carried out, including toy preference (Eisenberg Murray & Hite 1982), knowledge of cultural sex-role stereotypes (Kuhn, Nash & Brucken 1978), activity preferences (Connor & Serbin 1977), play interests (Fling & Manosevitz 1972), and so on (see also Chapter 6). It seems safe to conclude that preschool children possess an extensive knowledge of the characteristics of gender roles in adults as well as in children, and that they evaluate themselves in terms of these roles. *Gender constancy* gradually emerges during this period: children come to realize that a girl remains a girl regardless of her dress or choice of toys, for example (DeVries 1969). The further development of gender identity in childhood, adolescence and adulthood (cf. Ullian 1976) hinges on the *organization* of roles in the developing self-concept. Sociological role theorists such as Mead, Linton, Sarbin and others have devoted considerable effort to the definition of roles and role-taking, so it is useful to draw on some of their conclusions here. Individuals can be thought of as being at the centre of a complex network of interlinking roles: and the sex role is one of the primary features of this network. There are two distinctions that can usefully be made: the first is between different *levels of assimilation* of roles, and the second is between their *learning* and *performance*.

We can distinguish between three levels of assimilation of a given role: *identity*, *taking*, and *enactment*. Applying this distinction to sex roles, *sex-role identity* is that which operates at the most basic, unconscious level. People are not usually conscious of acting in a way which is 'masculine' or 'feminine', even though this may clearly be the case to an outside observer. *Sex-role enactment*, in contrast, is very self-conscious and superficial; a male actor in a female part on stage, for example, is unlikely to assimilate or retain many aspects of that part when the play is over. In between these two is *sex-role taking*, which refers to the way in which people take on prescribed sex roles in everyday life. A policewoman, for example, might be called upon at different times of her working day to display 'feminine' behaviour when dealing with children, as well as 'masculine' behaviour when dealing with a male offender.

The distinction between the *learning* and *performance* of sex roles has been made by Mischel (1966, 1970), amongst others. It seems clear from the evidence reviewed earlier in this section that children *learn* the attitudes and behaviour patterns associated with both sex roles; and yet they largely *perform* only that which is associated with the same sex role. Some of my own research (Hargreaves 1976, 1977, 1979) has shown that 10–11-year-old children can display 'opposite-sex' behaviour on a neutral task with remarkable ease if they are given a simple instruction to do so. Some subsequent research (Hargreaves, Bates & Foot 1985) shows furthermore that consistent sex differences in performance on objective perceptual-motor ability tests can be unambiguously reversed when the tasks are labelled sex-inappropriately. In other words, it appears as though boys and girls tend not to perform the 'opposite-sex' parts of their behavioural repertoires under normal, everyday circumstances. This state of affairs is regarded as undesirable by some theorists; and some of the proposed alternatives are outlined in the next section.

Masculinity, femininity and psychological androgyny

The concept of 'psychological androgyny' has become increasingly prevalent over the last decade or so, and now forms an essential part of any discussion of masculinity and femininity. The term is from the Greek *andro*, male and *gyne*, female — it refers to the extent to which an individual displays both masculine and feminine characteristics. The work of Sandra Bem and her associates, which will be reviewed in this section, has exerted a considerable influence in this field. She was the first to challenge the widely accepted belief that it was most appropriate for males to behave in a typically 'masculine' manner — displaying aggression, dominance, ambition and so on — and for females to be correspondingly 'feminine', displaying characteristics such as nurturance, submissiveness, and compassion (e.g. Bem 1975).

All of us have both masculine and feminine elements in our psychological make-up; and Bem proposed that a more 'psychologically healthy' state of affairs was for people of both sexes to be *psychologically androgynous*; to be capable of displaying both masculine *and* feminine characteristics in different situations. She suggested that women unconsciously stifle the masculine parts of their characters; that they are potentially quite capable of being competitive, assertive and independent if they can overcome cultural expectations. Similarly, 'keeping a stiff upper lip' and not displaying emotion, for example, are ways in which males suppress potentially valuable aspects of their personalities. It is easy to see that this proposal is at one with the idea of sexual equality; and this is probably why the notion of androgyny rapidly gained wide currency.

Central to Bem's research is the *Bem Sex Role Inventory* (BSRI; Bem 1974), an instrument which has become the most widely used measure of sex-role stereotyping in adults. Its original form consists of sixty seven-point self-rating scales; twenty of these refer to 'masculine' personality traits such as 'forceful', 'competitive' and 'willing to take risks'; twenty refer to 'feminine' traits such as 'affectionate', 'gentle' and 'sensitive to the needs of others'; and twenty refer to neutral characteristics such as 'adaptable', 'moody' and 'truthful'. These traits were selected on the basis of the consensual opinions of groups of undergraduate judges about their desirability 'for a man' or 'for a woman' in American society. Subjects are asked to indicate how well each of the sixty traits describes them on the scales, which range from one ('never or almost never true of me') to seven ('always or almost always true of me'). A variety of indices of sex-typing and androgyny can be derived from these ratings, as we shall see in the next section. Bem (1979) has developed a short form of the scale, and there are several others available which assess sex-role stereotyping along similar lines (see review by Heilbrun 1981).

Bem's research strategy was to assess subjects' sex-typing by means of the BSRI, and then to relate this to behaviour in real-life situations. In one such experiment, for example, Bem and Lenney (1976) asked subjects to indicate which of a series of paired activities they would prefer to perform for pay whilst being photographed. Twenty of these were stereotypically masculine (e.g. 'nail two boards together'); twenty were stereotypically feminine (e.g. 'iron cloth napkins'); and twenty were neutral (e.g. 'play with a yo-yo'). When the subjects' preferences were compared with their scores on the BSRI, it was found that sex-typed subjects expressed clear preferences for sex-appropriate and against sex-inappropriate activities, even though such choices cost them money.

A whole series of studies has subsequently been carried out in this vein, by Bem's associates as well as by others, in which the relationships between psychological androgyny and a wide range of different positive psychological attributes have been investigated. These include sex-role adaptability across situations (Bem 1975); high levels of self-esteem (Spence, Helmreich & Stapp 1975); performance on ability tests (Antill & Cunningham 1982); effectiveness as a parent (Baumrind 1982); subjective feelings of emotional well-being (Lubinski, Tellegen & Butcher 1981), and so on. The results of these studies by no means make it clear that psychological androgyny is a good predictor of psychological well-being: indeed, a recent review of the literature by Taylor and Hall (1982) suggests that masculinity in both males and females may be a better predictor than certain measures of androgyny. Since the different techniques employed in assessing androgyny presuppose different theoretical views of its relationship with masculinity and femininity, and since this issue is at the core of the topic of sex-role stereotyping, it is worth looking at some of the methodological issues in more detail.

In her earliest formulation, Bem (1974) defined androgyny as the Student's t ratio for the difference between a person's masculine and feminine self-endorsements on the BSRI rating scales. A high positive score on this measure indicated femininity, a high negative score indicated masculinity, and the proximity of the score to zero indicated the degree of androgyny. This technique was soon abandoned because of the confounding of two different types of androgyny score; a t ratio of near zero could be obtained by a subject scoring high on both masculinity and femininity scales, as well as by a subject scoring low on both. Another important limitation of this technique was that it implied that masculinity and femininity occupy opposite ends of a single bipolar dimension, with androgyny falling somewhere in between.

The method that succeeded this involved distinguishing between high and low scorers on the masculinity and femininity scales considered separately, and forming four subjects groups on the basis of the resulting 2×2 classification (see Bem 1977). Subjects in the high masculine-high feminine group were designated as 'androgynous'; those in the high masculine-low feminine and high feminine-low masculine groups were designated as 'masculine' and 'feminine' respectively; and those in the low masculine-low feminine group were designated as 'undifferentiated'. The confounding of 'androgynous' and 'undifferentiated' subjects was thereby avoided; and the strategy of many research studies which followed was to compare the scores of the four groups on different dependent variables using 2×2 analysis of variance designs. It is very important to realize that this revised scoring method implies a different underlying view of the relationship between masculinity and femininity: namely, that these are now regarded as independent, orthogonal dimensions rather than as two poles of a single scale.

Various detailed discussions of these methodological issues have appeared in the literature (e.g. Bem 1979; Locksley & Colten 1979; Pedhazur & Tetenbaum 1979); and I have pointed out elsewhere (Hargreaves *et al.* 1981) that there are two major problems associated with the four-way classification procedure in androgyny research. In brief, these are the loss of information that occurs when subjects are divided into groups on the basis of median splits, and the need to assume that masculinity and femininity are independent dimensions. The implication of the second point is that it is invalid to carry out 2×2 analyses of variance with Bem's four subject groups as the independent variable if the dimensions of masculinity and femininity are themselves correlated in the population. One solution to these problems lies in the application of multiple regression analysis; Bem (1977) has indeed suggested this possibility herself.

My own proposal (Hargreaves *et al.* 1981) is that androgyny is most parsimoniously assessed as the *product* of a subject's masculinity and femininity scores. Cohen (1978) has demonstrated that it is possible to regard such products as measures of the degree of interaction between the two variables; and so the theoretical implication is that we regard masculinity and femininity as conceptually distinct, yet interacting variables. It is quite possible to construct simple linear regression equations in which the value of different dependent variables (ideational fluency was investigated in my own study) can be predicted from masculinity (M) and femininity (F) scores, and from androgyny defined as $M \times F$. Lubinski *et al.* (1981) have taken this approach further by incorporating the sex of the subject as a further variable in the regression equation that interacts with all the others. Though a good deal of effort needs to be put into the development of this approach – in developing techniques to refine the discrimination between 'sex-typed' and 'undifferentiated' subjects, for example – there seems little doubt that it will be a most promising way forward.

Gender schema theory

Gender schema theory (Bem 1981a) represents what might be called a cognitive, or information-processing approach to sex-role stereotyping. The starting point of the theory is the definition of the degree of sex-typing of males and females as the extent to which they are socialized into masculine and feminine behaviour patterns; and it is assumed that this can be measured directly in terms of scores on the BSRI. The theory holds that this degree of sex-typing determines *gender-based schematic processing*, which is the individual's 'generalised readiness to process information on the basis of the sex-linked associations that constitute the gender schema' (Bem 1981a, p. 354).

Schemas, or schemata, are not new in psychology. They are fundamental to Piaget's theory, as well as to some cognitive psychological theories of perception (e.g. Neisser 1976): and Hampson employs them in her constructivist analysis of personality (see Chapter 3). Schemas form the internal conceptual frameworks that individuals build up as a result of past experiences; and new information is assimilated to them.

Bem holds that the *gender schema* is a network of associations that forms a fundamental and basic part of an individual's conceptual framework, such that 'gender-based schematic processing' is a central characteristic of perception. Furthermore, she proposes that the self-concept itself eventually becomes assimilated to the gender schema, such that self-evaluation becomes organized around the degree to which the self is perceived as congruent with the gender schema. There are individual differences in the strength of this assimilation: sex-typed individuals are seen to differ from non-sex-typed individuals according to the degree to which their self-concepts are organized around the gender schema.

This view puts the concept of androgyny into an interesting new perspective. Gender schema theory does not primarily emphasize the degree to which an individual is masculine or feminine, that is the *content* of sex-typing, but rather its *process*, that is the extent to which the individual codes new information in terms of sex roles. This change of perspective has broader political implications as far as feminist ideals are concerned. Bem suggests that the power of the individual's gender schema derives from 'society's ubiquitous insistence on the functional importance of the gender dichotomy' (Bem 1981, p. 354); and her prescription for the future is that we should strive to oppose this. In other words, the lesson to be learnt is not that individuals should be more or less masculine or feminine, but that they should be less ready to explain actions and intentions in terms of gender schemata. This is an interesting alternative to the ideal of an 'androgynous society', which some authors (e.g. Archer & Lloyd 1982) in any case regard as unrealistic.

It is easy to see the appeal of an information-processing approach to sex-role stereotyping in that this is in tune with the zeitgeist of other areas of psychology; and so it is not very surprising that other, essentially similar models of gender-schematic processing have emerged almost simultaneously (e.g. Markus *et al.* 1982; Martin & Halverson 1981). The empirical support for these models, however, is so far rather weak.

In Bem's (1981a) own research, subjects' sex-typing is first assessed by means of the BSRI, and the scores are then compared with performance on measures of gender-schematic processing. One study investigated the extent to which the free recall of a set of stimulus words was 'clustered by gender', defined in terms of the occurrence of same-gender sequential pairs. A second investigated the speed of processing of schema-consistent and schema-inconsistent self-ratings; and a third looked at individuals' readiness to interact with members of the opposite sex as a function of physical attractiveness. Bem found support for gender schema theory in the results of all these studies. More strongly sex-typed individuals as defined by scores on the BSRI were more likely to exhibit gender clustering in free recall; to make schema-consistent self-judgements more quickly than schema-inconsistent ones; and to be influenced by physical attractiveness in interacting with members of the opposite sex.

There may be a certain degree of circularity in this argument in that the attributes used for the dependent variable in the second experiment (speed of gender-schematic processing) were actually taken from the

BSRI. In other words, subjects' self-ratings on a set of personality characteristics were compared with their speed of processing of the same characteristics. Bem's results would carry much more weight if the independent and dependent variable measures were demonstrably drawn from different stimulus domains. This point raises the wider issue of the *validity* of measures of masculinity and femininity on scales like the BSRI: what exactly is being measured?

Spence and Helmreich (1981), who have had a long-standing debate with Bem about the nature and measurement of masculinity and femininity, have made some specific criticisms of gender schema theory that address this crucial question. They claim that there is a logical contradiction between the BSRI as a measure of the two independent dimensions of masculinity and femininity, and as a measure of gender-schematic processing, which they see as a unidimensional construct. Further, they suggest that 'the BSRI and other similar instruments measure primarily self-images of instrumental and expressive personality traits and that these trait clusters show little or no relationship to global self-images of masculinity and femininity' (Spence & Helmreich 1981, p. 365). Bem's (1981b) reply is that there is no contradiction in the use of the two-dimensional BSRI for research on the unidimensional concept of gender-schematic processing because the BSRI is only a tool for identifying sex-typed individuals. The concept of gender-schematic processing, in other words, is not based on the *content* of the behaviour in question.

Bem replies to the second of Spence and Helmreich's points by suggesting that the instrumental and expressive traits tapped by the BSRI may or may not correspond to masculinity and femininity according to the degree of an individual's sex-typing; the scale 'taps different things for different people'. In other words, the scale measures instrumentality and expressiveness in non-sex-typed people, and masculinity and femininity in sex-typed people: and this highlights a fundamental conceptual problem in androgyny research.

Researchers have defined subjects' masculinity and femininity in terms of their self-ratings with respect to culturally-defined patterns of behaviour: and have then tested these definitions by comparing them with experimental measures of the same behaviour patterns. Experimental research on androgyny may thus be partly circular, or tautological, because the dependent variables are likely to be causally related to the independent variables. Sex-role stereotypes, that is consensual beliefs about the behaviour of males and females, are very likely to influence that very behaviour of males and females, that is the nature of the roles themselves. Archer (1980, 1984) and Stoppard and Kalin (1978, 1981) have disagreed about whether or not this distinction corresponds to that between *descriptive* ('men and women *are* like this') and *prescriptive* beliefs (men and women *ought to be* like this'): and their argument almost certainly stems from the same problem of circularity. Fortunately, as we have seen, gender schema theory holds out the promise of overcoming this problem by analysing the *process*, as well as the *content*, of sex-role stereotyping.

Conclusion

There is a considerable amount of common ground between the theories reviewed in this chapter, as well as some conflict which primarily arises from the emphases placed on different aspects of behaviour. The psychoanalytic approach probably stands furthest apart from the others, although its developmental orientation, and its stress on the process of identification, are common to all. Social learning theory and cognitive-developmental theory, although apparently espousing precisely opposite views of the process of sex-typing, also have a good deal in common; many of the concepts that distinguish the former from a purely behaviouristic approach could essentially be characterized as 'cognitive'. The role theory approach also shares this orientation in the sense that it is primarily concerned with the description and explanation of *internalized* sets of rules and attitudes.

Gender schema theory is most closely related to the cognitive developmental approach. The concepts of 'gender schema' and 'gender identity', and the way in which the two theories describe their functions, are indeed virtually identical. The mechanisms of sex-role stereotyping, in terms of concepts such as these, are the subject of a considerable amount of current research. I believe that this attention is justified on theoretical grounds, since these mechanisms are central to our understanding of individual behaviour, as well as on broader social and political grounds. Practical solutions to the problems raised by sexism should be based on the best available explanations of the processes of sex-role stereotyping.

References

Antill, J. K. & Cunningham, J. D. (1982) Sex differences in performance on ability tests as a function of masculinity, femininity, and androgyny. *Journal of Personality and Social Psychology*, 42, 718–728.

Archer, J. (1980) The distinction between gender stereotypes and sex-role concepts. *British Journal of Social and Clinical Psychology*, 19, 51.

Archer, J. (1984) Gender stereotype and sex-role concepts: a reply to Stoppard and Kalin. *British Journal of Social Psychology*, 23, 89–91.

Archer, J. & Lloyd, B. B. (1982) *Sex and gender*. Harmondsworth: Penguin.

Bandura, A. (1977). *Social learning theory*. Englewood Cliffs, N. J.:Prentice-Hall.

Bandura, A. & Walters, R. H. (1963) *Social learning and personality development*. New York: Holt, Rinehart & Winston.

Bandura, A., Ross, D. & Ross, S. A. (1961) Transmission of aggression through imitation of aggressive models. *Journal of Abnormal and Social Psychology*, 63, 575–582.

Bandura, A., Ross, D. & Ross, S. A. (1963) A comparative test of the status envy, social power, and secondary reinforcement theories of identification learning. *Journal of Abnormal and Social Psychology*, 67, 527–534.

Baumrind, D. (1982) Are androgynous individuals more effective persons and parents? *Child Development*, 53, 44–75.

Bem, S. L. (1974). The measurement of psychological androgyny. *Journal of Consulting and Clinical Psychology*, 42, 155–162.

Bem, S. L. (1975) Sex role adaptability: one consequence of psychological androgyny. *Journal of Personality and Social Psychology*, 31, 634–643.

Bem, S.L. (1977) On the utility of alternative procedures for assessing psychological androgyny. *Journal of Consulting and Clinical Psychology*, 45, 196–205.

Bem, S. L. (1979) Theory and measurement of androgyny: a reply to the Pedhazur-Tetenbaum and Locksley-Colten critiques. *Journal of Personality and Social Psychology*, 37, 1047–1054.

Bem, S. L. (1981a) Gender schema theory: a cognitive account of sex typing. *Psychological Review*, 88, 354–364.

Bem, S. L. (1981b) The BSRI and gender schema theory: a reply to Spence and Helmreich. *Psychological Review*, 88, 369–371.

Bem, S.L. & Lenney, E. (1976) Sex typing and the avoidance of cross-sex behaviour. *Journal of Personality and Social Psychology*, 33, 48–54.

Cohen, J. (1978) Partialed products *are* interactions: partialed powers *are* curve components. *Psychological Bulletin*, 85, 858–866.

Connor, J. M. & Serbin, L. A. (1977) Behaviourally based masculine- and feminine-activity-preference scales for preschoolers: correlates with other classroom behaviours and cognitive tests. *Child Development*, 48, 1411–1416.

Danziger, K. (1971) *Socialization*. Harmondsworth: Penguin.

DeVries, R. (1969) Constancy of gender identity in the years three to six. *Monographs of the Society for Research in Child Development*, 34 (127).

Eisenberg, N., Murray, E. & Hite, T. (1982) Children's reasoning regarding sex-typed toy choices. *Child Development*, 53, 81–86.

Fagot, B. I. (1977) Consequences of moderate cross gender behavior in preschool children. *Child Development*, *48*, 902–907.

Fling, S. & Manosevitz, M. (1972) Sex typing in nursery school children's play interests. *Developmental Psychology*, *7*, 146–152.

Freud, S. (1925) Some psychical consequences of the anatomical distinction between the sexes. *Standard Edition*, *19*, 243–258. London: Hogarth Press (1961).

Hargreaves, D. J. (1976) What are little boys and girls made of? *New Society*, *37*, 542–544.

Hargreaves, D. J. (1977) Sex roles in divergent thinking. *British Journal of Educational Psychology*, *47*, 25–32.

Hargreaves, D. J. (1979) Sex roles and creativity. *In* O. Hartnett, G. Boden & M. Fuller (eds) *Sex-role stereotyping*. London: Tavistock.

Hargreaves, D. J., Bates, H. M. & Foot, J. M. C. (1985) Sex-typed labelling affects task performance. *British Journal of Social Psychology*, *24*, 153–155.

Hargreaves, D. J., Stoll, L., Farnworth, S. & Morgan, S. (1981) Psychological androgyny and ideational fluency. *British Journal of Social Psychology*, *20*, 53–55.

Heilbrun, A. B. (1981) *Human sex-role behavior*. New York: Pergamon Press.

Horney, K. (1924) On the genesis of the castration complex in women. *International Journal of Psychoanalysis*, *5*, 50–65.

Kohlberg, L. (1966), A cognitive developmental analysis of children's sex role concepts and attitudes. *In* E. E. Maccoby (ed.) *The development of sex differences*. Stanford: Stanford University Press.

Kuhn, D., Nash, S. C. & Brucken, L. (1978) Sex role concepts of two- and three-years-olds. *Child Development*, *49*, 445–451.

Lewis, M. (1975). Early sex differences in the human: studies of socio-emotional development. *Archives of Sexual Behaviour*, *4*, 329–335.

Locksley, A. & Colten, M. E. (1979). Psychological androgyny: a case of mistaken identity? *Journal of Personality and Social Psychology*, *37*, 1017–1031.

Lubinski, D., Tellegen, A. & Butcher, J. N. (1981) The relationship between androgyny and subjective indicators of emotional well-being. *Journal of Personality and Social Psychology*, *40*, 722–730.

Maccoby, E. E. (ed.) (1966) *The development of sex differences*. Stanford: Stanford University Press.

Markus, H., Crane, M., Bernstein, S. & Siladi, M. (1982). Self-schemas and gender. *Journal of Personality and Social Psychology*, *42*, 38–50.

Martin, C. L. & Halverson, C. F. (1981) A schematic processing model of sex typing and stereotyping in children. *Child Development*, *52*, 1119–1134.

Miller, P. H. (1983) *Theories of developmental psychology*. San Francisco: W. H. Freeman.

Mischel, W. (1966) A social learning view of sex differences. *In* E. E. Maccoby (ed.) *The development of sex differences*. Stanford: Stanford University Press.

Mischel, W. (1970) Sex-typing and socialization. *In* P. H. Mussen (ed.) *Carmichael's manual of child psychology*, 3rd edn, vol. 2. New York: John Wiley.

Mitchell, J. (1974) *Psychoanalysis and feminism*. Harmondsworth: Penguin.

Neisser, U. (1976) *Cognition and reality*. San Francisco: W. H. Freeman.

Pedhazur, E. J. & Tetenbaum, T. J. (1979) Bem Sex Role Inventory: a theoretical and methodological critique. *Journal of Personality and Social Psychology*, *37*, 996–1016.

Serbin, L. A., O'Leary, K. D., Kent, R. N. & Tonick, I. J. (1973) A comparison of teacher response to the preacademic problems and problem behavior of boys and girls. *Child Development*, *44*, 796–804.

Spence, J. T. & Helmreich, R. L. (1981) Androgyny versus gender schema: a comment on Bem's gender schema theory. *Psychological Review*, *88*, 365–368.

Spence, J. T., Helmreich, R. L. & Stapp, J. (1975) Ratings of self and peers on sex role attributes and their relation to self-esteem and conceptions of masculinity and femininity. *Journal of Personality and Social Psychology*, *32*, 29–39.

Stoppard, J. M. & Kalin, R. (1978) Can gender stereotypes and sex-role concepts be distinguished? *British Journal of Social and Clinical Psychology*, *17*, 211–217.

Stoppard, J. M. & Kalin, R. (1981) Gender stereotype and sex-role concepts: a comment on Archer. *British Journal of Social Psychology*, *20*, 224–225.

Taylor, M. C. & Hall, J. A. (1982) Psychological androgyny: theories, methods, and conclusions. *Psychological Bulletin*, *92*, 347–366.

Ullian, D. Z. (1976) The development of conceptions of masculinity and femininity. In B. B. Lloyd & J. Archer (eds) *Exploring sex differences*. London: Academic Press.

CHAPTER THREE Sex Roles and Personality
Sarah Hampson

> When you meet a Gethenian you cannot and must not do what a bisexual naturally does which is to cast him in the role of Man or Woman, while adopting towards him a corresponding role depending on the patterned or possible interactions between persons of the same or the opposite sex. Our entire pattern of socio-sexual interaction is nonexistent here. They cannot play the game. They do not see one another as men or women. This is almost impossible for our imagination to accept. What is the first question we ask about a newborn baby? (LeGuin 1979, pp. 69–70)

It is virtually impossible to understand someone's personality without knowing the person's sex. This point is well-illustrated in the science fiction story *The Left Hand of Darkness* (LeGuin 1979), in which the planet Winter is populated with human-like beings who, most of the time, exist in a sexless state. In writing her story, LeGuin used the male pronoun when referring to these beings and, inevitably, the reader forms an impression of them as male personalities. The alternative would have been to invent a pronoun which did not discriminate between the sexes. However, to do so would have created enormous problems for the development of characterization in the novel. The reader would have had great difficulty in forming an impression of a personality for which no gender information was available despite the presence of other sorts of information. Why is this so? There is no straightforward answer to this question, and the issues it raises constitute the subject matter of this chapter.

The purpose of this chapter is to explore the connections between sex roles and personality. But before looking at the connections, it is important to be clear about what is being linked with what. Williams and Best (1982) provided a sensible set of distinctions between the various terms: *sex roles* refer to the activities in which each sex participates; *sex stereotypes* refer to beliefs about men and women; hence *sex-role stereotypes* refer to beliefs about the appropriate activities for men and women; and *sex-trait stereotypes* refer to the beliefs about the traits differentially associated with men and women. For present purposes, a slight modification of Williams and Best's definitions will be adopted. Instead of restricting the definition of sex roles to activities only, it will be extended to include personality traits and behaviours, as well as the activities characterizing each sex. This chapter will consider both sex roles (that is differences between the sexes in traits, behaviours, and activities) and sex-role stereotypes (that is beliefs about these differences).

In defining personality, a constructivist view will be adopted (Hampson 1982, 1984). Personality is regarded as the combination of three elements: the individual's behaviour; the meaning of that behaviour as constructed by other people; and the meaning of that behaviour as constructed by the individual her or himself. The underlying rationale of the constructivist view is that studying personality outside its social context is bound to provide an incomplete account. Behaviour alone does not amount to personality. It is only when that behaviour is imbued with social meaning that it becomes personality. For example, it may be possible to use various psychophysiological recordings to measure arousal level, but arousal is not personality. Extraversion refers to a variety of behaviours through which arousal level is expressed, but there is a social world of difference between extraversion and arousal. Behaviour has to be overlaid with social meaning before it may be said to constitute personality. We share a set of understandings about the social meaning of behaviour and we use traits as a way of summarizing and communicating this meaning. The language of personality description − trait language − is the vehicle for personality construction.

The constructivist approach to personality is well-suited for an analysis of the connections between sex roles and personality. As will soon be apparent, the actual differences in sex roles (as defined above) are very few. However, sex-role stereotypes attribute distinctly different sex roles to each sex. The existence of sex-role stereotypes, and their effects on behaviour, despite their tenuous connections with reality, demands a constructivist approach. To illustrate, it is widely believed that women have a lower sex drive than men despite the lack of evidence to support this claim. A definition of personality which focused exclusively on individual behaviour would produce a tremendously boring account of human sexuality, as indeed, strictly biological accounts of sexual intercourse tend to be. Where sexuality and personality unite is in the beliefs about sex held by the participants about each other and themselves.

This chapter is organized in three main sections. The first, and the shortest, provides a brief review of the findings on sex roles. It examines the evidence for sex differences across a range of personality traits, behaviours, and activities. This section constitutes the first element of constructed personality: the action the individual brings to the social arena. The second section discusses the second element: the beliefs people hold about sex roles (i.e. sex-role stereotypes). It looks at the form these beliefs take, and examines some of the empirical work from social cognition on sex-role stereotyping. The third section completes the constructivist circle by examining the influence of sex-role stereotypes on people's beliefs about themselves.

Acting sex roles

The first component of constructed personality to be considered is that provided by the actor. In making connections between sex roles and personality, a major issue is the extent to which women and men differ on personality characteristics. If it should be the case that sex, as a subject variable, has powerful main effects, then answering the question posed at the beginning of this chapter would be relatively simple. A person's biological sex would be a valuable piece of information that would reliably predict a sex-role pattern of activities, traits and behaviours. Not surprisingly, reality turns out to be more complicated.

From a scientific point of view, the case that women differ psychologically from men has yet to be proven. When Maccoby and Jacklin (1974) reviewed the research on sex differences, they were only able to identify four areas where anything like reliable differences between men and women had been established: women are superior in verbal abilities; men are superior in mathematical and visual-spatial abilities; and men are more aggressive. Only the last of these differences is of direct relevance to personality.

Aggression can be assessed in several ways. The majority of studies in which men were observed to be more aggressive than women used behavioural measures such as physical violence. In studies where verbal measures were used, the findings are less clear-cut. Under certain conditions, women have been observed to be just as aggressive as men, and sometimes more so (Frieze *et al.* 1978). For example, women are more aggressive in private than public situations (Mallik & McCandless 1966) and they are more aggressive when they are given permission to be so by the experimenter (Leventhal, Shemberg & Schoelandt 1968).

These caveats for one of the more solid of the sex differences are indicative of the methodological and conceptual problems in this research. It is extremely difficult to manipulate sex as an independent variable while simultaneously holding other potentially relevant variables constant. Since so much of human behaviour is believed to be differentially associated with one sex or the other, it is hard to choose a dependent variable that is free from such associations and hence free from the implicit expectations they imply. The problematic nature of this research area makes for controversy over the correctness of conclusions drawn in literature reviews, and Block (1976) was critical of Maccoby and Jacklin's (1974) emphasis on the absence of sex differences. She argued that they had underestimated the presence of sex differences by, for example, giving too much weight to the non-significant results from studies with small samples, and ignoring the developmental trend towards a greater sex difference with increasing age of the sample.

Block's critique has to some extent been borne out by the last decade of research into sex differences. Deaux (1984) concluded that there is evidence for more sex differences now than were acknowledged by Maccoby and Jacklin (1974). For example, women are more conforming and more susceptible to persuasion, and they are better than men at decoding non-verbal messages. Nevertheless, it is still widely concluded by reviewers today that women and men actually differ far less than people believe they differ (e.g. Nicholson 1984).

All this emphasis on the similarities between the sexes must be set against the backdrop of the social facts of life where the reality of sex roles is undisputed. Despite the absence of actual personality differences, sex is undeniably used as a marker for the appropriateness of a vast range of behaviours and activities. Other chapters in this book discuss the sex-role differentiation of occupations (Chapter 11) and sport and leisure (Chapter 12). In addition, some other social realities should be noted such as the inequitable distribution of social power, status, and hence influence – to the male's advantage.

These social facts may provide the solution to the puzzle of the prevalence of sex-role stereotypes in the absence of actual sex differences (Eagly 1983; Eagly & Steffan 1984). Eagly has argued that sex-role stereotypes are the result of the segregation of women and men into different occupations and social roles. The characteristics of these jobs and roles (for example influence for politicians, nurturance for parents) are then attributed to the group typically found occupying these positions (that is more men than women are politicians, and more women than men are full-time parents). From this perspective, sex-role stereotypes are a prominent example of role bias: the tendency to attribute to particular role-players the characteristics associated with the social role they are playing (Ross, Amabile & Steinmetz 1977).

Observing sex roles in others

In the previous section the actual differences in the roles acted by women and men were briefly examined and found to lie more in activities than psychological characteristics. In this section, the links between sex roles and personality are explored via the observer-component of constructed personality. The concern here is with the beliefs people hold about sex roles, and the part these beliefs play when people attempt to understand one another's personalities.

The measurement of sex-role stereotypes

The recent history of research on sex-role stereotypes began with the now classic study by Broverman and her colleagues conducted in the 1960s (cf. Broverman *et al.* 1972). They established the existence of consensual beliefs about sex-role stereotypes at that time (see Chapter 13). A few years later, the first stage of the construction of the Bem Sex Role Inventory (BSRI) incorporated an investigation of sex-role stereotypes which largely confirmed the pattern of beliefs described by Broverman *et al.* (Bem 1974). The BSRI contains items chosen on the basis of their perceived sex-typed social desirability. Subjects rated a large pool of personality traits either in terms of how desirable they were for a woman in American society or for a man. Those items judged by both male and female subjects as significantly more desirable for a woman were used for the Femininity scale, and similarly those items judged as significantly more desirable for a man constituted the Masculinity scale. The Femininity scale incorporates warmth, emotionality and expressiveness, and the Masculinity scale refers to dominance, assertiveness and aggression.

A slightly different approach to the study of beliefs about sex-role stereotypes is illustrated by the work of Williams and Best and their colleagues (c.f. Williams & Best 1982). They used Gough's Adjective Check List (ACL) as a way of measuring what they called sex-trait stereotypes. The ACL is used in personality research as a self-assessment instrument, but Williams and Best changed the instructions and asked subjects to decide, for each of the 300 items, whether it was more frequently associated with men than with women, or neither. They found substantial agreement between male and female college students on the sex-trait stereotypes which largely corresponded to the male-instrumental and female-expressive distinction obtained in previous research.

Additionally, they obtained extensive cross-cultural data which indicated the pan-cultural nature of these beliefs.

All of the above studies focused predominantly on the personality traits that are differentially ascribed to either sex. However, sex-role stereotypes contain more than traits: there are also beliefs about behaviours, occupations and physical appearance. Deaux and Lewis (1984) demonstrated that these elements constitute relatively independent components of sex-role stereotypes, and knowledge about one component, particularly physical appearance, is used to make inferences about the others. There may also be non-verbal components to sex-role stereotypes, in particular, affective reactions to the stereotype may be an important element of the stereotype itself (Ashmore & Del Boca 1979).

The research described so far in this section has established the existence of social or cultural stereotypes about the differences between women's and men's personalities. These stereotypes are social in the sense that they represent a widely shared consensus about the characteristics associated with the typical man and the typical woman. In contrast, at the individual level of analysis, stereotypes may be studied as cognitive structures constructed by the individual to assist in the complex task of social information processing. The individual level of analysis is the focus of the present discussion since the purpose of this section is to examine the influence of the sex-role stereotypes held by individuals on their understanding of other people. The study of social stereotypes is suggestive of the content of individual's stereotypes, but is not informative about the nature of the representation of the stereotype in the individual, or the way the stereotype affects the individual's social information processing (Ashmore & Del Boca 1979).

Within social cognition, stereotypes are viewed by some investigators as cognitive schemata (e.g. Snyder & Uranowitz 1978), and by others as cognitive categories (e.g. Rothbart 1981). These alternative approaches to the representation of stereotypes are, in the main, complementary and their similarities rather than differences will be emphasized here.

Sex-role schemata

Schemata are cognitive structures which represent organized knowledge in memory (Fiske & Taylor 1984). This knowledge may include specific instances or episodes, but in the main it is composed of abstract, generic knowledge which has been distilled from past experience (Taylor &

Crocker 1980). Schemata serve two major functions. First, as the tools of top-down processing, they are used in the active construction of perception: schemata guide the encoding and representation of incoming information. Second, schemata contain recipes for action: they determine what inferences can be made from incoming data and they provide guidelines for subsequent behaviour.

In exploring the connections between sex roles and personality from a constructivist point of view, sex-role schemata provide a way of conceptualizing the differences between observers in their reliance on sex-role stereotypes for the processing of gender-related information about others. (The use of sex-role schemata for processing information about the self is discussed in the next section). The investigation of the effects of individual differences in sex-role schemata is based on the assumption that relatively stable perceiver characteristics affect information processing. Two forms of these individual differences have been investigated with respect to sex-role schemata. First, there are many schemata with which the observer can process social information, so there will be differences between individuals simply in terms of the extent to which they use sex-role schemata. Second, there will be individual differences in the content of those schemata. The power of casting an individual difference in schematic form is that the schema provides a structure for representing this aspect of a person, and a mechanism by which this characteristic influences perception and behaviour.

One way of determining which schema an individual uses for processing information about others is to discover which schemata have self-relevance for the person. Self-relevant schemata, known more simply as self-schemata, are knowledge structures about the self (Markus 1977). It is assumed that they have significant consequences not only for processing information about the self, but also for processing information about other people (Markus 1983). Bem (1981) argued that the BSRI can be used as a measure of the degree to which an individual engages in gender-based schematic processing. She hypothesized that those people who are highly 'sex-typed' (that is score high on either the Masculinity or the Femininity scales) would be more likely to use a sex-role schema in the encoding and representation of gender-related information than people who are androgynous or undifferentiated. She found that sex-typed individuals produced more gender-based clustering in free recall than did androgynous, undifferentiated, and cross-typed individuals.

Markus *et al.* (1982) pursued the effects of individual differences in schema-content by comparing four kinds of self-relevant sex-role schemata: masculine sex-typed, feminine sex-typed, high androgynous, and low androgynous. In a comparison of amount of recall and clustering of masculine, feminine and neutral words, they found some evidence that recall of words congruent with the self-schema was advantaged.

However, neither of these studies directly addresses the issue of how a sex-typed person processes information about others. One example of such a study is Mills and Tyrell's (1983) investigation of the effects of sex of subject and sex-typing of subject on the encoding of occupations varying on a gender-related dimension. Whereas sex of subject was related to differential use of the masculine–feminine dichotomy for encoding occupations (women used it more consistently than men), no effects of sex-typing were observed.

The use of sex-role schemata will depend in part on perceiver characteristics and in part on the situation. It may be that studies of the effects of sex-role schemata have failed to pay sufficient attention to situational or contextual variables. There will be some unambiguous contexts where sex-role schemata will be highly appropriate and, regardless of the exact form a person's sex-typing takes, the knowledge embedded in the sex-role schema will be used. It may only be in relatively ambiguous contexts that sex-typing effects will emerge (Mills & Tyrell 1983).

These studies relate to the first function of schemata referred to above: their perceptual function. There has been less work to date on the second function of schemata: their role as recipes for action. One such study is an investigation into the relation between sex-typing and values (Feather 1984). In a correlational study, endorsing feminine items on questionnaire measures of self-relevant sex-role schemata was related to seeing communal and expressive values as more important than agentic and instrumental values, whereas endorsing masculine items was related to the reverse pattern of values (that is seeing agentic and instrumental values as more important than communal and expressive values). Androgyny was not related to any distinct set of values. In so far as a person's values will enter into behavioural choice, this study is suggestive of a link between sex-role schemata and behaviour.

To conclude this section on the schematic approach to sex roles, a number of limitations of these studies should be mentioned. First, using the BSRI as a measure of sex-typing may be misguided since it was designed as a measure of two dimensions (masculinity and femininity), and not as a measure of strength of gender schema (Spence & Helmreich 1981): this issue is discussed in Chapter 2. Second, these laboratory experiments are highly artificial and may be failing to mimic what actually goes in real social life. Third, it may be that the level at which sex roles operate in the processing of information about others is somewhat broader than is implied by schema research. Sex-role stereotypes combine a range of elements which together suggest an entire life-style for a person, not merely which trait words might be appropriate. The research to be described next, in which sex roles are conceptualized as cognitive categories, has been more illuminating and this may be because it is typically more ecologically valid, it incorporates a broader view of sex roles, and it has not attempted to investigate individual differences.

Sex-role categories

We usually register a person's sex easily and automatically. Indeed, it is only when we find ourselves taking second glances at an ambiguous case that we become conscious of making this judgement. Sex, like race and age, provides a readily available basis for deciding between mutually exclusive (albeit crude) categories: female versus male; black versus white; old versus young (Rothbart, Dawes & Park 1984) since each of us is either female or male, black or white, and old or young.Therefore, making this categorization inevitably sets up an ingroup versus an outgroup, which has important implications.

For example, Park and Rothbart (1982) established that men see other men as more variegated and complex than women, whereas women see other women as more variegated and complex than men. Rothbart, Dawes and Park (1984) discussed how ingroup versus outgroup categorization affects the interpretation of behaviour. Men and women differ in the way they perceive the same conversation between a couple (Abbey 1982), with men emphasizing the sex role and sexual connotations of the interaction more than women.

Awareness of the ingroup versus outgroup distinction may actually produce more stereotyped behaviour by the participants. For example, women may become more 'feminine' in the presence of men, but the evidence for this is mixed. Skrypnek and Snyder (1982) demonstrated that knowledge of a target's sex affected the way a perceiver divided up some job-like tasks. These tasks were sex-typed, and the male perceivers allocated the tasks according to the sex of the target. Other studies have shown that people will change their behaviour to conform to others' expectations (e.g. Snyder, Tanke & Berscheid 1977; Swann 1984).

In summary, when an observer categorizes another into male versus female, an ingroup versus an outgroup distinction is established which can affect the way the observer perceives the target and the way the observer behaves towards the target. In turn, the observer's behaviour may elicit behaviour from the target that is consistent with the observer's stereotypic beliefs. From these conclusions, it is apparent that the observer can play an active role in personality construction along sex-role stereotypic lines, remaining remarkably oblivious to any aspect of the target's input to the construction process other than the target's sex.

Although the target's sex can be the most salient cue and the only one used in personality construction (cf. Taylor *et al.* 1978) obviously this is not always the case, since we are capable of making far more complex categorical distinctions between people than the crude sexual dichotomy. Sex provides the basis for allocating a person into one of two extremely broad or superordinate categories which are used when sex is the only information we have about a person, or when it is particularly salient.

Observing sex roles in ourselves

The last element of constructed personality to be considered is the self-observer component. It has been argued by some (e.g. D. J. Bem 1967) that we learn about our own personality in the same way that we learn about other people's, by observing our behaviour and drawing the appropriate inferences. Others (e.g. Singer 1984) emphasize the unique contribution of the self perspective in the form of private information to which only we have access. The human capacity to be self-reflective permits us to try to see ourselves as other people see us. So the impressions we construct of our own personalities are formed from three sources: our behaviour, our private thoughts and feelings, and our beliefs about how other people see us.

Recently, the self has become the focus of some new directions in personality research (Markus 1977, 1983). The self has been conceptualized both as a schema (e.g. Markus 1977) and as a social category (e.g. Kihlstrom & Cantor 1984), but the concept of a self-schema has generated more research. As was noted in the previous section (see also Chapter 2), the BSRI has been used by Bem (1981) and others as a measure of the extent to which an individual thinks of her or himself in sex-typed terms (i.e. has a self-relevant gender schema). Despite the lack of powerful evidence that individual differences in strength of sex-role schemata play an important role in the perception of others, there is a case to be made for their influence on self-perception.

Bem (1981) found that sex-typed subjects made faster schema-consistent judgements and slower schema-inconsistent judgements than cross-sexed, androgynous, or undifferentiated subjects. Markus *et al.* (1982) found that feminine schematics remembered more feminine items, and judged their self-relevance more rapidly and confidently than masculine items. They obtained equivalent findings for male schematics. Together, these studies suggest that self-perceived sex-role stereotyping has important consequences for self-perception. However, both studies have an inherent circularity. The stimulus items to be judged for self-relevance were taken from the BSRI, the same measure used to identify the schematic nature of the subjects initially. It is hard to see how these studies may be interpreted as anything other than a set of converging operations to measure a person's self-perceived sex-role stereotype. They do not step outside the circularity by exploring how these same subjects processed different, self-relevant, gender-related information.

Sex is at the root of sex roles. As obvious as this may seem, when psychologists are lost in the white-coated world of science, it is something they tend to forget. The one form of human behaviour widely believed to be where we come closest to being and finding our true selves unfettered by social norms and expectations, is in sexual relationships. But is this really true? Hollway's studies of men and women's experience of heterosexual relationships (Hollway 1984) suggested that romantic relationships are powerfully influenced by social roles. She identified three 'discourses' which dictate heterosexual sexuality: the male sex drive discourse (men possess an insatiable biological drive to copulate); the have/hold discourse (woman are happy with monogamy and family life even though men are inevitably sexually incontinent); the permissive discourse (both men and women can enjoy sex without love).

The inconsistencies that arise from the simultaneous influences of all three discourses cause problems of both self and other-understanding for heterosexual couples. Whereas Hollway regarded discourses as external to the individual, in the language of social cognition, discourses contain knowledge which is internalized in the form of sex-role schemata. The forays of Hollway and others (e.g. Segal 1983) into the very real world of sexual relationships have exposed the complexities and inconsistencies of sex-role beliefs which have been glossed over in social cognition.

Conclusions

In the preceding sections, the connections between sex roles and personality have been traced from three perspectives: the evidence for sex differences, the beliefs about sex differences as applied to others, and as applied to the self. Despite the lack of objective evidence for psychological differences between the sexes, sex-role stereotypes permeate just about every aspect of social life. It is in the context of social life that personality is constructed and therefore sex roles and personality are inextricably entwined. One last complication should be noted. The tendency to oversimplify sex roles has already been observed, and another aspect of this oversimplification is the failure to consider sex roles and personality over the lifespan. There is a growing appreciation of the importance of studying personality in the context of life histories (e.g. Runyon 1982). An important feature of sex roles, like all social roles, it their sensitivity to age. Young men and women are not expected to behave in the same way as old women and men. Constructed personality is an elaborate interplay of social roles, and there will be phases in the lifespan when sex roles will be emphasized more strongly than other roles (Erdwins & Mellinger 1984).

Finally, to return to the question raised at the beginning of this chapter by LeGuin's provocative novel: why is gender information so central to personality? In answer, it appears that of all the categories with which we can divide up the world of people sex roles, like other dichotomies such as age and colour, are the broadest. They are superordinate in the sense that other categories are included in them. As a result of the breadth and inclusiveness of sex roles, gender information is the basis for an enormous number and range of inferences, even though these will be riddled with inaccuracy for specific individuals. On the basis of gender, we can set up a hypothetical impression to be refined by subsequent information. In the absence of gender information we have no such default impression. The difficulty experienced by the reader of LeGuin's novel in forming personality impressions suggest that we do need these broad social categories as starting points in personality construction. This suggests that if our society does one day achieve a release from the sex roles then another (but let us hope less oppressive) dichotomy may fill the vacuum.

Acknowledgement

I would like to thank my colleague Stephen Frosh for his helpful comments and discussion on an earlier draft of this chapter.

References

Abbey, A. (1982) Sex differences in attribution for friendly behaviour: do males misperceive females' friendliness? *Journal of Personality and Social Psychology, 42,* 830–838.

Ashmore, R. D. & Del Boca, F. K. (1979) Sex stereotypes and implicit personality theory: toward a cognitive-social psychological conceptualization. *Sex Roles, 5,* 219–248.

Bem, D. J. (1967) Self-perception: an alternative interpretation of cognitive dissonance phenomena. *Psychological Review,* 74, 183–200.

Bem, S. L. (1974) The measurement of psychological androgyny. *Journal of Consulting and Clinical Psychology, 42,* 155–162.

Bem, S. L. (1981) Gender schema theory: a cognitive account of sex typing. *Psychological Review, 88,* 354–364.

Block, J. H. (1976) Debatable conclusions about sex differences. *Contemporary Psychology, 11,* 517–522.

Broverman, I. K., Vogel, S. R., Broverman, D. M., Clarkson, F. E. & Rosenkrantz, P. S. (1972) Sex-role stereotypes: a current appraisal. *Journal of Social Issues, 28,* 59–78.

Deaux, K. (1984) From individual differences to social categories: an analysis of a decade's research on gender. *American Psychologist, 39,* 105–116.

Deaux, K. & Lewis, L. L. (1984) Structure of gender stereotypes: interrelationships among components and gender label. *Journal of Personality and Social Psychology, 46,* 991–1004.

Eagly, A. H. (1983) Gender and social influence: a social psychological analysis. *American Psychologist, 38,* 971–981.

Eagly, A. H. & Steffan, V. J. (1984) Gender stereotypes stem from the distribution of women and men into social roles. *Journal of Personality and Social Psychology, 46,* 735–754.

Erdwins, C. J. & Mellinger, J. C. (1984). Mid-life women: relation of age and role to personality. *Journal of Personality and Social Psychology, 47,* 390–395.

Feather, N. T. (1984). Masculinity, femininity, psychological androgyny, and the structure of values. *Journal of Personality and Social Psychology, 47,* 604–620.

Fiske, S. T. & Taylor, S. E. (1984) *Social cognition.* Reading, MA: Addison-Wesley.

Frieze, I. H., Parsons, J. E., Johnson, P. B., Ruble, D. N. & Zellman, G. L. (1978) *Women and sex roles.* New York: Norton.

Hampson, S. E. (1982) *The construction of personality: an introduction.* London: Routledge & Kegan Paul.

Hampson, S. E. (1984) The social construction of personality. *In* H. Bonarius, G. Van Heck & N. Smid (eds) *Personality psychology in Europe: theoretical and empirical developments.* Lisse, Holland: Swets & Zeitlinger.

Hollway, W. (1984) Gender difference and the production of subjectivity. *In* J. Henriques, W. Hollway, C. Urwin, C. Venn & V. Walkerdine *Changing the subject.* London: Methuen.

Kihlstrom, J. F. & Cantor, N. (1984) Mental representations of the self. In L. Berkowitz (ed.) *Advances in experimental social psychology,* vol. 17. New York: Academic Press.

LeGuin, U. K. (1979). *The left hand of darkness*. London: Panther Books.

Leventhal, D. B., Shemberg, K. M. & Schoelandt, S. K. (1968) Effects of sex role adjustment upon the expression of aggression. *Journal of Personality and Social Psychology, 8*, 393–396.

Maccoby, E. E. & Jacklin, C. N. (1974) *The psychology of sex differences*. Stanford, CA: Stanford University Press.

Mallick, S. K. & McCandless, B. R. (1966) A study of catharsis of aggression. *Journal of Personality and Social Psychology, 4*, 591–596.

Markus, H. (1977) Self-schemas and processing information about the self. *Journal of Personality and Social Psychology, 35*, 63–78.

Markus, H. (1983) Self-knowledge: an expanded view. *Journal of Personality, 51*, 543–565.

Markus, H., Crane, M., Bernstein, S. & Siladi, M. (1982) Self-schemas and gender. *Journal of Personality and Social Psychology, 42*, 38–50.

Mills, C. J. & Tyrell, D. J. (1983) Sex-stereotypic encoding and release from pro-active interference. *Journal of Personality and Social Psychology, 45*, 772–778.

Nicholson, J. (1984) *Men and women: how different are they?* Oxford: Oxford University Press.

Park, B. & Rothbart, M. (1982). Perception of out-group homogeneity and levels of social categorization: memory for the subordinate attributes of in-group and out-group members. *Journal of Personality and Social Psychology, 42*, 1051–1068.

Ross, L., Amabile, T. M. & Steinmetz, J. L. (1977) Social roles, social control, and biases in social perception processes. *Journal of Personality and Social Psychology, 35*, 485–494.

Rothbart, M. (1981) Memory processes and social beliefs. *In* D. Hamilton (ed.) *Cognitive processes in stereotyping and intergroup behavior*. Hillsdale, NJ: Erlbaum.

Rothbart, M., Dawes, R. & Park, B. (1984) Stereotyping and sampling bias in intergroup perception. *In* J. R. Eiser (ed.) *Attitudinal judgment*. Berlin: Springer-Verlag.

Runyon, W. M. (1982) *Life histories and psychobiography: explorations in theory and method*. New York: Oxford University Press.

Segal, L. (1983) Sensual uncertainty, or why the clitoris is not enough. *In* S. Cartledge & J. Ryan (eds) *Sex and love*. London: The Women's Press.

Singer, J. L. (1984) The private personality. *Personality and Social Psychology Bulletin, 10*, 7–30.

Skrypnek, B. J. & Snyder, M. (1982) On the self-perpetuating nature of stereotypes about men and women. *Journal of Personality and Social Psychology, 18*, 277–291.

Snyder, M., Tanke, E. D. & Berscheid, E. (1977) Social perception and interpersonal behavior: on the self-fulfilling nature of social stereotypes. *Journal of Personality and Social Psychology, 35*, 656–666.

Snyder, M. & Uranowitz, S. W. (1978) Reconstructing the past: some cognitive consequences of person perception. *Journal of Personality and Social Psychology, 36*, 941–950.

Spence, J. J. & Helmreich, R. L. (1981) Androgyny versus gender schema: a comment on Bem's gender schema theory. *Psychological Review, 88*, 365–368.

Swann, W. B. (1984) Quest for accuracy in person perception. *Psychological Review, 91,* 457–477.

Taylor, S. E. & Crocker, J. (1980) Schematic bases of social inference processing. In E. T. Higgins, C. P. Herman & M. P. Zanna (eds) *Social cognition: the Ontario symposium,* vol. 1. Hillsdale, NJ: Erlbaum.

Taylor, S. E., Fiske, S. T., Etcoff, N. L. & Ruderman, A. J. (1978) Categorical and contextual bases of person memory and stereotyping. *Journal of Personality and Social Psychology, 36,* 778–793.

Williams, J. E. & Best, D. L. (1982) *Measuring sex stereotypes.* Beverly Hills, CA: Sage.

CHAPTER FOUR Sex Roles in Cognition
C. H. Singleton

Introduction

Do men and women think differently? Our sex-role stereotypes frequently embody the assumption, implicitly or explicitly, that they do. Men, for example, are widely believed to be the more logical sex, their thought processes untrammelled by emotions. Women are thought by many to be more intuitive, and to prefer dealing with personal, social and verbal problems rather than with the scientific, mathematical and mechanical problems to which men may aspire. These stereotypes of cognitive functioning are reflected in occupational differences between the sexes and in the career preferences and expectations expressed by children and young people. In clerical occupations women predominate, while men are substantially in the majority in scientific and technological occupations (Mackie & Pattullo 1977). Regardless of whether or not these occupational differences are justified by biological differences between men and women, sex-role stereotypes clearly play a major part in the shaping of cognitive abilities during development and their translation into occupational opportunities and achievements in adulthood.

Stereotyped concepts of sex-appropriate characteristics, beliefs and adult roles are displayed very early in life, sometimes as early as two or three years of age (Kuhn, Nash & Brucken 1978). Throughout their school life, most children set highly sex-typed occupational goals (Hewitt 1975; Looft 1971; Papalia & Tennent 1975; Schlossberg & Goodman 1972) and generally agree that social, verbal and artistic abilities are 'feminine' while spatial, mechanical and athletic skills are 'masculine' (Nash 1975). By adolescence, scientific and mathematical abilities are also stereotyped as 'masculine', boys predicting that these subjects will probably be relevant in their careers and girls disclaiming them as irrelevant to their future lives (Stein 1971). As one might expect, these attitudes and predictions take on the character of self-fulfilling prophecies, and as they grow up boys and girls diverge in their cognitive abilities. Girls develop greater proficiency in language and verbal tasks, while boys become more adept in tasks which have spatial or mathematical components. Sex-role stereotypes not only affect performance on cognitive tasks by the constraints they exercise over the processes of learning and socialization, but also by influencing the perception of the task itself. Performance is generally superior on tasks perceived as sex-appropriate, and inferior on tasks perceived as sex-inappropriate, regardless of the content of the task. In some cases these effects will swamp the normally expected sex differences, in other cases they will only moderate them. Overall, these findings are in accord with the prediction from Kohlberg's (1966) cognitive-developmental theory of sex-role acquisition that the child will strive to act consistently with his or her gender self-classification.

The purpose of this chapter is to examine the relationship between sex roles and cognition. The first objective is to outline the current state of knowledge about sex-related differences in cognitive abilities. Rather than attempting a complete survey of the field, however, the principal focus will be on those areas in which the strongest evidence for cognitive sex differences has emerged, and these are the areas of verbal, spatial, mathematical and creative abilities. Some emphasis will be given to developmental aspects, for these are of critical importance in evaluating the alternative explanations for sex differences in cognition. Before considering how sex roles contribute to these processes we will discuss the potential biological factors involved (genetic, hormonal and neurological) and assess their relevance to our understanding of the phenomena. Finally, we shall examine the various ways in which sex roles appear to influence cognition, considering the contributions of differential expectation, causal attribution of success and failure, and of differential socialization. The mechanisms at work here are very complex indeed and their elucidation calls for interactional or transactional models; the possibilities in these respects will be explored in the conclusions.

Critical issues in the investigation of sex differences

The investigation of psychological differences between the sexes is a highly controversial matter, particularly where the issue of cognitive differences is concerned. Many female researchers in this area believe that male psychologists have often interpreted data on sex differences in accordance with their own personal stereotyped expectations, thus not only perpetuating popular myths but also giving them scientific credence (Griffiths & Saraga 1979). Kaplan (1980) has pointed out that one effect of this has been the inclination to classify the specific parameters of whatever one is studying under the rubrics of 'feminine' or 'masculine' according to a priori notions of what is appropriate for each sex, and also the tendency to seek out or emphasize those findings which most clearly discriminate between males and females. Researchers' choice of traits to be investigated tend to be determined by stereotyped and preconceived notions of what behaviours one might expect to be exhibited by each sex. Underlying such investigations one frequently discovers the assumption that masculine and feminine characteristics are polar ends of a single continuum, such that males and females must necessarily be opposite in interests and abilities. This view has been criticized by Bem (1974), Constantinople (1973), Fedigan (1982) and others, who argue that masculinity and femininity are better conceptualized as independent, orthogonal constructs; this issue is discussed in Chapter 2.

In assessing studies of sex differences one inevitably has to contend with an equivocal state of affairs. In any given behavioural area there is likely to be a considerable number of investigations, some of which may report significant sex differences, and others which may find no significant sex differences. If significant differences are found, the mean scores for males may be higher than those for females, or vice versa. To resolve the dilemma this creates one could adopt the simple strategy of counting up the number of confirming and disconfirming results and come to a conclusion purely on the basis of frequency. Few researchers would accept such a strategy as scientifically adequate. One must take into account that significant results are going to emerge by chance on a number of occasions, and that sometimes these will replicate by chance. One must also consider the nature and size of the samples used, and the scientific merits of the individual studies. Unfortunately, reports in the journals do not necessarily tell us everything we would like to know in order to evaluate the empirical research. Experimental and control groups are often matched for sex as a matter of routine, but only if significant sex differences emerge is the researcher likely to consider the matter worth reporting. Negative results are not usually the subject of great interest, and editors typically eschew their publication except in very special circumstances. For many reasons, therefore, we simply do not know how many negative findings regarding hypothesized sex differences have never been published. If it were possible somehow to take these into account, our contemporary scientific picture of psychological differences between the sexes might be very different.

Sex differences in cognition

General intelligence and variability

Surveys of tests of general intellectual and developmental abilities indicate that although girls may have a slight advantage in the early years (up to seven or thereabouts), males and females are not generally found to differ in average ability (Maccoby 1966; Maccoby & Jacklin 1975; Tyler 1965). The critical factor seems to be the mixture of items in the test. A test comprising mainly verbal items will tend to favour females, while a test requiring predominantly spatial or numerical skills will tend to favour males. Consequently, most widely used tests of intelligence are standardized in such a way as to minimize sex differences. The slight advantage which a small number of studies have found for girls in the early years may be due to more advanced verbal ability or possibly to faster general maturation of girls compared to boys. Both these possibilities will be considered later.

The most controversial issue regarding sex differences in intelligence has concerned the postulated greater variability of male scores, which is seen by some as a manifestation of a general tendency to greater variability in the male (Heim 1970). According to this view, more males than females are found at both ends of the distribution of intelligence with the result that there are more male geniuses in the population, but also more mentally subnormal males. However, while there is some evidence for these beliefs there is no reason why we should pursue a single explanation for them. It is indisputably true that there is a predominance of males amongst the outstandingly successful persons in many walks of life, but evidence strongly suggests social and cultural causes for this phenomenon. Its antecedents can be seen in studies of precocity, in which more boys than girls tend to present themselves or be presented by others as outstanding, and in which boys have been found to have experienced greater opportunities or encouragement for the development of their talents (Astin 1974). On the other hand, for school achievement in most subjects, girls tend to obtain higher grades and are overrepresented in the upper ability ranges (Maccoby & Jacklin 1975). Evidence points to motivational factors being important here: girls are usually found to be more compliant with adult demands and to display greater concern about doing well as school (Morris, Finkelstein & Fisher 1976). Moreover, most school subjects are heavily loaded with verbal activities, and this might be expected to give girls an advantage.

Because of the problems of selection bias, large-scale surveys provide the most satisfactory evidence of sex-related variation in intelligence. Those conducted in Scotland in the 1930s and 1940s revealed small but statistically greater variance for boys, findings which are largely attributable to an excess of boys with very low scores (Scottish Council for Research in Education 1949). These findings are congruent not only with evidence for an excess of male mental defectives (Abramovicz & Richardson 1975; Freire-Maia, Freire-Maia & Morton 1974; Lapouse & Weitzner 1970; Lehrke 1978) but also with the accepted views that boys are more vulnerable to a variety of pre- and post-natal abnormalities of development, and more vulnerable to virtually all of the psychopathological conditions of childhood (Eme 1979; Singer, Westphal & Niswander 1968). Biological factors would seem to be of particular importance here: for example, the greater head size of the male neonate increases the risk of birth injury, and the XY chromosomal pattern of the male carries with it the risk of X-linked genetic disorders which can affect intellectual functioning (Mosely & Stan 1984).

The greater physical vulnerability of males has been suggested by some as being indicative of their greater susceptibility to environmental influence (Bayley & Schaefer 1964; Glucksmann 1974; Hutt 1972; Ounsted & Taylor 1972). However, apart from the over-representation of males at the very low end of the ability range due to handicap, contemporary surveys have failed to reveal any consistent evidence for a wider range of intellectual abilities in males compared to females, and hence support for both the variability and the environmental susceptibility hypothesis from this source is rather weak (Maccoby & Jacklin 1975; Wilson & Vandenberg 1978). An alternative approach has been to look more directly for evidence of sex differences in the effects of the environment. For example, Bayley and Schaefer (1964) maintained that whereas the intelligence of adopted girls is found to correlate significantly with that of their natural mothers, this relationship does not hold for boys. However, more recent studies have not supported this view (Kamin 1978; McAskey & Clarke 1976; McCall, Appelbaum & Hogarty 1973). Bayley and Schaefer also contended that there are higher correlations between indices of maternal behaviour and indices of child behaviour for boys than for girls. These contentions have been challenged on various grounds (Kamin 1978; Maccoby & Jacklin 1975), although perhaps the principal consideration is that current knowledge of sex differences in child-rearing (Block 1984) points to an explanation based on differential socialization rather than differential environmental susceptibility.

The hypothesis of greater male variability in intelligence as an all-encompassing explanation for the phenomena discussed here has therefore little to commend it. Our understanding of the evidence indicates that there are different processes at work at the two ends of the intellectual scale, with both biological and socio-cultural factors involved.

Verbal abilities

It has consistently been reported in the psychological literature that, on average, females are superior to males on verbal tasks (Maccoby & Jacklin 1975). Whilst this is a generally accepted conclusion in the field at the present time, the matter is much more complex than commonly imagined (Fairweather 1976). There is a vast range of different tasks and skills that attract the general label 'verbal', despite wide variation in other abilities necessary for their performance, such as concept formation, reasoning, learning and memory. Mode of presentation of verbal material may affect results as well, for May and Hutt (1974) found that when learning lists of nouns boys performed better if the list was presented visually while girls did better when it was presented orally.

There is some disagreement as to when, developmentally, girls begin to manifest their verbal superiority. Maccoby and Jacklin (1975) concluded that it is from about ten or eleven years that girls begin to come into their own in verbal performance, but in fact there is a good deal of evidence for verbal superiority of females much earlier than this (Bayne & Phye 1977; Koenigsknecht & Friedman 1976; McGuinness 1976). In the early stages of speech acquisition girls are generally ahead of boys in many respects (Harris 1977). For example, Nelson (1973) found that girls had acquired an average of fifty words by eighteen months of age, whereas boys had not achieved this until twenty-two months. Nearly all the boys in her sample were slower than the slowest girl, and over the subsequent two years girls' speech was more complex than that of boys.

The issue of female verbal precocity is particularly interesting because if it is indeed the case that girls have an early advantage in language this may incline them to a preference for verbal rather than spatial modes of problem solving. This has been referred to as the 'bent twig hypothesis' (Sherman 1967, 1971, 1978). Sherman argues that as girls grow up the twig is bent progressively further by the verbal emphasis of the educational system and by sex-role stereotypes which discourage development of their spatial skills. It is also known that mothers talk to their daughters from early infancy onwards more than they do to their sons (Cherry & Lewis 1976).

Many authorities cite sex differences in reading ability as important evidence of continuing verbal superiority in females during the middle period of childhood. Although girls have been found to be better at reading than boys in a large number of studies, this finding is by no means universal (Fairweather 1976; Thompson 1975). The evidence suggests that sex differences in reading are largely a function of the child's perception of reading as sex-appropriate or sex-inappropriate, and thus one would expect there to be inconsistent findings owing to variation in teaching styles. School reading materials have often been found to be of less interest to boys, and boys tend to perform particularly badly in comparison with girls on low-interest material; overall, boys are inclined to view reading as a feminine activity (Asher & Markell 1974; Dwyer 1974). However, biological factors probably cannot be ruled out entirely, for boys substantially outnumber girls in dyslexia and reading retardation (Rutter & Yule 1975; Singleton 1975, 1977).

Spatial abilities

Spatial abilities include finding your way around a town or building, recognizing upside-down objects, playing chess, map-reading, solving mazes and doing jigsaw puzzles. From adolescence onwards, males are consistently superior in these tasks, and some studies indicate male superiority amongst younger subjects also (Fairweather 1976; Harris 1981; Maccoby & Jacklin 1975; McGee 1979; Richmond 1980). Two major types of spatial ability – spatial visualization and spatial orientation – have been identified in factor analytic studies (e.g. McGee 1979). The former involves comprehension of imaginary movements of objects in three-dimensional space (e.g. in mental rotation tasks) while the latter involves perception of the position and configuration of objects in space with the observer as the reference point (e.g. in navigation). Many psychological tests of spatial ability involve both these factors in varying degrees, and it is often difficult to differentiate them and interpret their relative significance in spatial processes (Carroll & Maxwell 1979). The evidence suggests that where male superiority is found before adolescence it is largely confined to tasks employing orientation ability (Harris 1978).

Arguably, a third type of cognitive ability – perceptual disembedding – may also be regarded as essentially spatial in nature. The embedded figures test, in which the subject must locate a simple geometric form hidden in a complex design, provides a good illustration of perceptual disembedding, and from adolescence onwards males have generally been reported to be better at this type of task. Sherman (1967, 1974) argued that these sex differences are due to the spatial component of the tasks, but Witkin and Berry (1975) rejected this view, maintaining that perceptual disembedding is a measure of cognitive style discrete from spatial ability. There is a substantial body of evidence to show that the former view is the correct one (Hyde, Geiringer & Yen 1975; Vernon 1972; Widiger, Knudson & Rorer 1980; Witkin *et al.* 1968). Findings of sex differences on some other cognitive style variables have also turned out to be dependent on differences in spatial ability. For example, it has been contended that males are superior at solving problems which require set-breaking (inhibition of a dominant response) or restructuring (re-arranging problem components to reach a solution) (Broverman, Klaiber & Vogel 1980; Broverman *et al.* 1968; Parlee 1972). However, restructuring and set-breaking tasks which are relatively low in spatial loading generally do not yield the expected sex differences (Maccoby & Jacklin 1975).

The age at which sex-related differences in spatial ability first appear is of considerable theoretical importance. The conclusion that they first appear in adolescence (e.g. Maccoby & Jacklin 1975) has been taken as supporting both environmental (e.g. Nash 1979) and hormonal (e.g. Waber 1977a, 1977b) explanations. However, the appearance of sex-related differences earlier in childhood does not necessarily indicate a biological basis to the phenomenon, because there is evidence that children's play activities are sex-typed from very early in life (Connor & Serbin 1977; Serbin & Connor 1979). Furthermore, during childhood, adolescence and early adulthood, sex differences in spatial ability are generally found to increase in magnitude (Wilson *et al.* 1975).

A study by Keogh (1971) provides an interesting insight into pre-adolescent sex differences in spatial orientation ability. Children aged eight and nine were asked to copy simple designs by drawing, by walking the shapes on the unmarked floor of a large room, and by walking on either a mat or in a sandbox in which footprints were left. Boys and girls were equally accurate at drawing the patterns, and in walking them on an unmarked floor, but in the remaining two conditions the boys were significantly more accurate than the girls. This suggests that the boys were better at utilizing available visual cues to orient themselves in space (Vasta, Regan & Kerley 1980). Boys' relatively more sophisticated awareness of space has been demonstrated in even younger children by Siegel and Schadler (1977). In this experiment $4\frac{1}{2}$–6-year-olds were asked to construct a three-dimensional scale model of their classroom by placing various items in the correct positions. The boys were much more accurate than the girls.

Although the evidence is not entirely consistent (see Herman 1980; Siegel *et al*. 1979) there are strong indications that reconstruction or reproduction is a critical factor contributing to findings of early sex differences in spatial ability. The illustrative studies of Keogh (1971) and Siegel and Schadler (1977), discussed above, depend on the child's ability to reconstruct a spatial pattern. Spatial tasks which do not rely so heavily on this skill have not generally shown sex-related differences in childhood (e.g. Allen *et al*. 1979; Cohen *et al*. 1979; Feldman & Acredolo 1979).

It seems apparent that before we can expect to understand the nature and implications of sex-related differences in spatial ability, more experimentation is required in order to identify the cognitive components of different spatial tasks with greater precision. Many such tasks demand representation of spatial information in memory together with mental transformation of that information. Do sex differences extend to both these components equally? The present evidence on this issue is equivocal. Several commentators have argued that male superiority is largely confined to mental transformation rather than spatial memory (e.g. Harris 1978) but Kail and Siegel (1977) found that spatial memory was superior in pre-adolescent, adolescent and college males. The task employed involved the presentation of letters in a sixteen cell grid. Females had better memory for the positions of letters. On the other hand, Kail, Pellegrino and Carter (1980) found that although males were superior in mental transformation of spatial stimuli, they did not appear to excel at encoding spatial stimuli. These studies suggest that the complexities and multiple demands of spatial tasks are not well understood at the present time. The relative significance of memory, mental transformation, visualization, orientation and task difficulty requires further elucidation before a satisfactory account of spatial processes can be formulated.

Mathematical abilities

Until fairly recently it was generally accepted that males are superior to females in mathematical abilities, particularly from about twelve onwards (Maccoby & Jacklin 1975). This belief was reinforced by the fact that large numbers of girls avoid mathematics and science subjects in the latter years of high school and in further and higher education (Fennema & Sherman 1978). Of course, females' avoidance of mathematics and related subjects might simply be an expression of preference or a reflection of social constraints, rather than a consequence of lack of mathematical potential. Whilst it is true that empirical studies have usually found males to be better at mathematics than females, earlier research generally used random samples of secondary school pupils in which the males will often have had greater experience at mathematics because of their subject choices. If the number of mathematics courses taken is controlled for, the sex difference in mathematics achievement is significantly diminished although not eradicated (Fennema & Carpenter 1981).

Sex differences in mathematical achievement vary considerably from country to country, and some of these differences may be attributed to the opportunities the students have to learn mathematics (Harnisch 1984; Keeves 1973). Finn (1980) found that sex differences in science achievement were smaller among single-sex schools. Findings of this type lend support to the view that there are strong social factors contributing to mathematics and science achievement, a conclusion reached by three independent analyses of the problem from different perspectives, commisioned by the US National Institute of Education (Fennema 1977; Fox 1977; Sherman 1977).

Although males, during the school years, do not report liking mathematics more than females, they do generally perceive mathematics as being more useful (Fox, Tobin & Brody 1979; Sherman & Fennema 1977). This belief in the value of mathematics is in turn related to curriculum interests and career aspirations. Such attitudes are powerfully shaped by the sex-typing of mathematics and sciences as male domains, with the consequence that many girls associate achievement in these fields as 'masculine' and thus as a potential threat to their social relationships with boys (Fennema & Sherman 1977). The comparative lack of scientific and mathematical career opportunities for females may further reinforce their disinclination to study these subjects (Sells 1980). By adolescence boys tend to rate themselves as having more ability in mathematics than girls, despite the fact that the sexes perform about equally up to that time (Parsons 1984), which suggests that sex-role stereotypes have a deleterious effect on girls' expectations for success in mathematics and on their confidence in their mathematical abilities generally.

There is also some evidence that sex differences in mathematical abilities are in part due to sex differences in spatial ability (Burnett, Lane & Dratt 1979; Fennema 1983; Sherman 1967). While it is easy to appreciate the importance of spatial visualization in such subjects as geometry and engineering, its relevance to other areas of mathematics and science is not so obvious. However, it may be argued that the fundamental concepts in modern science, relating to the structure of atoms, molecules, DNA, etc. are essentially spatial, and similarly, that the concepts underlying all of modern mathematical thinking beyond the level of simple computation may be spatial/geometrical in nature. Hyde, Geiringer and Yen (1975) and Fennema and Sherman (1977) have demonstrated that no sex differences in arithmetical ability are found when spatial ability is statistically controlled. These findings have been supported by Burnett, Lane and Dratt (1979), who also reported that the pattern of intercorrelations between performance on spatial visualization tests and a test of quantitative ability revealed a real link between the two. Whilst there is room for further research here, it may turn out that boys' achievement in mathematics and science is a spin-off from their spatial superiority, either directly, or perhaps indirectly in the sense that girls' verbal proficiency might enhance their interest and achievement in subjects in which verbal rather than spatial modes of problem-solving are more effective.

Creative thinking

In empirical studies neither males nor females show a consistent superiority in creative thinking ability, although creative tasks which depend more on verbal skills tend to favour females (Helson 1978; Kogan 1974; Maccoby & Jacklin 1975). However, amongst the creative occupations such as painting, sculpture, literature and music, men far outnumber women, especially within the ranks of the most successful. While these latter findings imply, above all, that women's opportunities in creative occupations do not approach those of men, the difficulty in defining and measuring 'creativity' precludes any settled verdict on the issue at the present time. Hargreaves (1979) suggests that a more fruitful approach might be to examine the qualitative aspects of creative performance. On a divergent thinking task involving the generation of drawings based on blank circles, Hargreaves (1977) found no differences between boys and girls on conventional measures of creativity such as fluency and originality, but there were significant sex differences in the content of the creative responses of the children. Boys produced more drawings classed a 'mechanical-scientific', but girls produced more drawings classed as 'domestic'. Furthermore, when the children were asked to switch sex roles while carrying out a similar creativity task, the sex differences in creative content were found to be reversed. This finding has implications for the theory that creativity is enhanced in persons able to adopt opposite-sex roles, for which there is some tentative evidence (Hargreaves 1979; Helson 1978), although this relaionship may signify no more than a greater fluidity or flexibility of thinking amongst androgynous individuals, as indeed one might expect.

Biological explanations

The primary concern of this chapter is with the extent to which sex roles can provide us with a basis for understanding sex-related differences in cognition. However, this issue must be considered in the light of the competing biological explanations of the phenomena we have been discussing. The treatment here will be brief: for fuller accounts see Fairweather (1976), Maccoby & Jacklin (1975), Parsons (1980), Sherman (1978) and Wittig & Petersen (1979).

Genetic factors

Stafford (1961) reported a pattern of family intercorrelations for spatial ability which suggested transmission from mother to son and from father to daughter, but not from father to son, thus implying a sex-linked genetic mechanism. Later investigations gave only limited support for this (Bock & Kolakowski 1973; Hartlage 1970) and a large-scale survey by De Fries and his co-workers gave none at all (De Fries *et al.* 1976). There is some doubt as to whether the distribution of spatial scores within each sex matches the predictions of the X-linked recessive major gene theory (Yen 1975), and also certain genetic-hormonal anomalies show a pattern of cognitive abilities which contradicts the genetic explanation. Females with Turner's syndrome (XO), despite possessing, like males, only one X chromosome, have been found to exhibit exceptionally poor spatial ability (Garron 1970). Genetic males (XY) with androgen-insensitivity syndrome, raised as girls, tend to show the usual female pattern of verbal superiority over spatial skill (Masica *et al.* 1969).

(Both these syndromes are discussed in Chapter 1.) These findings indicate that a simple genetic basis to sex-related cognitive differences in general is unlikely, although there is some evidence for genetic transmission of disturbances of verbal ability such as dyslexia (Singleton 1976), and it has been estimated that approximately 20 per cent of mental retardation amongst males is caused by genes on the X chromosome (Turner 1982). However, there are several more complex possible mechanisms of genetic transmission which signal the need for further research (Vandenberg & Kuse 1979).

Hormonal factors

The fact that both the androgen-insensitivity syndrome and Turner's syndrome exhibit hormone abnormalities invites the speculation that sex hormones may influence the brain and so affect cognitive functioning. The mechanism might be one of continuous hormone action from puberty onwards, or alternatively one in which cognitive potentials are 'set' by hormone action during prenatal development. The Broverman hypothesis is probably the best-known example in this area. Broverman and his co-workers hypothesize that the gonadal hormones, estrogen and testosterone, affect the CNS by influencing the metabolism of neuro-transmitters (Broverman, Klaiber & Vogel 1980). Their results suggested that males with more 'masculine' physiques (which were presumed to correlate with higher levels of male hormones) were superior at simple repetitive tasks rather than at tasks which require set-breaking or restructuring. Petersen (1976) also studied the relationship of somatic measures of hormone influence (for example muscle versus fat distribution) to cognitive performance in both males and females aged 16–18 years. Amongst males the results broadly supported the Broverman pattern: males with more extremely masculine somatic characteristics were better at 'fluent production' (that is the rapid and accurate production of symbolic codes or names) than on spatial ability tasks, while the reverse was true for males who were less stereotypic in physical appearance. In females, physical androgyny was related to spatial ability, but there were no significant relationships with fluency of production. These studies suffer from the lack of direct measures of hormone levels and from their adoption of correlational designs. However, subsequent studies by Broverman and his co-workers involving more direct assaying of blood-hormone levels and experimental manipulation of hormone infusion, have failed to yield consistent results. Petersen (1979) concludes that this research is limited at the present time by lack of satisfactory methods of hormone measurement. More recently, Woodfield (1984) reported an interesting approach to the problem. He investigated women's performance on the EFT and another spatial test before and after childbirth, when hormone changes are marked. Two separate groups showed significant increases in field independence and spatial ability over a period during which estrogen levels decreased dramatically.

An alternative hormonal theory has been put forward by Waber (1976, 1977a, 1977b), who explains sex-related differences in cognition as functions of maturation rate, which is under hormonal control. She argues that the later the individual matures, the greater the relative superiority of spatial over verbal ability. Since girls mature physically about two years earlier than boys, they will tend to be verbally superior and spatially inferior. However Petersen (1976) found that early *and* late maturing males tend to be relatively better at spatial tasks than fluent production, whereas early *and* late maturing females tended to show the opposite pattern.

The menstrual cycle has been the focus of much research on hormonal factors in cognitive functioning. Based on her studies of the examination performance of teenage girls, Dalton (1968) claimed that a decline in intellectual performance was associated with the premenstrual and menstrual phases of the female cycle. However, the analysis and interpretation of these data were very unsatisfactory and independent reviews of the many studies carried out since then concur that despite a powerful folklore to the contrary there is no empirical evidence to support a general conclusion of cognitive changes during the menstrual cycle. Various CNS measure do appear to vary in some fashion with the hormonal fluctuations of the cycle, but further research is necessary to identify the significance of these in the light of considerable individual variation. There is also evidence that cognitive variables influence the perception of and response to menstruation, so that individual variability may interact in a complex manner with personal adaptation (Dan 1979; Parlee 1982; Sommer 1982).

Neurological factors

Clinical and experimental studies have revealed that in most right-handed individuals the left hemisphere of the brain governs language functions, while visual-spatial information is largely processed by the right hemisphere (Nebes 1974). Since we also know that females are generally superior in verbal abilities and males in spatial abilities it is but a small step to speculate that these cognitive sex differences might be attributable to relative specialization of the two hemispheres. Two main theories have emerged. Buffery and Gray (1972) argued that linguistic skills are enhanced by strong, early lateralization of function in the left hemisphere, but spatial skills benefit from a more bilateral representation across both hemispheres. By contrast, Levy (1972) maintained that strong lateralization of function in the right hemisphere enhances spatial skills. The bulk of the evidence supports the latter of these two views (Bryden 1979; Harris 1978, 1981; McGlone 1980; Petersen 1980). For example, Witelson (1976) tested right-handed children aged 6–13 for visual recognition of meaningless shapes which had been felt with either the right or left hand. Girls did equally well with either hand, but boys performed better with the left. Similar findings have been reported in other studies, both with children (Affleck & Joyce 1979) and with adults (Flanery & Balling 1979), suggesting stronger lateralization in males. Witelson's results indicate that the right hemisphere becomes specialized for spatial perception earlier in boys than in girls, which supports an earlier finding by Rudel, Denckla and Spalten (1974).

For over two decades dichotic listening tests have been regarded as a convenient method for establishing lateralization of language function. Different sounds are presented simultaneously to both ears, and it is assumed that the sound reported first is the one processed by the dominant, contralateral hemisphere. A right-ear advantage is found with verbal material, and a left-ear advantage with melodies or environmental sounds. For visuospatial functions, a comparable tachistoscopic task can be used, and on this a right visual field advantage is manifested with words and letters, while a left visual field superiority is found when recognizing faces or determining orientation. With regard to sex differences in brain lateralization, however, the evidence from studies employing these techniques is not altogether consistent, although it does indicate that in adult samples, males are much more likely than females to show left-hemisphere superiority for verbal tasks, and to show greater asymmetry than females on visuospatial tasks; with child subjects results have been inconclusive (Bryden 1979). Overall, these findings lend some support to Levy's hypothesis, although Bryden (1978) has criticized these approaches for failing to control for individual differences in attention and strategy. When attentional biases are reduced to a minimum, sex differences in dichotic listening tend to disappear, suggesting that such differences result from the subjects' strategy rather than from cerebral lateralization.

It is tempting to conclude, therefore, that the phenomena under consideration here are purely a matter of subjects' strategy. However, such a conclusion would be unwarranted for there is clear evidence of sex-related differences in cerebral anatomy (Wada, Clark & Hamm 1975), and we know from studies of the patterns of impairment in males and females following unilateral brain lesions that brain function is more strongly lateralized in males (McGlone 1977, 1978). We must, in consequence, shift our focus to a more interactionist perspective, as Bryden (1979), Harris (1978) and Petersen (1980) have advocated. In order to gain a proper understanding of sex differences in cognitive abilities we must consider not only what cognitive mechanisms (memory, attention, information-processing style, etc.) could be brought about by different kinds of brain organization, but also, given the likely sex differences in the underlying neurological bias, what is the nature and effect of the relevant environmental inputs into these processes. It is this issue to which we now turn.

The contributions of sex roles

It has already been pointed out that the perceived sex appropriateness of a cognitive task affects both attitudes to and performance on that task. For example, the way in which adults characterize tasks for children can be shown to have differential effects on performance by boys and girls. Labelling an activity 'for girls' produces a higher level of activity by girls compared to boys, while labelling the same activity 'for boys' elicits a comparatively higher level of activity from boys (Montemayor 1974). When given a choice of tasks , boys are more likely than girls to choose to spend more time on tasks labelled as appropriate for their own sex and less time on opposite-sex tasks (Stein, Pohly & Mueller 1971), and sex-typing influences children's evaluation of the appeal of a task (Etaugh & Ropp 1976). In adults, sex roles can have similar effects on attitudes and performance. For example, describing problems in feminine terms can improve the problem-solving performance of females and reduce that of males (Milton 1957, 1959). Naditch (1976, quoted by Nash 1979) demonstrated a sex-typing effect using a test of spatial field-independence: males were more field-independent on a masculine version of the test, and females on a feminine one.

A number of studies have reported findings which suggest that an intricate relationship exists between belief in or adoption of stereotypic sex-role characteristics and intellectual functioning. Male gender preference is generally found to be associated with superior spatial performance in both males and females (Nash 1975, 1979; Serbin & Connor 1979). However, although high spatial ability is often strongly associated with relatively high masculinity in females, it tends to be associated (somewhat less strongly) with relatively *low* masculinity in males (Kagan & Kagan 1970; Maccoby & Jacklin 1975; Newcombe 1982; Petersen 1976). These findings seem consistent with the view that the relationship between sex-typing and spatial ability may to some extent be explained in terms of experience. Boys' toys and activities are more likely to be spatial in nature (Harris 1978; Newcombe 1982) and yet engaging in such pursuits is less stereotypically 'masculine' than more boisterous pastimes. The success of some efforts to reduce sex differences in spatial ability by training supports this view (Connor, Schackman & Serbin 1978; Harris 1978; Maxwell, Croake & Biddle 1975; Vandenberg 1975). However, in cultures where boys do not have this experience, one would expect the magnitude of the expected sex difference in spatial ability to be reduced, but this does not appear to be the case (Jahoda 1980).

Differential expectations

A further mechanism of influence in this process is that of differential expectation. Labelling a task appears to influence a person's expectations of success on that task. Expectations tend to be highest when a task is labelled as appropriate for the sex of the subject, and lowest when labelled as appropriate for the opposite sex (Stein, Pohly & Mueller 1971). Males are more likely to expect to do well on 'masculine' tasks or in male-typed intellectual areas such as science and mathematics, whereas females tend to do less well on 'masculine' tasks and on spatial and mathematical tasks, but anticipate better performance on verbal tasks (Deaux & Emswiller 1974; Frieze 1975; Lenney 1977).

Differential expectations can be created in several ways. To some extent, individuals might be expected to be aware of their own abilities and shortcomings as a result of personal experience, but it is also probable that they will have acquired certain (possibly stereotyped) beliefs about them during socialization. The sex of the experimenter, examiner or teacher can also affect performance. Pedersen, Shinedling and Johnson (1975) found that arithmetic test performance in girls was higher with female examiners, and in males with male examiners. Although this study was on primary schoolchildren, who experience mostly female teachers, it is worth reflecting on the fact that in secondary schools male teachers of mathematics predominate while for English and languages there are much larger proportions of female teachers. Could the origins of the sex differences in verbal and mathematical ability lie here to some degree? The expectations of others can also affect performance. Dickstein and Kephart (1972) found that females who were told they were expected to perform well on the Performance Scale of the Wechsler Adult Intelligence Scale not only enhanced their own level of achievement but also did better than females who had not been told this.

Success and failure

Causal attributions for success and failure in cognitive tasks also differ between the sexes. Males are more inclined than females to attribute their success to ability, and females are more likely to attribute both success and failure to luck (Bar-Tal & Frieze 1977; Frieze 1975; Viaene 1979). Deaux & Farris (1977) have proposed a general expectancy model to account for these findings. In this model, performance consistent with expectations is attributed to a stable internal factor (e.g. ability), while performance which is inconsistent with expectations is attributed to one or more temporary factors (e.g. luck or effort). Since the expectancies of males and females differ, the attribution patterns will differ also. Although this model seems to fit much of the data, there are other factors involved, including the pattern of success and failure encountered and the nature and pattern of reinforcement received (Altshuler & Kassinove 1975; Dweck & Gilliard 1975; Feather 1969; Feather & Simon 1971a, 1971b; Simon & Feather 1973). Generally speaking, it appears that the greater the difference between an outcome and expectations, the greater the tendency to attribute it to luck, and the lesser the difference the more likely is it to be attributed to ability. Some of these issues are explored in greater depth in Chapter 8.

An alternative theory which has been the focus of considerable attention has concerned the 'motive to avoid success' (Horner 1979). Horner suggested that women learn to expect negative consequences from success because of incongruence with expected sex-role standards. Many studies have reported that females express more avoidance of success than males, and Horner's theory might explain females' avoidance of mathematics and the sciences and their feelings about this (Fennema & Sherman 1977). However, the theory is not widely accepted, mainly because it is associated with projective techniques for motivational assessment which have been severely criticized on grounds of reliability and validity (Condry & Dyer 1976; Tresemer 1977; Ward 1979; Zucker-man & Wheeler 1975). Furthermore, the results may be more satisfactorily explained in terms of both men and women expressing the cultural stereotype that success is often aversive for women, rather than in terms of a stable personality disposition to avoid success (Feather 1975; Monahan, Kuhn & Shaver 1974).

Differential socialization

It is widely believed that boys and girls are socialized differently and in ways which encourage the development of sex-appropriate behaviours. However, in their major analysis of the field, Maccoby and Jacklin (1975) concluded that there was surprisingly little differentiation in parental behaviour according to the sex of the child, a conclusion which has been forcefully challenged by Block (1978). Serious methodological inadequacies and naive models of socialization have led to inconsistent rather than null findings, but a more critical analysis of the evidence gives strong indications that differential socialization plays an important part in creating sex differences in cognition (Block 1981).

The growth of the child's cognitive abilities rests upon his understanding of the physical and social environment as meaningful. To a very large extent, this process is dependent on the responses which other people (especially the parents) make to the child's behaviour. Considerable evidence now exists that boys experience significantly more contingent responding than girls (Block 1981; Lewis 1972; Maccoby & Jacklin 1975; Margolin & Patterson 1975; Murphy & Moriarty 1976) and that in comparison with girls the toys and play behaviours of boys encourage the development of independent and exploratory problem solving and spatial awareness rather than verbal fluency (Carpenter 1983; Carpenter & Huston-Stein 1980; Fagot & Littman 1975; Rheingold & Cook 1975; Yarrow 1972). These issues are dealt with in greater depth in Chapters 5 and 6.

The process by which the child progresses from one level of understanding to another is mediated by the experience of 'disequilibration' (Block 1981, 1982; Hunt 1961; Piaget 1953). The crux of this concept is the idea of confronting events which challenge the cognitive *status quo*, resulting in the restructuring of understanding. The relatively restricted environment, limited toys and protective relationship with the parents which girls typically experience, do not encourage disequilibration (Sigel & Cocking 1976), whereas the child-rearing orientations boys usually encounter have the effects of distancing them from their parents and forcing them to develop cognitive strategies for coping with the disequilibrating experiences which, as a result, they are more likely to have to contend with (Block 1981; Lamb 1976; Singleton 1978).

Conclusions

The state of knowledge in this area does not warrant any grand conclusions at the present time, nor will any simple causal models suffice. It is clear that the biological explanations for sex-related differences in cognition do not do justice to the complexity of the findings, although the biological evidence is quite strong, especially with regard to cerebral lateralization. Whether such biological differences will ultimately turn out to be trivial in comparison with social and environmental factors remains to be seen.

Researchers in this field are increasingly coming to recognize the need for interactional or transactional theories to encompass the complicated network of factors involved (see Chapter 1). For example, Singleton (1978) outlined an amplification model whereby subtle sex differences in infant behaviour can become magnified in the child-rearing process. The emphasis here is on the reciprocal patterns of influence within the family situation, and this foreshadows a shift in the focus of research towards understanding the dynamic and fluid processes within the family which shape cognitive development. In this chapter I have tried to show that as children grow up their cognitive development is influenced not only by processes within the family, but also by societal norms and stereotypes of sex-role behaviour. As Kohlberg (1966) has argued, all these factors shape the child's developing self-concept. The urge to define the self in a fashion which is meaningful and consistent in relation to the perceived social world is very strong (Bem & Lenney 1976; Mischel 1970; Tresemer & Pleck 1976) and creates a framework within which sex roles can mediate cognitive functioning (Nash 1979). A transactional model of sex differences in cognition must incorporate this process as well as the processes by which family and societal influences work on the biological substrate. Whilst the undoubted complexity of the factors involved here is a disincentive to the generation and testing of unifying theories, the alternative is the continuation of the present empirical fragmentation and conceptual disorganization. Progress towards an integrative bio-psychosocial perspective at least holds out the promise of a richer understanding in this complex field, albeit in the long term.

References

Abramovicz, H. K. & Richardson, S. A. (1975) Epidemiology of severe mental retardation in children: community studies. *American Journal of Mental Deficiency*, *80*, 18–39.

Affleck, G., & Joyce, P. (1979) Sex differences in the association of cerebral hemispheric specialisation of spatial function with conservation task performance. *Journal of Genetic Psychology*, *134*, 271–280.

Allen, G. L., Kirasic, K. C., Siegel, A. W. & Herman, J. F. (1979) Developmental issues in cognitive mapping: the selection and utilisation of environmental landmarks. *Child Development*, *50*, 1062–1070.

Altshuler, R. & Kassinove, H. (1975) The effects of skill and chance instructional ꙩs, schedule of reinforcement, and sex on children's temporal persistence. *Child Development*, *46*, 258–262.

Asher, S. R. & Markell, R. A. (1974) Sex differences in comprehension of high- and low-interest reading materials. *Journal of Educational Psychology*, *66*, 680–687.

Astin, H. S. (1974) Sex differences in mathematical and scientific precocity. *In* J. C. Stanley, D. P. Keating & L. H. Fox (eds) *Mathematical talent: discovery, description and development*. Baltimore: Johns Hopkins Press.

Bar-Tal, D. & Frieze, I. H. (1977) Achievement motivation and gender as a determinant of attributions for success and failure. *Sex Roles*, *3*, 301–313.

Bayley, N. & Schaefer, E. S. (1964) Correlations of maternal and child behaviours with the development of mental abilities: data from the Berkeley Growth Study. *Monographs of the Society for Research in Child Development*, *29*, No. 97.

Bayne, N. E. & Phye, G. D. (1977) Age and sex differences in induced hierarchical organisational ability. *Journal of Genetic Psychology*, *130*, 191–200.

Bem, S. L. (1974) The measurement of psychological androgyny. *Journal of Consulting and Clinical Psychology*, *42*, 155–162.

Bem, S. L. & Lenney, E. (1976) Sex typing and the avoidance of cross-sex behaviour. *Journal of Personality and Social Psychology*, *33*, 48–54.

Block, J. H. (1978) Another look at sex differentiation in the socialisation behaviours of mothers and fathers. *In* J. A. Sherman & F. L. Denmark (eds)

The psychology of women: future directions in research. New York: Psychological Dimensions, pp. 29–87.

Block, J. H. (1981) Gender differences in the nature of orientations developed about the world. *In* E. K. Shapiro & E. Weber (eds) *Cognitive and affective growth: developmental interaction.* Hillsdale, N.J.: Erlbaum.

Block, J. H. (1982) Assimilation, accommodation and the dynamics of personality development. *Child Development, 53,* 281–295.

Block, J. H. (1983) Differential premises arising from differential socialisation of the sexes: some conjectures. *Child Development, 54,* 1335–1354.

Block, J. H. (1984) *Sex role identity and ego development.* San Francisco: Jossey-Bass.

Bock, D. R. & Kolakowski, D. (1973) Further evidence of major-gene influence on human spatial visualising ability. *American Journal of Human Genetics, 25,* 1–14.

Broverman, D. M., Klaiber, E. L., Kobayashi, Y. & Vogel, W. (1968) Roles of activation and inhibition in sex differences in cognitive abilities. *Psychological Review, 75,* 23–50.

Broverman, D. M., Klaiber, E. L. & Vogel, W. (1980) Gonadal hormones and cognitive functioning. In J. E. Parsons (eds) *The psychobiology of sex differences and sex roles.* New York: McGraw-Hill, pp. 57–80.

Bryden, M. P. (1978) Strategy effects in the assessment of hemispheric asymmetry. In G. Underwood (ed) *Strategies of information processing.* London: Academic Press, pp. 117–149.

Bryden. M. P. (1979) Evidence for sex-related differences in cerebral organisation. *In* M. A. Wittig & A. C. Peterson (eds) *Sex-related differences in cognitive functioning: developmental issues.* New York: Academic Press, pp. 121–143.

Buffery, A. & Gray, J. (1972) Sex differences in the development of spatial and linguistic skills. *In* C. Ounsted & D. Taylor (eds) *Gender differences: their ontogeny and significance.* Edinburgh: Churchill Livingstone, pp. 123–158.

Burnett, S. A., Lane, D. M. & Dratt, L. M. (1979) Spatial visualisation and sex differences in quantitative ability. *Intelligence, 3,* 345–354.

Carpenter, C. J. (1983) Activity structure and play: implications for socialisation. *In* M. Liss (ed.) *Social and cognitive skills: sex roles and children's play.* New York: Academic Press.

Carpenter, C. J. & Huston-Stein, A. (1980) Activity structure and sex-typed behaviour in preschool children. *Child Development, 51,* 862–872.

Carroll, J. B. & Maxwell, S. E. (1979) Individual differences in cognitive abilities. *Annual Review of Psychology, 30,* 603–640.

Cherry, L. & Lewis, M. (1976) Mothers and two-year-olds: a study of sex-differentiated aspects of verbal interaction. *Developmental Psychology, 12,* 278–282.

Cohen, R., Weatherford, D. L., Lomenick, T. & Koeller, K. (1979) Development of spatial representations: role of task demands and familiarity with the environment. *Child Development, 50,* 1257–1260.

Condry, J. & Dyer, S. (1976) Fear of success: attribution of cause to the victim. *Journal of Social Issues, 32,* 63–83.

Connor, J. M., Schackman, M. & Serbin, L. A. (1978) Sex-related differences in response to practice on a visual-spatial test and generalisation to a related test. *Child Development, 49,* 24–29.

Connor, J. M. & Serbin, L. A. (1977) Behaviourally-based masculine- and feminine-activity-preference scales for preschoolers: correlates with other classroom behaviours and cognitive tests. *Child Development, 48,* 1411–1416.

Constantinople, A. (1973) Masculinity-femininity: an exception to the famous dictum. *Psychological Bulletin, 80,* 389–407.

Dalton, K. (1968) Menstruation and examinations. *Lancet, 2,* 1752–1753.

Dan, A. J. (1979) The menstrual cycle and sex-related differences in cognitive variability. *In* M. A. Wittig and A. C. Petersen (eds) *Sex-related differences in cognitive functioning: developmental issues.* New York: Academic Press, pp. 241–260.

Deaux, K. & Emswiller, T. (1974) Explanations of successful performance on sex-linked tasks: what's skill for the male is luck for the female. *Journal of Personality and Social Psychology, 29,* 80–85.

Deaux, K. & Farris, E. (1977) Attributing causes for one's own performance: the effects of sex, norms and task outcome. *Journal of Research in Personality, 11,* 59–72.

De Fries, J. C., Ashton, G. C., Johnson, R. C., Kuse, A. R., McClearn, G. E., Mi, M. P., Rashad, M. N., Vandenberg, S. G. & Wilson, J. R. (1976) Parent-offspring resemblance for specific cognitive abilities in two ethnic groups. *Nature, 261,* 131–133.

Dickstein, L. & Kephart, J. (1972) Effect of explicit examiner expectancy upon WAIS performance. *Psychological Reports, 30,* 207–212.

Dweck, C. S. & Gilliard, D. (1975) Expectancy statements as determinants of reactions to failure: sex differences in persistence and expectancy change. *Journal of Personality and Social Psychology, 32,* 1077–1084.

Dwyer, C. A. (1974) Influence of children's sex-role standards on reading and arithmetic achievement. *Journal of Educational Psychology, 66,* 811–816.

Eme, R. F. (1979) Sex differences in childhood psychopathology: a review. *Psychological Bulletin, 86,* 574–595.

Etaugh, C. & Ropp, J. (1976) Children's self-evaluation of performance as a function of sex, age, feedback, and sex-type task. *Journal of Psychology, 94,* 115–122.

Fagot, B. I. & Littman, I. (1975) Stability of sex-role and play interests from preschool to elementary school. *Journal of Psychology, 89,* 285–292.

Fairweather, H. (1976) Sex differences in cognition. *Cognition, 4,* 231–280.

Feather, N. T. (1969) Attribution of responsibility and valence of success and failure in relation to initial confidence and task performance. *Journal of Personality and Social Psychology*, *13*, 129–144.

Feather, N. T. (1975) Positive and negative reactions to male and female success and failure in relation to the perceived status and sex-typed appropriateness of occupations. *Journal of Personality and Social Psychology*, *31*, 536–548.

Feather, N. T. & Simon, J. G. (1971a) Attribution of responsibility and valence of outcome in relation to initial confidence and success and failure of self and other. *Journal of Personality and Social Psychology*, *18*, 173–188.

Feather, N. T. & Simon, J. G. (1971b) Causal attributions for success and failure in relation to expectations of success based upon selective and manipulative control. *Journal of Personality*, *39*, 527–541.

Fedigan, L. M. (1982) *Primate paradigms: sex roles and social bonds*. Montreal: Eden Press.

Feldman, A. & Acredolo, L. (1979) The effect of active versus passive exploration on memory for spatial location in children. *Child Development*, *50*, 698–704.

Fennema, E. (1977) Influences of selected cognitive, affective and educational variables on sex-related differences in mathematics learning and studying. *In* J. Shoemaker (ed.) *Women and mathematics: research perspectives for change*. Washington, DC: US Government Printing Office.

Fennema, E. (1983) Success in mathematics. *In* M. Marland (ed.) *Sex differentiation and schooling*. London: Heinemann, pp. 163–180.

Fennema, E. & Carpenter, T. P. (1981) Sex-related differences in mathematics: results from national assessment. *Mathematics Teacher*, *74*, 554–566.

Fennema, E. & Sherman, J. (1977) Sex-related differences in mathematics, achievement, spatial visualisation and affective factors. *American Educational Research Journal*, *14*, 51–71.

Fennema, E. & Sherman, J. (1978) Sex-related differences in mathematical achievement and related factors: a further study. *Journal of Research in Mathematics Education*, *9*, 189–203.

Finn, J. D. (1980) Sex differences in educational outcomes: a cross-national study. *Sex Roles*, *6*, 9–26.

Flannery, R. C. & Balling, J. D. (1979) Developmental changes in hemispheric specialisation for tactile spatial ability. *Developmental Psychology*, *15*, 364–372.

Fox, L. H. (1977) The effects of sex-role socialisation on mathematics participation and achievement. *In* J. Shoemaker (ed.) *Women and mathematics: research perspectives for change*. Washington, DC: US Government Printing Office.

Fox, L. H., Tobin, D. & Brody, L. (1979) Sex role socialisation and achievement in mathematics. *In* M. A. Wittig and A. C. Petersen (eds) *Sex-related differences in cognitive functioning: developmental issues*. New York: Academic Press, pp. 303–332.

Freire-Maia, A., Freire-Maia, D. V. & Morton, N. E. (1974) Sex effect on intelligence and mental retardation. *Behaviour Genetics, 4*, 269–272.

Frieze, I. H. (1975) Women's expectations for causal attributions of success and failure. *In* M. T. S. Mednick, S. S. Tangri & L. W. Hoffman (eds) *Women and achievement*. New York: John Wiley, pp. 158–171.

Garron, D. C. (1970) Sex-linked, recessive inheritance of spatial and numerical abilities, and Turner's syndrome. *Psychological Review, 77*, 145–152.

Glucksmann, A. (1974) Sexual dimorphism in mammals. *Biological Review, 49*, 423–475.

Griffiths, D. & Saraga, E. (1979) Sex differences and cognitive abilities: a sterile field of enquiry? *In* O. Hartnett, G. Boden and M. Fuller (eds) *Sex-role stereotyping*. London: Tavistock, pp. 17–45.

Hargreaves, D. J. (1977) Sex roles in divergent thinking. *British Journal of Educational Psychology, 47*, 25–32.

Hargreaves, D. J. (1979) Sex roles and creativity. *In* O. Hartnett, G. Boden, & M. Fuller (eds) *Sex-role stereotyping*. London: Tavistock, pp. 185–199.

Harnisch, D. L. (1984) Females and mathematics: a cross-national perspective. *In* M. W. Steinkamp & M. L. Maehr (eds) *Women in science*. Greenwich, Connecticut: JAI Press, pp. 73–91.

Harris, L. J. (1977) Sex differences in the growth and use of language. *In* E. Donelson & J. Gullahorn (eds) *Women: a psychological perspective*. New York: John Wiley, pp. 79–94.

Harris, L. J. (1978) Sex differences in spatial ability: possible environmental, genetic and neurological factors. *In* M. Kinsbourne (ed.) *Asymmetrical functions of the brain*. Cambridge: Cambridge University Press, pp. 405–522.

Harris, L. J. (1981) Sex-related variations in spatial skill. *In* L. S. Liben, A. H. Patterson & N. Newcombe (eds) *Spatial representation and behaviour across the life span*. New York: Academic Press, 83–125.

Hartlage, L. C. (1970) Sex-linked inheritance of spatial ability. *Perceptual and Motor Skills, 31*, 610.

Heim. A. (1970) *Intelligence and personality*. Harmondsworth: Penguin.

Helson, R. M. (1978) Creativity in women. *In* J. A. Sherman & F. L. Denmark (eds) *The psychology of women: future directions in research*. New York: Psychological Dimensions, pp. 553–604.

Herman, J. F. (1980) Children's cognitive maps of large-scale places: effects of exploration, direction and repeated experience. *Journal of Experimental Child Psychology, 29*, 126–143.

Hewitt, L. S. (1975) Age and sex differences in the vocational aspirations of elementary school children. *Journal of Social Psychology, 96*, 173–177.

Horner, M. S. (1970) Femininity and successful achievement: a basic inconsistency. *In* J. M. Bardwick (ed.) *Feminine personality and conflict*. Belmont, California: Brooks/Cole.

Hunt, J. McV. (1961) *Intelligence and experience*. New York: Ronald Press.

Hutt, C. (1972) *Males and females*. Harmondsworth: Penguin.

Hyde, J. S., Geiringer, E. R. & Yen, W. M. (1975) On the empirical relation between spatial ability and sex differences in other aspects of cognitive performance. *Multivariate Behavioural Research, 10,* 289–310.

Jahoda, G. (1980) Sex and ethnic differences on a spatial-perceptual task: some hypotheses tested. *British Journal of Psychology, 71,* 425–431.

Kagan, J. & Kogan, N. (1970) Individuality and cognitive performance. *In* P. H. Mussen (ed.) *Carmichael's manual of child psychology,* 3rd edn. New York: John Wiley.

Kail, R. V., Pellegrino, J. & Carter, P. (1980) Developmental changes in mental rotation. *Journal of Experimental Child Psychology,* 29, 102–116.

Kail, R. V. & Siegel, A. W. (1977) Sex differences in retention of verbal and spatial characteristics of stimuli. *Journal of Experimental Child Psychology, 23,* 341–347.

Kamin, L. J. (1978) Sex differences in susceptibility of IQ to environmental influence. *Child Development, 49,* 517–518.

Kaplan, A. (1980) Human sex-hormone abnormalities viewed from an androgynous perspective: a reconsideration of the work of John Money. *In* J. E. Parsons (ed.) *The psychobiology of sex differences and sex roles.* New York: McGraw-Hill, pp. 81–91.

Keeves, J. (1973) Differences between the sexes in mathematics and science courses. *International Review of Education, 19,* 47–64.

Keogh, B. K. (1971) Pattern copying under three conditions of an expanded spatial field. *Developmental Psychology, 4,* 25–31.

Koenigsknecht, R. A. & Friedman, P. (1976) Syntax development in boys and girls. *Child Development, 47,* 1109–1115.

Kogan, N. (1974) Creativity and sex differences. *Journal of Creative Behaviour, 8,* 1–14.

Kohlberg. L. A. (1966) A cognitive-developmental analysis of children's sex-role concepts and attitudes. *In* E. E. Maccoby (ed.) *The development of sex differences.* Stanford, California: Stanford University Press.

Kuhn, D., Nash, S. C. & Brucken, L. (1978) Sex-role concepts of two- and three-year-olds. *Child Development, 49,* 445–451.

Lamb, M. E. (ed.) (1976) *The role of the father in child development.* New York: John Wiley.

Lapouse, R. & Weitzner, M. (1970) Epidemiology. *In* J. Wortis (ed.) *Mental retardation: an annual review,* vol. 1. New York: Grune & Stratton, pp. 197–223.

Lehrke, R. G. (1978) Sex linkage: a biological basis for greater male variability in intelligence. *In* R. T. Osborne, C. E. Noble & N. Weyl (eds) *Human variation: the biopsychology of age, race, and sex.* New York: Academic Press, pp. 171–198.

Lenney, E. (1977) Women's self-confidence in achievement settings. *Psychological Bulletin, 84,* 1–13.

Levy, J. (1972) Lateral specialisation of the human brain: behavioural manifestation and possible evolutionary basis. *In* J. A. Kiger (ed.) *The biology of behaviour.* Corvalis: Oregon University Press.

Lewis, M. (1972) State as an infant-environment interaction: an analysis of mother–infant interaction as a function of sex. *Merrill-Palmer Quarterly, 18,* 95–121.

Looft, W. R. (1971) Sex differences in the expression of vocational aspiration by elementary school children. *Developmental Psychology, 5,* 366.

McAskie, M. & Clarke, A. M. (1976) Parent-offspring resemblances in intelligence: theories and evidence. *British Journal of Psychology, 67,* 243–273.

McCall, R. B., Applebaum, M. I. & Hogarty, P. S. (1973) Developmental changes in mental performance. *Monographs of the Society for Research in Child Development, 38(3),* Serial No. 150.

McGee, M. G. (1979) Human spatial abilities: psychometric studies and environmental, genetic, hormonal, and neurological influences. *Psychological Bulletin, 86,* 889–918.

McGlone, J. (1977) Sex differences in the cerebral organisation of verbal functions in patients with unilateral brain lesions. *Brain, 100,* 775–793.

McGlone, J. (1978) Sex differences in functional brain asymmetry. *Cortex, 14,* 122–128.

McGlone, J. (1980) Sex differences in human brain asymmetry. *Brain and Behavioural Sciences, 3,* 215–264.

McGuinness, D. (1976) Sex differences in the organisation of perception and cognition. *In* B. Lloyd & J. Archer (eds) *Exploring sex differences.* London: Academic Press, pp. 123–156.

Maccoby, E. E. (1966) Sex differences in intellectual functioning. *In* E. E. Maccoby (ed.) *The development of sex differences.* Stanford, California: Stanford University Press.

Maccoby, E. E. & Jacklin, C. N. (1975) *The psychology of sex differences.* Oxford: Oxford University Press.

Mackie, L. & Pattullo, P. (1977) *Women at work.* London: Tavistock.

Margolin, L. & Patterson, G. R. (1975) Differential consequences provided by mothers and fathers for their sons and daughters. *Developmental Psychology, 11,* 537–538

Masica, D. N., Money, J., Ehrhardt, A. A. & Lewis. V. G. (1969) IQ, fetal sex hormones, and cognitive patterns: studies in the testicular feminising syndrome of androgenic insensitivity. *Johns Hopkins Medical Journal, 124,* 34–43.

Maxwell, J. W., Croake, J. W. & Biddle, A. P. (1975) Sex differences in the comprehension of spatial orientation. *Journal of Psychology, 91,* 127–131.

May, R. B. & Hutt, C. (1974) Modality and sex differences in recall and recognition memory. *Child Development, 45,* 228–231.

Milton, G. A. (1957) The effects of sex-role identification upon problem-solving skill. *Journal of Abnormal and Social Psychology, 55,* 208–212.

Milton, G. A. (1959) Sex differences in problem solving as a function of role appropriateness of the problem content. *Psychological Reports, 5,* 705–708.

Mischel, W. (1970) Sex-typing and socialisation. *In* P. H. Mussen (ed.) *Carmichael's manual of child psychology,* 3rd edn. New York: John Wiley.

Monahan, L., Kuhn, D. & Shaver, P. (1974) Intrapsychic versus cultural explanations for the 'Fear of Success' motive. *Journal of Personality and Social Psychology, 29,* 60–64.

Montemayor, R. (1974) Children's performance in a game and their attraction to it as a function of sex-typed labels. *Child Development, 45,* 152–156.

Morris, L. W. Finkelstein, C. S. & Fisher, W. R. (1976) Components of school anxiety: developmental trends and sex differences. *Journal of Genetic Psychology, 128,* 49–57.

Mosley, J. L. & Stan, E. A. (1984) Human sexual dimorphism: its cost and benefit. *In* H. W. Reese (ed.) *Advances in child development and behavior,* vol. 18. New York: Academic Press, pp. 147–185.

Murphy, L. B. & Moriarty, A. E. (1976) *Vulnerability, coping and growth.* Newhaven, Conn.: Yale University Press.

Naditch, S. F. (1976) Sex differences in field dependence: the role of social influence. Paper presented at a Symposium of the American Psychological Association on Determinants of Gender Differences in Cognitive Functioning, Washington, DC.

Nash, S. C. (1975) The relationship among sex-role stereotyping, sex-role preference, and sex differences in spatial visualisation. *Sex Roles, 1,* 15–32.

Nash, S. C. (1979) Sex role as a mediator of intellectual functioning. *In* M. A. Wittig & A. C. Petersen (eds) *Sex-related differences in cognitive functioning: developmental issues.* New York: Academic Press, pp. 263–302.

Nebes, R. D. (1974) Hemipheric specialisation in commissurotomized man. *Psychological Bulletin, 81,* 1–14.

Nelson, K. (1973) *Structure and strategy in learning to talk.* Monographs of the Society for Research in Child Development, No. 38.

Newcombe, N. (1982) Sex-related differences in spatial ability: problems and gaps in current approaches. *In* M. Potegal (ed.) *Spatial abilities: development and physiological foundations.* New York: Academic Press, pp. 223–250.

Ounsted, C. & Taylor, D. C. (1972) The Y chromosome message: a point of view. *In* C. Ounsted & D. C. Taylor (eds) *Gender differences: their ontogeny and significance.* London: Churchill.

Papalia, S. E. & Tennent, S. S. (1975) Vocational aspirations in preschoolers: a manifestation of early sex-role stereotyping. *Sex Roles, 1,* 197–199.

Parlee, M. B. (1972) Comments on D. M. Broverman, E. L. Klaiber, Y. Kobayashi & W. Vogel: Roles of activation and inhibition in sex differences in cognitive abilities. *Psychological Review, 79,* 180–184.

Parlee, M. B. (1982) The psychology of the menstrual cycle: biological and physiological perspectives. *In* R. C. Friedman (ed.) *Behaviour and the menstrual cycle.* New York: Marcel Dekker, pp. 77–99.

Parsons, J. E. (ed.) (1980) *The psychobiology of sex differences and sex roles*. New York: McGraw-Hill.

Parsons, J. E. (1984) Sex differences in mathematics participation. *In* M. W. Steinkamp & M. L. Meehr (eds) *Women in science* (Advances in Motivation and Achievement, vol. 2). Greenwich, Connecticut: JAI Press.

Pederson, D. M., Shinedling, M. M. & Johnson, D. L. (1975) Effects of examiner and subject of children's quantitative test performance. *In* R. K. Unger & F. L. Denmark (eds) *Woman: dependent or independent variable*. New York: Psychological Dimensions, pp. 409–416.

Petersen, A. C. (1976) Physical androgyny and cognitive functioning in adolescents. *Developmental Psychology*, *12*, 524–533.

Petersen, A. C. (1979) Hormones and cognitive functioning in normal development. *In* M. A. Wittig & A. C. Petersen (eds) *Sex-related differences in cognitive functioning: developmental issues*. New York: Academic Press, pp. 189–214.

Petersen, A. C. (1980) Biopsychosocial processes in the development of sex-related differences. *In* J. E. Parsons (ed.) *The psychobiology of sex differences and sex roles*. New York: McGraw-Hill, pp. 31–55.

Piaget, J. (1953) *The origin of intelligence in the child*. London: Routledge & Kegan Paul.

Rheingold, H. L. & Cook, K. V. (1975) The contents of boys' and girls' rooms as an index of parents' behaviour. *Child Development*, *46*, 459–463.

Richmond, P. G. (1980) A limited sex difference in spatial test scores with a preadolescent sample. *Child Development*, *51*, 601–602.

Rudel, R., Denckla, M. & Spalten, E. (1974) The functional asymmetry of Braille letter learning in normal sighted children. *Neurology*, *24*, 733–738.

Rutter, M. & Yule W. (1975) The concept of specific reading retardation. *Journal of Child Psychology and Psychiatry*, *16*, 181–197.

Schlossberg, N. K. & Goodman, J. A. (1972) A woman's place: children's sex stereotyping of occupations. *Vocational Guidance Quarterly*, *20*, 266–270.

Scottish Council for Research in Education (1949) *The trend of Scottish intelligence*. London: University of London Press.

Sells, L. W. (1980) The mathematical filter and the education of women and minorities. *In* L. H. Fox, L. Brody & D. Tobin (eds) *Women and the mathematical mystique*. Baltimore: Johns Hopkins University Press.

Serbin, L. A. & Connor, J. M. (1979) Sex-typing of childrens' play preferences and patterns of cognitive performance. *Journal of Genetic Psychology*, *134*, 315–316.

Sherman, J. (1969) Problem of sex differences in space perception and aspects of intellectual functioning. *Psychological Review*, *74*, 290–299.

Sherman, J. (1971) *On the psychology of women: a survey of empirical studies*. Springfield, Illinois: C. C. Thomas.

Sherman, J. (1974) Field articulation, sex, spatial visualisation, dependency, practice, laterality of the brain and birth order. *Perceptual and Motor Skills*, *38*, 1223–1235.

Sherman, J. (1977) The effect of genetic factors on women's achievement in mathematics. *In* J. Shoemaker (ed.) *Women and mathematics: research perspectives for change*. Washington, DC: US Government Printing Office.

Sherman J. (1978) *Sex-related cognitive differences*. Springfield, Illinois: C. C. Thomas.

Sherman, J. & Fennema, E. (1977) The study of mathematics by high school girls and boys: related variables. *American Educational Research Journal*, *14*, 51–71.

Siegel, A. W., Herman, J. F., Allen, G. L. & Kirasic, K. C. (1979) The development of cognitive maps of large- and small-scale places. *Child Development*, *50*, 582–585.

Siegel, A. W. & Schadler, M. (1977) The development of young children's spatial representations of their classrooms. *Child Development*, *48*, 388–394.

Sigel, I. E. & Cocking, R. R. (1976) Cognition and communication: a dialectical paradigm for development. *In* M. Lewis & L. Rosenblum (eds) *Communication and language: the origins of behaviour*, vol. 5. New York: John Wiley.

Signorella, M. L. & Jamison, W. (1978) Sex differences in the correlations among field dependence, spatial ability, sex-role orientation, and performance on Piaget's water-level task. *Developmental Psychology*, *14*, 689–690.

Simon, J. G. & Feather, N. T. (1973) Causal attribution for success and failure at university examinations. *Journal of Educational Psychology*, 64, 46–56.

Singer, J. E., Westphal, M. & Niswander, K. R. (1968) Sex differences in the incidence of neonatal abnormalities and abnormal performance in early childhood. *Child Development*, *32*, 103–111.

Singleton, C. H. (1975) The myth of specific developmental dyslexia: part I History, incidence and diagnosis of the syndrome. *Remedial Education*, *10*, 109–113.

Singleton, C. H. (1976) The myth of specific developmental dyslexia: part II Aetiology. *Remedial Education*, *11*, 13–17.

Singleton, C. H. (1977) Dyslexia or specific reading retardation: a psychological critique. *In* J. Gilliland (ed.) *Reading: improving classroom practice and research*. London: Ward Lock.

Singleton, C. H. (1978) Sex differences. *In* B. M. Foss (ed.) *Psychology Survey 1*. London: George Allen & Unwin, pp. 116–130.

Sommer, B. (1982) Cognitive behaviour and the menstrual cycle. *In* R. C. Friedman (ed.) *Behaviour and the menstrual cycle*. New York: Marcel Dekker, pp. 101–127.

Stafford, R. E. (1961) Sex differences in spatial visualisation as evidence of sex-linked inheritance. *Perceptual and Motor Skills*, *13*, 428.

Stein, A. H. (1971) The effects of sex-role standards for achievement and sex-role preference on three determinants of achievement motivation. *Developmental Psychology*, *4*, 219–231.

Stein, A. H., Pohly, S. R. & Mueller, E. (1971) The influence of masculine, feminine and neutral tasks on children's achievement behaviour, expectancies of success, and attainment values. *Child Development*, *42*, 195–207.

90 *Part I Theoretical Background*

Thompson, G. B. (1975) Sex differences in reading attainments. *Educational Research*, 18, 16–23.

Tresemer, D. W. (1977) *Fear of success*. New York: Plenum.

Tresemer, D. W. & Pleck, J. (1976) Sex-role boundaries and resistance to sex-role change. *In* F. L. Denmark (ed.) *Women*, vol. 1. New York: Psychological Dimensions.

Turner, G. (1982) X-linked mental retardation. *Psychological Medicine, 12*, 471–473.

Tyler, L. E. (1965) *The psychology of human differences*, 3rd edn. New York: Appleton.

Vandenberg, S. G. (1975) Sources of variation in performance on spatial tasks. *In* J. Eliot & N. J. Salkind (eds) *Children's spatial development*. Springfield, Illinois: C. C. Thomas.

Vandenberg, S. G. & Kuse, A. R. (1979) Spatial ability: a critical review of the sex-linked major gene hypothesis. *In* M. A. Wittig & A. C. Petersen (eds) *Sex-related differences in cognitive functioning: developmental issues*. New York: Academic Press, pp. 67–95.

Vasta, R., Regan, K. G. & Kerley, J. (1980) Sex differences in pattern copying: spatial cues or motor skills? *Child Development, 51*, 932–934.

Vernon, P. E. (1972) Sex differences in personality structure at age 14. *Canadian Journal of Behavioural Science, 4*, 283–297.

Viaene, N. (1979) Sex differences in explanations of success and failure. *In* O. Hartnett, G. Boden & M. Fuller (eds.) *Sex-role stereotyping*. London: Tavistock, pp. 117–139.

Waber, D. P. (1976) Sex differences in cognition: a function of maturation rates? *Science, 192*, 572–574.

Waber, D. P. (1977a) Biological substrates of field dependence: implications of the sex difference. *Psychological Bulletin*, 84, 1076–1087.

Waber, D. P. (1977b) Sex differences in mental abilities, hemispheric lateralisation and rate of physical growth at adolescence. *Developmental Psychology*, 13, 29–38.

Wada, J. A., Clarke, R. & Hamm, A. (1975) Cerebral hemispheric asymmetry in humans. *Archives of Neurology, 32*, 239–246.

Ward, C. (1979) Is there a motive in women to avoid success? *In* O. Hartnett, G. Boden & M. Fuller (eds) *Sex-role stereotyping*. London: Tavistock, pp. 140–156.

Widiger, T. A., Knudson, R. M. & Rorer, L. G. (1980) Convergent and discriminant validity of measures of cognitive styles and abilities. *Journal of Personality and Social Psychology, 39*, 116–129.

Wilson, J. R., De Fries, J. C., McClearn, C. E., Vandenberg, S. G., Johnson, R. C. & Rashad, M. N. (1975) Cognitive abilities: use of family data to assess sex and age differences in two ethnic groups. *International Journal of Aging and Human Development, 6*, 261–276.

Wilson, J. R. & Vandenberg, S. G. (1978) Sex differences in cognition: evidence from the Hawai family study. *In* T. E. McGill, D. A. Dewsbury, B. D. Sachs (eds) *Sex and behaviour: status and prospects*. New York: Plenum Press.

Witelson, S. F. (1976) Sex and the single hemisphere: specialisation of the right hemisphere for spatial processing. *Science, 193*, 425–427.

Witkin, H. A. & Berry, J. W. (1975) Psychological differentiation in cross-cultural perspective. *Journal of Cross-Cultural Psychology*, *6*, 4–87.

Witkin, H. A., Birnbaum, J., Lomonaco, S., Lehr, S. & Herman, J. L. (1968) Cognitive patterning in congenitally blind children. *Child Development*, *39*, 768–786.

Wittig, M. A. & Petersen, A. C. (eds) (1979) *Sex-related differences in cognitive functioning: developmental issues*. New York: Academic Press.

Woodfield, R. L. (1984) Embedded figures test performance before and after childbirth. *British Journal of Psychology*, *75*, 81–88.

Yarrow, L. J. (1972) Dimensions of early stimulation and their differential effects on infant development. *Merrill-Palmer Quarterly*, *18*, 205–218.

Yen, W. M. (1975) Sex linked major-gene influence on selected types of spatial performance. *Behaviour Genetics*, *5*, 281–298.

Zuckerman, M. & Wheeler, L. (1975) To dispel fantasies about the fantasy-based measure of fear of success. *Psychological Bulletin*, *82*, 932–946.

PART II

DEVELOPMENTAL ISSUES

CHAPTER FIVE   Early Sex-Role Socialization
Charlie Lewis

Our survey of data has revealed a remarkable degree of uniformity in the socialisation of the two sexes.... existing evidence has not revealed any consistent process of 'shaping' boys and girls toward a number of behaviours that are normally part of our sex stereotypes. (Maccoby & Jacklin 1974, p. 348)

In their monumental review of the literature on sex differences, Maccoby and Jacklin (1974) came to the conclusion that socialization pressures (those influences exerted by parents and others upon the child) have little impact upon the child's sex-role development. However, their assertion gave rise to a wave of criticism and renewed speculation about the effect of parental handling upon boys and girls (Birns 1976; Block 1976). In this chapter I will examine the evidence which has accumulated mainly since Maccoby and Jacklin's work was published.

Within the past decade or so developmental psychology has undergone a number of changes which should be mentioned here. As the above quotation suggests, Maccoby and Jacklin were working within a theoretical framework where it was felt that socialization is a process of 'shaping' the child's behaviours in a somewhat mechanical fashion. Since then two substantial changes have occurred. In the early 1970s it became accepted that this model of interaction was too simple, and developmentalists now admit firstly that interaction is a two-way affair − each participant influences the others (Lewis & Rosenblum 1974). Secondly, and more recently, it has become apparent that development is influenced by a variety of social factors and that we need to understand the child in his or her 'ecological' context (Bronfenbrenner 1979).

These changes necessarily alter our understanding of sex-role development and this discussion will be primarily concerned with the effects of these general theoretical moves. The chapter will be divided into two main parts. The first examines recent data which suggests that parents treat their boys and girls in different ways and points out the methodological shortcomings in measuring parental 'behaviour'. The second section examines the possible influences which parents may have upon their children.

Parental influences on early sex-role development

The obvious time to look for differences in the behaviour and development of males and females might seem to be very early in life. In the late 1960s many researchers became preoccupied with such a task. At first their results suggested clear differences between the sexes. While males are more muscular in build (Tanner 1974) they were found to be less resistant to disease or injury (Garai & Scheinfeld 1968), more irritable (Moss 1967) and less attentive to both auditory (Lewis 1972) and visual stimuli (Hittleman and Dickes 1979).

However, these investigations produced numerous problems. For a start, some studies may well have confounded early sex differences with the effects of circumcision, since significant differences were more likely to be reported in countries where circumcision rates were higher (Richards, Bernal & Brackbill 1975). Second, research into early sex differences is noted for its lack of replication (Birns 1976; Ruble 1984). Moss (1974), for example, failed to repeat his earlier findings that male infants are more irritable in the first month of life. Third, recent work suggests that sex differences are complex. Differences at two days after delivery have been found to disappear at four days (Hwang 1978). Even during one activity, like breast feeding, sex differences in the behaviour are influenced by factors like the infant's state of wakefulness and the behaviour of the mother (Rosenthal 1983).

A second area of research has examined how parents react to 'stranger babies' introduced either as boys or girls. Some studies (Frisch 1977; Smith & Lloyd 1978) suggest that adults are predisposed to treat labelled infant boys and girls differently, irrespective of any subtle feedback they might receive from the baby him/herself. How generalizable data such as these really are is hard to assess. Leaving aside that most researchers study middle-class people and test only a few aspects of adult behaviour, it is very possible that we resort to such sex-typed activities only when faced by strange babies for the first time or perhaps only when being observed by psychologists. Frisch (1977) readily admits these reservations.

We appear to handle 'stranger babies' in sex-typed ways, but to what extent is this matched in the ways parents treat their own children? No one denies that young girls and boys are dressed differently (Maccoby & Jacklin 1980), nor that they are provided with sex-appropriate belongings. Rheingold and Cook (1975), for example, examining ninety-six preschoolers' bedrooms, found that boys' rooms contained significantly more vehicles, sports equipment, zoo animals and 'spatial-temporal toys' (e.g. clocks). Girls' rooms were decorated with 'floral furnishings' and 'ruffles', and contained more dolls.

Given these obvious differences it may seem surprising that Maccoby and Jacklin (1974) concluded that there is no clear evidence to show that parents treat their boys and girls differently. Maccoby and Jacklin's argument about the data collected before 1974 is compelling since few trends in the data were apparent. However, they pointed out that whole areas of potential research had not been carried out, particularly on fathers. Their critics were also quick to record the fact that they compared a disparate number of studies over a wide range of ages (Birns 1976; Block 1976).

In the last ten years many of the gaps in research have been filled. As developmentalists have become increasingly interested in the child's ecological niche, they have involved fathers in research. This has given rise to renewed speculations about the socialization of sex roles. From birth parents appear to map out their infant's present and future in terms of its sex. In one study 82 per cent of parents' comments within twenty minutes of the baby's arrival were made about the infant's sex (Woollett, White & Lyon 1982). A much-discussed interview study of parents' attitudes after delivery, for example, found that they described their daughters as 'softer' and 'finer featured', and their sons as 'firmer', 'more alert' and 'stronger' (Rubin, Provenzano & Luria 1974). Men used such terms more frequently than their wives. This has led many to suggest that fathers play a major role in sex typing. Before we make such a hasty conclusion we should consider two rarely discussed aspects of this study which might also account for the discrepancy between mothers' and fathers' accounts. First, the fathers were interviewed in the heat of the moment − just after delivery − while their wives were questioned up to twenty-four hours later. Second, none of the fathers had been allowed to handle their babies. Like those introduced to 'stranger babies', the fathers may have resorted to stereotypical responses simply because they had less experience of the child.

With this type of caution in mind I will now discuss the literature which suggests that mothers and fathers contribute to sex-role development in distinctive ways. Broadly there are two related themes which recur. First, in keeping with the ideas of both psychoanalysts (Burlingham 1973) and social learning theorists (Mischel 1966) it is suggested that mothers and fathers have different relationships with their children and serve as sex-typed models to them throughout development. The second and more central theme is that mothers and fathers exert different influences upon sons and daughters. Each of these issues will be discussed in turn.

Mothers and fathers as role models

Evidence from many sources shows that in most families children have qualitatively different types of relationship with each parent. While there are many family types in contemporary society (Rapoport, Rapoport & Strelitz 1977), most children are cared for most of the time by women. Interview studies suggest that while nearly all men play regularly with their child, few involve themselves in child care on a daily basis, particularly the 'dirty jobs' (Kotelchuck 1972; Lewis, in press; Newson & Newson 1963). In all these studies over 40 per cent of fathers never changed a nappy. Similarly, when psychologists observe families going about their daily routines, mothers do far more care-giving even when both parents are available (Belsky 1979; Belsky, Gilstrap & Rovine 1984; Fagot 1978; Lamb 1976a, 1976b).

It is hard to say what effect such role differences have upon the developing infant. Observations of parent–infant interaction at home suggest that despite these differences parents adopt similar styles of interaction (Pedersen 1980). For example, Clarke-Stewart (1980), observing children between fifteen and thirty months, found that both spouses tended to play and give affection in similar ways.

Despite these similarities, some differences between mothers and fathers have been found. When observed fathers are more likely to get involved in rough and tumble play with younger children (Parke 1979), their styles of interaction are less smoothly modulated than those of mothers (Yogman 1977), and they may appear to be less skilled at keeping their child's attention on a toy (Power 1981). Such behavioural differences may influence the development of the child's social understanding. For example, recent studies of parent–child communication suggest that fathers use more complex utterances and terms than their wives and may stretch the child's developing linguistic competence (Gleeson 1975; McLoughlin *et al.* 1983; Rondal 1980).

Differential socialization of girls and boys

Recent evidence suggests that mothers and fathers handle their boys and girls in subtly different ways. As research has become increasingly home-based, fathers have stepped into the limelight because, more than mothers, they appear to treat their young infants in sex-appropriate ways. Such a view was central to reciprocal role theory in sociology (Johnson 1963) and has filtered into psychology in the last ten years. Power (1981), reviewing the interaction literature, found that in sixteen projects involving mothers, seven found that boys and girls were treated differently. In fifteen studies of fathers, fourteen revealed such patterns. Power suggests that mothers do treat sons and daughters differently, but only during the first three months and later on in the second year. Fathers appear to do so consistently.

As mentioned above, very early in the child's life both mothers and fathers show sex-preferential behaviour towards sons and daughters. In one English delivery room fathers stayed longer, made six times more comments about the baby (Woollett, White & Lyon 1982), and held their baby twice as long (Woollett, personal communication) when it was a boy. American research suggests similar patterns in the few days after delivery with first-born but not later-born children. Fathers touched their sons more. Mothers touched their daughters more, but only when their husbands were not present (Parke & O'Leary 1976).

Within the first three months similar patterns have been recorded. The most comprehensive data come from Parke and Sawin's (1980) sample of fifty children followed from birth to three months. Parents exhibited similar styles to one another, especially in the ways they gave routine care to the child. However, two aspects of their interaction appeared to differ. Parents tended to cuddle opposite-sex children and to offer toys to and stimulate same-sex children.

The observation studies suggest that after about three months fathers continue to differentiate between boys and girls (Rendina & Dickerschied 1976; White, Woollett & Lyon 1982), while this is not so for mothers. On an Israeli kibbutz fathers visited their four-month-old sons more than daughters (Gewirtz & Gewirtz 1968). Field (1978) filmed mothers and fathers at play with their four-month-olds. Fathers engaged in more interaction games with their sons. Such observations have led to numerous propositions about the influence of mothers and fathers. Lewis and Weinraub (1974) suggested that parents, especially fathers, encourage their daughters to remain close to them while their sons are increasingly made to develop their independence. While Parke and Sawin's data with younger children support this view and, as I shall show later, male and female toddlers do often show such differences, the overall evidence is mixed. Indeed Belsky (1979) found that fathers were more likely to show affection to their sons than daughters at fifteen months.

In contrast to the view proposed by Lewis and Weinraub, Lamb (1977b, 1978, 1980) suggested that fathers are important contributors to sex-role development because they make themselves salient to their sons during the second year of life. He observed twenty children at home on four occasions between fifteen and twenty-four months and found that mothers and fathers played in different ways with their children. Mothers tended to initiate toy-based play and 'conventional' games like 'pat-a-cake' or 'peep-bo'. Fathers were far more likely to engage in rough and tumble or idiosyncratic play, especially towards their sons. In return sons were far more likely to seek out their fathers to play.

Lamb's data are interesting, although hard to assess as they are contradicted by other evidence. In a further study I shall discuss later, Lamb *et al.* (1983) failed to obtain similar results. Other evidence suggests that we cannot infer the causes of such patterns of interaction. For example, Snow, Jacklin and Maccoby (1983), examining 107 father–twelve-month-old pairs in a room in which toys and breakable objects had been arranged, found that while fathers tended to treat their sons and daughters differently, so too were there sex differences in the children's behaviour. The fathers gave dolls to their sons less frequently and tended to prohibit them more. However, when given dolls, boys played with them less than did girls. Boys were also more naughty and needed reprimanding more.

Evidence from research on children from about two years has yielded the same patterns as those with younger children. As Power (1981) pointed out, both mothers and fathers appear to treat boys and girls differently from about this age. Home-based observations have indicated that parents are more likely to leave boys to play (Fagot 1974, 1978) and to interfere in order to stop their activities (Fagot 1978) especially those which are forbidden, like tampering with electric sockets (Smith & Daglish 1977). As with studies of younger children, fathers appear to encourage sex differences more than mothers (McGuire 1982). Fagot's (1978) five-hour observations in twenty-four homes revealed that fathers encouraged their daughters to stay near them and were especially critical of doll play in sons. Studies of children aged between three and five continue to suggest that men, more than their wives, differentiate between boys and girls. For example, they appear to be far more critical of sex-inappropriate play (Langlois & Downs 1980) and initiate sex-appropriate activities, especially rough and tumble play with sons

(Jacklin, DiPietro & Maccoby 1984). Such findings have suggested that fathers continue to play a key role in sex-role differentiation.

Why we must be cautious about data on early sex-role socialization

Before moving on to consider just how the observed and reported patterns of socialization might influence boys and girls in early development, it is necessary to reflect upon the evidence I have discussed above. As models of psychological development have become increasingly complex, so too have our ideas about the limits of the methods we use. Authors like Maccoby and Jacklin (1980) have pointed out the problems in interpreting interview material and have suggested that these point to the value of observational studies. However, the validity of observational data has also been frequently questioned (Bronfenbrenner 1973, 1979), particularly those concerning parent–infant interaction (Lewis 1982; Parke 1978; Pedersen *et al.* 1979).

Cautions about methods apply particularly to studies of sex roles. In a recent review Ruble (1984) points out that the sex of the experimenter can have an influence on the way adults behave:

> There are many features of a study that may elicit differential reactions of males and females, which are irrelevant to the focus of study, but nevertheless contaminate its findings. The experimenter's sex, familiarity with the situation, or interest in the topic of the experiment are all aspects of the methods of study that can interact with the sex of the subject and can influence the results. (p. 335)

Do such cautions carry over to work on parent–infant relationships? In order to answer this question we need to consider the possible reasons why mothers and fathers appear to interact with sons and daughters in particular ways. Many authors simply accept any differences without considering their origins (Lewis 1982). However, Power (1981) has suggested three possible causes. First, mothers and fathers may have different child-rearing goals. Second, fathers may have more stereotypical perceptions of their offspring. Third, by virtue of the paucity of father–child contact in most families, men may be demonstrating their lack of experience when they resort to stereotypical interaction patterns with their children.

While there is circumstantial evidence to support each of these possible influences upon parents, a fourth explanation is just as likely. Mothers and fathers may well be influenced in different ways by the very act of observation. In recent years efforts have been made to measure the changes in parents' activities in different contexts. It has been found in many studies that parents and infants interact less with one another when the other parent is present (Belsky 1979; Clarke-Stewart 1978). They also talk less (Golinkoff & Ames 1979; Killarney & McCluskey 1981). The influences of a third person on the interaction between two others are known as 'second order effects'.

While there is ample documentation about second order effects and some discussion about the influence of group size upon the interactions of parents and children depending on their sex (Parke & O'Leary 1976), little attention has been paid to the effect which an observer has upon the interaction between parent and child. However, the existing evidence suggests that mothers do behave differently when observed in a waiting room before an experiment (Zeigob, Arnold & Forehand 1975) and when a stooge observer is called out to a telephone call (Randall 1974). Indeed, Randall found that mothers tended to encourage their ten-month-old sons more when an observer was present recording their behaviour, and their daughters more when the observer left the room and they thought they were no longer being watched.

Adapting Randall's methodology, I recently studied the language of twenty mothers and fathers to their ten-month-old children when being observed and when the observer was called away to the telephone (Lewis, in preparation). Parents were told that the researcher was interested in children's play, so as to discourage them from attempting to display their linguistic skills in front of the observer. Nevertheless the structure and function of parent's language changed between the two conditions in a number of ways. On some measures mothers and fathers were differentially influenced by both the presence of the observer and the sex of their child. For example, Figure 5.1 shows the proportion of interrogatives used by parents in each condition – a measure taken to reflect the involvement of the parent in the child's activity. Statistical analysis showed that the mothers did not alter this aspect of their language in each context. Fathers, by contrast, appeared to ask more questions of their sons in the standard observational setting, as we might expect from the literature reviewed above. However, they used more interrogatives with their daughters after the observer left the room.

These results do not of course invalidate the data obtained in observational studies. They simply suggest that observed differences between

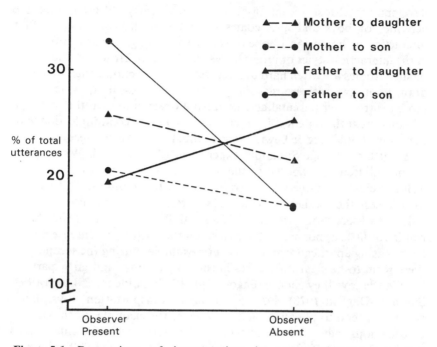

Figure 5.1 Proportions of interrogatives in parents' language to their ten-month-olds

mothers and fathers may not generalize to all settings. It seems highly likely that parents are under particular pressure to demonstrate their skills when being observed. Fathers may well act differently towards sons and daughters in this context, because they are less used to making such public displays. Certainly data such as these suggest that we should temper any generalizations we make from observational studies about the 'effects' of parental input on sex-role development. Such patterns may only occur when outsiders are present. This does not, however, rule out the possibility that parental influence on sex-role socialization may be important because they differentiate between boys and girls in public settings.

Sex roles in infants and toddlers

In the rest of this chapter I will consider whether the reported differences in the ways parents appear to act influence their children's sex-role development. Most recent discussion about early differences in the activities of boys and girls comes from the studies of parent–infant interaction at home. As I hope to show, these suggest many differences in the interaction styles of infant males and females. However, the results of such studies are often hard to interpret. In this section I shall therefore draw upon two other areas of parent–infant research, which exert more control over parental activity during observation. In the first type of experiment the parent is instructed not to initiate communication with the infant (Goldberg & Lewis 1969; Lamb 1976c). In the second, Mary Ainsworth's 'Strange Situation' experiment (Ainsworth & Wittig 1969) young children are exposed to the departure and return of a parent as well as being left alone with a stranger for a few minutes. This enables us to assess the toddler's reaction to a stressful circumstance.

Home observations are 'ecologically valid' – they disrupt the child's routine as little as possible – but as a result they often prevent researchers from teasing apart cause and effect. For example, during the second year there seem to be clear differences in the play of boys and girls, particularly in the toys they choose (Fagot 1974; 1978; Goldberg & Lewis 1969; Smith & Daglish 1978). Boys often push 'transportation' toys along, while girls tend to play with dolls or dance, for example. Such patterns of behaviour may arise out of biological differences in the children, as a result of parental influences, or, as Smith and Daglish (1978) point out, they may simply reflect the fact that males and females are usually provided with different toys.

In the home, other sex differences often arise within the first two years. Children have been found to direct more 'attachment behaviours' (Lamb 1977b) and be more affectionate towards (Belsky 1979) their same-sex parent. Both boys and girls are often found to approach their fathers for play (Belsky 1979; Hegland 1977) which might indicate that they are learning to equate masculinity with 'action' in the way reciprocal role theory suggests (Parsons & Bales 1955). Further, some evidence implies that girls show more social competence than boys (Klein & Durfee 1978).

However, these findings may not reflect inherent differences between boys and girls. Some of these studies have examined the activities of children in relation to those of their parents. This procedure, which uses parental behaviour as a 'covariate', often makes apparent significant differences between boys and girls disappear. For example, Belsky (1979) found that when paternal and maternal approaches were taken into account children were not more likely to approach their fathers for play. Likewise, when maternal behaviour was used as a covariate, Klein and

Durfee's (1978) sex difference in infant social competence was not significant – mothers apparently *invited* more social behaviour from their daughters.

These home-based studies have also produced contradictory evidence in the children's as well as the parent's activities. In a more recent study Lamb *et al.* (1983) failed to find that children sought out their same-sex parent in times of stress. Indeed both boys and girls approached their mothers more than fathers for play and comfort when both parents were at home. Just why Lamb obtained such different results in his two studies is unclear, but may well have something to do with the fact that the first took place in the United States and the second in Sweden. Lamb *et al.* (1983) suggested that cultural differences in men's fathering styles may be important, although these differences may only apply when observers are present.

Sociability in toddlers

Results from home-based studies are often difficult to interpret, but we should not reject them out of hand. Some of them correspond to those obtained in the experiments described above, where the parents and 'strangers' are instructed not to initiate communication with the child. In the 'Strange Situation' for example there is some support for the belief that, at least in the United States, one-year-old infants will seek their same-sex parent as an emotional haven. Some experiments have involved both mothers and fathers. These found that boys were more likely to show 'attachment behaviours' to their fathers (Kotelchuck 1972) and that girls sought the proximity of and talked more to their mothers (Spelke *et al.* 1973).

Both laboratory and home-based studies show that girls tend to stay closer to and are more sociable with their parents when being observed. In fifteen minutes of laboratory observation, for example, Goldberg and Lewis (1969) found that thirteen-month-old girls would return more and talk more to their mothers than would boys. This finding has been replicated in a study with both mothers and fathers (Lamb 1977a). In one home-based study, when maternal vocalization was taken into consideration, one-year-old girls made more attempts to communicate with their mothers (Klein & Durfee 1978).

Perhaps the most convincing test of boys' and girls' social responsivity comes from a laboratory study of 84 six-, nine- and twelve-month-olds.

Gunnar and Donahue (1980) divided parent and child actions into 'initiations' and 'responses', in order to check whether mothers were differentially reacting to boys' and girls' attempts to socialize. They found that mothers did not do this. At the same time, in all three age groups girls initiated more interactions and responded to more maternal initiations than did boys.

Perhaps even as young as six months, American girls seem to be more adult-centred than boys. As well as seeking the company of their parents, they also seem to be more friendly towards strangers – at least in more natural settings. Ross and Goldman (1977) modified the 'Strange Situation' experiment so that the stranger acted in a friendly way towards the child. They found that girls spent more time near the stranger and touched her sooner than did boys. Likewise, in the home, Klein and Durfee (1978) found that girls were more likely to approach the observer.

Sex differences in toddlers' responses to stress

It seems probable that these sex differences in proximity and sociability fit into more complex patterns of development. Attachment theory (Bowlby 1969) suggests that infants use their mothers as secure base, particularly in times of stress. Boys and girls may well develop different strategies when using their parents in this way. Lewis and Weinraub (1979) report that maternal separation in the 'Strange Situation' provokes more distress in boys. Examining children's response to stress, Maccoby and Jacklin (1973) carried out an experiment designed to evoke fear in one-year-olds playing with their mothers in a laboratory. At a set time a loud noise sounded. Girls tended to crawl to their mothers, as was expected. Boys on the other hand took far longer to begin crawling to their 'secure base' – they often froze at the sound of the noise.

Two further experiments examining infants' responses to potentially stress-provoking stimuli suggest that boys are more likely to be concerned about controlling these stimuli. In their study of infant play in the laboratory, Goldberg and Lewis (1969) erected a barrier between one-year-olds and their mothers. Girls tended to remain at the centre of the barrier and cry towards their mothers. Boys on the other hand made far greater effort to get round the barrier. This might imply that girls are simply more fearful. However, research by Gunnar (1978) suggest that boys' expressions of fear depend upon their ability to control aversive stimuli. She set up an experiment in which twelve-month-olds were exposed to a noisy toy – a cymbal-banging monkey. Half the children were taught how to stop the toy by pressing a panel. Girls and those boys who were shown how to terminate the noise did not usually react too strongly to it. In contrast most of the boys who were not taught how to control the stimuli dissolved quickly into tears.

Parental influences upon the development of early sex roles

Girls' sociability and boys' responses to stress may of course be caused by either biological or social factors. Perhaps because it is so hard to find adequate measures upon which the sexes are clearly differentiated in early life there have been few attempts to examine possible causal links in the chain of sex-role development. Even within research on how early attachments change over time – a field where much work has been carried out over the last few years – little attention has been paid to sex differences (Egeland & Farber 1984). However, some interesting findings have emerged. These suggest that sex-role development may be closely related to both social and cognitive growth and that parents seem to play a part in the shaping of these. Two areas of understanding may be particularly relevant in the child's early years.

The first is the role of the father in development. Research with older children has suggested that the father's involvement during early childhood correlates with the child's later academic performance (Lewis, Newson & Newson 1982) and that his closeness may help the intellectual development of boys, but not girls (Radin 1981). Some evidence has suggested that this pattern is evident in early childhood. For example, Clarke-Stewart (1980) correlated the child's cognitive level (as measured by standardized tests) at thirty months, with many aspects of observed and reported parental involvement. More advanced children of either sex tended to have mothers who stimulated them more and fathers who played more. In addition, sons who did well at the tests more often had fathers who attempted to stimulate them both intellectually and physically.

Perhaps the most intriguing finding concerning the influence of the father on son's early cognitive development comes from a study of families without fathers (Pedersen, Rubenstein & Yarrow 1979). Such studies have often been criticized for their failure to distinguish the effects of 'father absence' from the economic and social deprivation single-parent families often suffer. Pedersen and his colleagues were careful to exert adequate controls when selecting a comparison group. They found that as early as five months the cognitive and social development of fatherless sons was lagging behind both that of children of similar socio-economic standing and fatherless daughters. Not only did these boys score lower on the Bayley tests of development, but they also showed less interest in novel toys that were presented to them.

Results like these suggest that the sorts of involvement fathers were observed to show towards their sons in the studies discussed earlier may have an effect. However, we cannot be certain that such links can be made. In Clarke-Stewart's study (1980), for example, so many factors were investigated that the likelihood of significant correlations occurring by chance was very high. Even if valid, these significant correlations do not show us the direction of causality. Pedersen, Rubenstein & Yarrow's study (1979), while more controlled, does not necessarily show that the development of all fatherless boys is slower. For a start his sample was restricted to black Americans – the same patterns may not be found in other sub-cultural groups. In addition the tester in his study was male and no check was made to see whether the impaired performance of fatherless males generalized to different circumstances, in particular being tested by a female. More research needs to be carried out before we can be sure whether fathers influence the development of their sons more than their daughters, and if so how.

The second connection between parental styles and early sex-role development comes from a few longitudinal studies. These all suggest that maternal responsivity within the first year of life has differential 'effects' on boys and girls in the second year. More harmonious interaction between mother and son appears to correlate with the son's later social and cognitive performance. At the same time less involved mothering is often found to predict higher levels of skills in girls. Support for this proposition has often appeared in the literature on older children (e.g. Crandall *et al.* 1964) and in studies of early development (Clarke-Stewart 1980).

In order to examine the relationship between maternal style and later abilities in the child, Martin and his colleagues carried out two large studies which employed an interesting technique to measure maternal sensitivity (Martin 1981; Martin, Maccoby & Jacklin 1981). They set up an experiment designed to create a conflict of interest. Mothers were instructed to fill out questionnaires while their nine- or ten-month-old infants were placed in a high chair with no toys for five minutes. Martin and his colleagues correlated the responsivity of mothers to their infants' demands in this setting with the child's desire some months later to explore while the mother was being interviewed in one study (Martin, Maccoby & Jacklin 1981), and to a number of social and exploratory skills in the other (Martin 1981). These included their willingness to search out of sight behind a barrier where an interesting sounding toy was situated at twenty-two months, and their sensitivity to a stranger at forty-two months.

Martin's two studies produced similar results, suggesting a relationship between earlier maternal style and differential exploratory and social patterns in both boys and girls. Women who were highly responsive to their children at ten months tended to have sons who searched behind the barrier, and daughters who stayed close to them without searching, at twenty-two months (Martin 1981). Similar patterns were found in the interview setting (Martin, Maccoby & Jacklin 1981). At forty-two months Martin assessed the child's reaction to a strange experimenter and found that this was related to mother–infant interaction patterns at ten months. At the earlier age demanding boys whose mothers responded to their requests for attention were more likely over two years later to express warmth to the experimenter. Conversely, demanding girls whose mothers attended to them less were more likely to show warmth. These findings suggest that early sex differences in social behaviour may result from the interaction of complex internal and external factors.

Moves toward an ecological understanding of early sex-role development

The results from studies reported in the preceding section reveal the complexity of factors which may influence early sex-role development. Martin's research, in particular, may well support the previously stated belief that early in development boys need to have far greater control over events – their mother's responsiveness in this case. Studies like Martin's suggest at the same time that we are still far from understanding the relationships between influences, or even perhaps the variety of these influences. In this concluding section I will outline three areas of research which may lead us to extend our frames of reference beyond the parent–child relationship.

The first concerns our assumptions about the infant him/herself. The major theories of development propose that children are slow to develop powers of social awareness, let alone any notion of sex-role understanding. Recent evidence has started to open such belief to question. Lewis and Brooks (1975) showed that children aged between ten and eighteen months looked slightly, but significantly, longer at photographs of children of the same sex. Fifteen-month-olds also smiled more at photographs of their same-sex parent (Brooks-Gunn & Lewis 1979). Findings like these have led Lewis (1981) to suggest that early in the second year of life children are able to extract featural cues from such information and show a preference for those 'like me'. Such judgements are considered to be central to the child's early self concept. More recent experiments at the University of Edinburgh suggest that toddlers may well use higher order information like movement patterns to make these 'like me' preferences. They look more at film of same-sex children dressed in cross-sex clothing than opposite-sex children dressed in same-sex clothing (Aitken, cited in Bower 1982) and at one year even show such a preference when the only information given is twelve patch light displays attached to infant's joints (Kujawski 1984). Experiments like these suggest that we have still to discover much about early sex-role awareness.

A second area of research shows that if we are to come to terms with the infant's early socio-cognitive abilities we should go beyond studying parent–infant interaction, particularly at only one point in time. A clear example comes from a recent study of early sibling relationships which followed forty families for fourteen months after the arrival of the second child (Dunn & Kendrick 1982). Dunn and Kendrick found that when the younger child was fourteen months old, sex-linked patterns of relationship were apparent between siblings. Same-sex pairs were far more likely to be getting on well. In support of recent work on early sex-role awareness, younger children both initiated play with and approached their same-sex siblings more often. Relationships between brothers and sisters did not emerge suddenly. Dunn and Kendrick found that, at least among boys, friendship with younger siblings was positively correlated with the amount of interest shown towards them in the weeks after delivery. These relationships did not occur in isolation. Mothers were far more likely to spend time with their fourteen-month-old if the older sibling was of the opposite sex.

A third area of research adds a further dimension to the study of early sex roles. It suggests that the social organization of the family is important, particularly in the sex-role development of sons. For a start there is some evidence to suggest that boys may be more influenced by being placed in day care while their mothers work. Chase-Lansdale and Tresch

Owen (1981) found that boys whose mothers worked appeared to be more insecure in the 'Strange Situation'. Other studies of families where both parents work suggest that when observed, parents pay more attention to their daughters (Stuckey, McGhee & Bell 1982). When interviewed, mothers report a more glowing picture of their daughters than sons (Bronfenbrenner, Alvarez & Henderson 1984). Further evidence to suggest that young boys are susceptible in potentially stressful circumstances comes from research which shows that divorce tends to make them more disturbed and less sociable than girls (Hetherington, Cox & Cox 1982).

Conclusion

Given the large amount of research carried out since Maccoby and Jacklin (1974) came to the conclusion quoted at the start of this chapter, it now seems appropriate to reconsider their assertion that there is a 'remarkable degree of uniformity in the socialisation of the two sexes'. In contrast to Maccoby and Jacklin, the first half of this paper examined many studies which show that parents, especially fathers, do tend to treat boys and girls differently even during the first two years of life. However, such patterns might reflect ways in which men and women behave only in public or when being observed, so we cannot be certain that parental influences are paramount.

The second half of this chapter considered how socialization patterns might influence the child's early sex-role identity. Behavioural differences between boys and girls are apparent, even within the first year of life. In the United States, where most studies have taken place, girls seem to be more person-oriented. Boys tend to explore more, though they are also more susceptible to aversive stimuli and circumstances beyond their control. Just why such patterns have been found is not so clear. As developmental psychology has become increasingly broad in its orientation, so too has the list of potential influences upon the child grown. No doubt work in the coming years will show more about the complex interaction of these influences.

Acknowledgements

With thanks to Rosemary Smith, Phyllis Williams, Graham Luke, Alison Thomas and Jeanette Lilley.

References

Ainsworth, M. D. S. and Wittig, B. A. (1969) Attachment and exploratory behaviour in one-year-olds. *In* B. Foss (ed.) *Determinants of infant behaviour*. London: Methuen.

Belsky, J. (1979) Mother–father–infant interaction: a naturalistic observation study. *Developmental Psychology*, *15*, 601–607.

Belsky, J., Gilstrap, B. & Rovine, M. (1984). The Pennsylvania Infant and Family Development Project I: stability and change in mother–infant and father–infant interaction in a family setting at one, three, and nine months. *Child Development*, *55*, 692–705.

Berman, P. W. (1976) Social context as a determinant of sex differences in adults' attraction to infants. *Developmental Psychology*, *12*, 365–366.

Birns, B. (1976) The emergence and socialization of sex differences in the earliest years. *Merrill-Palmer Quarterly*, *22*, 229–254.

Blakemore, J., La Rue, A. & Olejkik, A. (1979) Sex appropriate toy reference and the ability to conceptualise toys as sex-role related. *Developmental Psychology*, *15*, 339–340.

Block, J. (1976) Issues, problems and pitfalls in assessing sex differences: a critical review of 'The Psychology of Sex Differences'. *Merrill-Palmer Quarterly*, *22*, 283–308.

Bower, T. G. R. (1982). *Development in infancy*. San Francisco: Freeman.

Bowlby, J. (1969) *Attachment and loss*, vol. 1. Harmondsworth: Penguin.

Bronfenbrenner, U. (1973) A theoretical perspective for research on human development. *In* H. P. Dreitzel (ed.) *Recent sociology*. New York: Macmillan. No. 5, Childhood and socialization, pp. 337–363.

Bronfenbrenner, U. (1979). *The ecology of human development*. Cambridge, Mass.: Harvard University Press.

Bronfenbrenner, U., Alvarez, W. & Henderson, C. (1984) Working and watching: maternal employment and parents' perceptions of their three year old children. *Child Development*, *55*, 1362–1378.

Brooks-Gunn, J. & Lewis, M. (1979) 'Why Mama and Papa?' The development of social labels. *Child Development*, *50*, 1203–1206.

Burlingham, D. (1973) The pre-Oedipal infant–father relationship. *Psychoanalytic Study of the Child*, *28*, 23–47.

Chase-Lansdale, L. & Tresch Owen, M. (1981) *Maternal employment in a family context*. Paper presented at the Society for Research in Child Development. Boston, April.

Clarke-Stewart, K. A. (1978) And Daddy makes three: the father's impact on mother and young child. *Child Development*, *49*, 466–479.

Clarke-Stewart, K. A. (1980) The father's contributions to children's cognitive and social development in early childhood. *In* F. A. Pedersen (ed.) *The father –infant relationship: observational studies in the family setting*. New York: Praeger.

Crandall, V., Dewey, R., Katkovsky, W. & Preston, A. (1964) Parent's attitudes and behaviours and grade school children's academic achievements. *Journal of Genetic Psychology*, *104*, 53–66.

Dunn, J. & Kendrick, C. (1982) *Siblings: love, envy and understanding*. London: Grant MacIntyre.

Egeland, B. & Farber, E. (1984) Infant: mother attachment: factors related to its development and changes over time. *Child Development, 55*, 753 –771.

Fagot, B. (1974) Sex differences in toddlers' behaviour and parental reaction. *Developmental Psychology, 10 (4)*, 554–558.

Fagot, B. (1978) The influence of sex of child on parental reactions to toddler children. *Child Development, 49*, 459–465.

Feldman, S. & Ingham, M. (1975) Attachment behaviour: a validation study in two age groups. *Child Development, 46*, 319–330.

Field, T. (1978) Interaction behaviours of primary vs. secondary caretaker fathers. *Developmental Psychology, 14*, 183–184.

Frisch, H. L. (1977) Sex stereotypes in adult infant play. *Child Development, 48*, 1671–1675.

Garai, J. & Scheinfeld, A. (1968) Sex differences in mental and behavioural traits. *Genetic Psychological Monographs, 77*, 169–299.

Gewirtz, H. & Gewirtz, J. (1968) Visiting and caretaking patterns for kibbutz infants: age and sex trends. *American Journal of Orthopsychiatry, 38*, 427–433.

Gleason, J. B. (1975). Fathers and other strangers. *In* D. Dato (ed.) *Developmental psycholinguistics: theory and applications*. Washington, DC: Georgetown Round Table.

Goldberg, S. & Lewis, M. (1969) Play behaviour in the year old infant: early sex differences. *Child Development, 40*, 21–31.

Golinkoff, R. & Ames, G. (1979) A comparison of fathers' and mothers' speech with their young children. *Child Development, 50*, 28–32.

Gunnar, M. (1978) Changing a frightening toy into a pleasant toy by allowing the infant to control its actions. *Developmental Psychology, 14(2)*, 157–162.

Gunnar, M. & Donahue, M. (1980) Sex differences in social reponsiveness between six and twelve months. *Child Development, 51*, 262–265.

Hetherington, M., Cox, M. & Cox R. (1982) Effects of divorce on parents and children. *In* M. E. Lamb (ed.) *Nontraditional families*. Hillsdale, New Jersey: Lawrence Erlbaum.

Hegland, S. M. (1977) Social interaction and responsiveness in parent–infant interaction. PhD Ohio State – *Diss. Abs*. 1978, May, vol. 38 (11-8).

Hittleman, J. & Dickes, R. (1979). Sex differences in neonatal eye contact time. *Merrill-Palmer Quarterly, 25(3)*, 171–184.

Hwang, C-P. (1978) Mother–infant interaction: effects of sex of infant on feeding behaviour. *Early Human Development, 2*, 341–349.

Jacklin, C. N., DiPietro, J. A. & Maccoby, E. E. (1984) Sex-typing behaviour and sex-typing pressure in child/parent interaction. *Archives of Sexual Behaviour, 13*, 413–425.

Johnson, M. M. (1963) Sex role learning in the nuclear family. *Child Development, 34*, 319–333.

Killarney, J. & McKluskey, K. (1981) Parent–infant conversations at age one: their length, reciprocity and contingency. Paper presented at the Society for Research in Child Development, Boston.

Klein, R. P. & Durfee, J. T. (1978) Effects of sex and birth order on infant social behaviour. *Infant Behaviour and Development, 1*, 106–117.

Kotelchuck, M. (1972) The nature of the child's tie to his father. Unpublished PhD diss., Harvard University.

Kujawski, J. (1984) Origins of gender identity. Unpublished PhD diss., University of Edinburgh.

Lamb, M. E. (1976a) Interactions between eight month old children and their fathers and mothers. *In* M. E. Lamb (ed.) *The role of the father in child development*. New York: John Wiley.

Lamb, M. E. (1976b) The one-year-old's interaction with its parents. Paper presented to Meeting of EPA, New York, April 1976.

Lamb, M. E. (1976c) Effects of stress and cohort on mother– and father–infant interaction. *Developmental Psychology, 12*, 435–443.

Lamb, M. E. (1977a) Infant social cognition and 'second order' effects. *Infant Behaviour and Development, 1(1)*.

Lamb, M. E. (1977b) The development of mother–infant and father–infant attachments in the second year of life. *Developmental Psychology, 13*, 637–648.

Lamb, M. E. (1978) Social interaction in infancy and the development of personality. *In* M. Lamb (ed.) *Sociopersonality development*. New York: Holt, Rinehart & Winston.

Lamb. M. E. (1980) The development of parent–infant attachments in the first two years of life. *In* F. A. Pedersen (ed.) *The father–infant relationship: observational studies in the family setting*. New York: Praeger.

Lamb. M. E., Frodi, M., Hwang, C-P. & Frodi, A. (1983) Effects of paternal involvement on infant preferences for mothers and fathers. *Child Development, 54*, 450–458.

Langlois, J. & Downs, C. (1980) Mothers, fathers and peers as socialisation agents of sex-typed play behaviour in young children. *Child Development, 51*, 1237–1247.

Lewis, C. (in press) *Becoming a father*. Milton Keynes: Open University.

Lewis, C. (in preparation) *The context of parent–infant interaction: effects of an observer on mothers' and fathers' language to their ten month olds*.

Lewis, C. (1982) The observation of father–infant relationships: an attachment to outmoded concepts? *In* L. McKee & M. O'Brien (eds) *The father figure*. London: Tavistock.

Lewis, C., Newson, J. & Newson, E. (1982) Father participation through childhood and its relation to career aspirations and delinquency. *In* N. Beail and J. McGuire (eds) *Fathers: psychological perspectives*. London: Junction.

Lewis, M. (1972) State as an infant–environment interaction: an analysis of mother–infant interaction as a function of sex. *Merrill-Palmer Quarterly, 18*, 95–121.

Lewis, M. (1981) Self-knowledge: a social cognitive perspective on gender identity and sex-role development. *In* M. Lamb & L. Sherrod (eds) *Infant social cognition*. Hillsdale, NJ: Lawrence Erlbaum.

Lewis, M. & Brooks, J. (1975) Infants' social perception: a constructional view. *In* L. Cohen & P. Salapatek (eds) *Perception in infancy*, vol. 2. New York: Academic Press.

Lewis, M. & Rosenblum, L. (1974) *The effect of the infant on its caregiver*. New York: John Wiley.

Lewis, M. & Weinraub, M. (1974) Sex of parent and sex of child: socio-emotional development. *In* R. C. Friedman, R. M. Richards & R. L. Van de Wiele (eds) *Sex differences in behaviour*. New York: John Wiley.

Lewis, M. & Weinraub, M. (1979) Origins of early sex role development. *Sex Roles*, *5*, 135–153.

Maccoby, E. & Jacklin, C. N. (1973) Stress, activity and proximity seeking: sex differences in the year old child. *Child Development*, *44*, 34–42.

Maccoby, E. & Jacklin C. N. (1974) *The psychology of sex differences*. Stanford: Stanford University Press. Published in the UK in 1975. London: Oxford University Press.

Maccoby, E. E. & Jacklin, C. N. (1980) Psychological sex differences. *In* M. Rutter (ed.) *Scientific foundations of child psychiatry*. London: Heinemann Medical.

McGuire, J. (1982) Gender-specific differences in early childhood: the impact of the father. *In* N. Beail and J. McGuire (eds) *Fathers: psychological aspects*. London: Junction.

McLoughlin, B., White, D., McDevitt, T. & Raskin, R. (1983) Mothers' and fathers' speech to their young children: similar or different? *Journal of Child Language*, *10*, 245–252.

Martin, J. (1981) A longitudinal study of the consequences of early mother–infant interaction: a microanalytic approach. *Monograph of the Society for Research in Child Development*, *42(3)*, serial no. 190.

Martin, J., Maccoby, E. & Jacklin, C. N. (1981) Mothers' responsiveness to interactive bidding and nonbidding in boys and girls. *Child Development*, *52*, 1064–1067.

Mischel, W. (1966) A social-learning view of sex differences in behaviour. *In* E. E. Maccoby (ed.) *The development of sex differences*. Stanford: Stanford University Press.

Moss, H. A. (1967) Sex, age and state as determinants of mother–infant interaction. *Merrill-Palmer Quarterly*, *13*, 19–36.

Moss, H. A. (1974) Early sex differences in mother–infant interaction. *In* R. C. Friedman, R. M. Rinhart & R. L. Van de Wiele (eds) *Sex differences in behaviour*. New York: John Wiley.

Newson, J. & Newson, E. (1963) *Infant care in an urban community*. London: Allen & Unwin.

Parke, R. D. (1978) Parent–infant interaction: progress, paradigms and problems. *In* G. B. Sackett & H. Hayward (eds) *Application of observational-ethological methods in the study of mental retardation*. Baltimore: University Park.

Parke, R. D. (1979) Perspectives on father–infant interaction. *In* J. D. Osofsky (ed.) *Handbook of infancy*. New York: John Wiley.

Parke, R. & O'Leary, S. (1976) Family interaction in the newborn period: some findings, some observations and some unsolved issues. *In* K. Riegal & J. Meacham (eds) *The developing individual in a changing world*, vol. 2. The Hague: Mouton.

Parke, R. & Sawin, D. (1980) The family in early infancy: social interaction and attitudinal analyses. *In* F. A. Pedersen (ed.) *The father–infant relationship: observational studies in the family setting.* New York: Praeger.

Parsons, T. & Bales, R. F. (1955) *Family, socialization and interaction process.* Glencoe: Free Press.

Pedersen F. A. (1980) Overview: answers and formulated questions. In F. A. Pedersen (ed.) *The father–infant relationship: observational studies in the family setting.* New York: Praeger.

Pedersen, F. A., Rubenstein, J. L. & Yarrow, L. J. (1979) Infant development in father-absent families. *Journal of Genetic Psychology, 135,* 51–61.

Pedersen, R. A., Yarrow, L., Anderson, B. & Cain, R. (1979) Conceptualization of father influences in the infancy period. *In* M. Lewis & L. Rosenblum (eds) *The social network of the developing infant.* New York: Plenum.

Power, T. (1981) Sex typing in infancy: the role of the father. *Infant Mental Health Journal, 2,* 226–240.

Radin, N. (1981) The role of the father in cognitive, academic and intellectual development. *In* M. E. Lamb (ed.) *The role of the father in child development.* New York: John Wiley.

Randall, T. M. (1974) An analysis of observer influence on sex and social class differences in mother–infant interaction. Unpublished PhD diss., State University of New York, Buffalo. University Microfilm no. 75-7788.

Rapoport, R., Rapoport, R. & Stretlitz, Z. (1977) *Fathers, mothers and others.* London: Routledge & Kegan Paul.

Rendina, I. & Dickerscheid, J. (1976) Father involvement with first born infants. *The Family Coordinator, 25,* 373–377.

Rheingold, H. & Cook, K. (1975) The contents of boys' and girls' rooms as an index of parents' behaviour. *Child Development, 46,* 459–463.

Richards, M., Bernal, J. & Brackbill, Y. (1975) Early behavioural differences: gender or circumcision? *Developmental Psychobiology, 9,* 89–95.

Rondal, J. A. (1980) Fathers' and mothers' speech in early language development. *Journal of Child Language, 7,* 353–369.

Rosenthal, M. K. (1983) State variations in the newborn and mother–infant interaction during breast feeding: some sex differences. *Developmental Psychology, 19,* 740–745.

Ross, H. S. & Goldman, B. D. (1977) Infants' sociability towards strangers. *Child Development, 48,* 638–642.

Rubin, J. L., Provenzano, F. J. & Luria, Z. (1974) The eye of the beholder: parents' views on sex of newborns. *American Journal of Orthopsychiatry, 4,* 512–519.

Ruble, D. (1984) Sex role development. *In* M. Bornstein & M. Lamb (eds) *Developmental psychology: an advanced textbook.* Hillsdale, NJ: Lawrence Erlbaum.

Seavey, C. A., Katz, P. A. & Zalk, S. (1975) The effect of gender label on adult response to infants. *Sex Roles, 1(2),* 103–109.

Smith, C. & Lloyd, B. (1978) Maternal behaviour and perceived sex of infants: revisited. *Child Development, 49,* 1263–1265.

Smith, P. K. & Daglish, L. (1977) Sex differences in parent and infant behaviour in the home. *Child Development, 48,* 1050–1054.

Snow, M. E., Jacklin, C. N. & Maccoby, E. E. (1983) Sex of child differences in father–child interaction at one year of age. *Child Development*, 54, 227–232.

Spelke, E., Zelazo, P., Kagan, J. & Kotelchuck, M. (1973) Father interaction and separation protest. *Developmental Psychology*, 9, 83–90.

Stuckey, M. F., McGhee, P. E. & Bell, N. J. (1982) Paternal–child interaction: the influence of maternal employment. *Developmental Psychology*, 18, 635–644.

Tanner, J. M. (1974) Variability of growth and maturity in newborn infants. *In* M. Lewis & L. Rosenblum (eds) *The effect of the infant on its caregiver*. New York: John Wiley.

White, D., Woollett, A. & Lyon L. (1982) Fathers' involvement with their infants: the relevance of holding. *In* N. Beail & J. McGuire (eds) *Fathers: psychological perspectives*. London: Junction.

Woollett, A., White, D. & Lyon, L. (1982) Observations of fathers at birth. *In* N. Beail & J. McGuire (eds) *Fathers: psychological perspectives*. London: Junction.

Yogman, M. (1977) The goals and structure of face to face interaction between infants and fathers. Paper presented to Society for Research in Child Development, New Orleans, March.

Zeigob, L. E., Arnold, S. & Forehand, R. (1975) an examination of observer effects in parent–child interaction. *Child Development*, 46, 509–512.

CHAPTER SIX   **Exploration, Play and Social Development in Boys and Girls**
Peter K. Smith

Through the preschool, infant school and middle school years, children are developing an understanding of sex and gender. Besides knowing that boys and girls are different physically, they know that they are typically different in their interests and behaviours. This chapter considers these latter differences, and the reasons for them. First there is a consideration of what children know about gender and sex roles. Then, there is a review of what social scientists have observed in the way of sex differences in behaviour. Finally, some of the reasons for the existence of differing sex roles are discussed, considering both immediate causal and functional/evolutionary explanations. The example of rough-and-tumble play is taken to illustrate an interactive developmental model for a typically sex-typed behaviour.

Children's understanding of gender, and of sex-role stereotypes

The evidence that children below two years of age make distinctions on the basis of sex, while not absent, is sparse (see Chapter 5). Not all two-year-olds even know if they are a boy or girl, in response to a verbal enquiry. By eight or nine years of age however a fairly mature understanding of gender is achieved. Three broad stages in the development of gender understanding have been described: gender identity, gender stability, and gender constancy (Eaton 1983; Slaby & Frey 1975).

Gender identity and labelling

Children at this stage know how to label correctly their own gender, or another person's gender. For example when using pictures of stereotypic males and females, Thompson (1975) found that 24-month-old children achieved 76 per cent correct responses, rising to 83 per cent by thirty months and 90 per cent by thirty-six months. Weinraub *et al.* (1984) found the ability to verbally label own and others' gender was present in the majority of children by twenty-six to thirty-one months of age.

(These tasks relied on verbal response; differential non-verbal responses to males and females can be observed at even earlier ages (see Chapter 5, and Fagot 1985).

Gender stability

This is achieved when children recognize that gender is a relatively stable attribute over time, in response to questions such as 'When you were a little baby, were you a little boy or a little girl?', or 'Are you going to be a mummy/daddy when you are older?'. Gender stability is shown by most four- and five-year-olds.

Gender constancy or consistency

This stage is attained when the child realizes that gender is constant and invariant, despite changes in appearance, clothes or activity. This is tested by questions such as 'Could you be a (opposite gender of subject) if you want to be?', or 'Suppose a child like that (picture of boy) lets their hair grow very long; is it a boy or a girl?' Gender constancy is achieved between seven and nine years. According to Marcus and Overton (1978), it is related to the ability to conserve in non-social domains, usually coming after the ability to conserve quantity.

Gender-typed perceptions

As early as two or three years children possess some knowledge of sex-role stereotypes, for example about boys' and girls' preferred activities. Knowledge of sex-role stereotypes is correlated with the degree of gender identity/stability/constancy achieved (Kuhn, Nash & Brucken 1978). By the early school years, all children possess sex-typed ideas of roles and behaviour, both of classmates, and of adults. In a study of English 5–8-year-olds, Hartley (1981) found that both boys and girls saw boys as being rough, noisy, untidy, immature and lacking concentration; girls saw themslves as being more gentle, and as having the positive qualities the boys lacked (though the boys did not perceive girls as different in this way). In a US sample of five- eight and ten year-olds, Williams, Bennett and Best (1975) compared the stereotypes held by children to those held by adults, using an adjective check-list. The five-year-olds showed appreciable similarity with the adults' ratings, and this increased by eight years, but no further by ten years. The male stereotype seemed to be learned at an earlier age than the female stereotype.

In a cross-cultural study, Goldman and Goldman (1982) examined children's knowledge of sex and gender in the United States, England, Sweden and Australia, from ages five through to fifteen. Knowledge about gender-related items inreased through the middle school years; but was appreciable even at five years. For example, some one-third of five-year-olds attributed distinctive employment roles to fathers ('Men can be doctors but a girl can't'), and over three-quarters saw the mother's role as being a distinctively domestic one.

Differences in the social and play behaviours of boys and girls

School-age children have some ideas of typical sex differences in their own behaviour, and these are quite similar to the perceptions adults have. Such perceptions are in effect 'common sense' views of sex differences. They are likely to be grounded in reality; but may nevertheless be imprecise or exaggerated, or out of date at a time when sex roles and socialization pressures may be changing quite rapidly. Social scientists have had a long history of observing and recording what the differences in boys' and girls' behaviour are, dating from the beginnings of systematic child study in the 1920s and 1930s. The results of many such studies are summarized in Maccoby and Jacklin (1974), and a collection of more recent reviews is in Liss (1983).

While more systematic and objective than the perceptions obtained from children or laypersons, the limitations of these studies must be borne in mind. Generalization from any particular study is constrained by the sample of children observed. This is often quite small; for example one or two nursery classes. In addition sex differences are influenced by such factors as class size, available equipment, social class and ethnic background, and of course the historical time at which the study was carried out. These provide an idiosyncratic aspect to any one small-scale study which also limits generalization, and may well explain many inconsistencies in results of apparently similar studies. Finally, the conceptions and expectations of the researcher may influence the published report, through for example the choice of methodology, categories used, and selection of and interpretation of results, and through possible sources of experimenter effect, such as unconscious bias in observation or scoring of data.

Activity level

It is a common perception that boys are more physically active than girls, and some evidence bears this out (Maccoby & Jacklin 1974), though differences are uncertain in the under-twos. In a longitudinal laboratory assessment, Feiring and Lewis (1980) failed to find sex differences in measures of vigour, or activity changes, at thirteen, twenty-five or forty-four months. Eaton and Keats (1982), however, in another laboratory study, found that 2–6-year-old boys were more active than girls, as measured by an actometer sensitive to rapid and vigorous movement. This sex difference was not found to interact with the presence or absence of same-sex peers.

In a more naturalistic study, Harper and Sanders (1975) found that 3–5-year-old boys in a nursery class used outdoor space more than girls did. However, in a study when both boys and girls were required to play outdoors, no sex difference in physical activity was found (Smith & Hagan 1980). In naturalistic studies of indoor nursery play, boys are usually found to engage in more large-muscle activities (Melson 1977), such as kicking, throwing and hitting (Smith & Connolly 1980). Through middle childhood, boys' development at ball throwing is in advance of girls', and boys report practising more overarm throwing than girls (Halverson, Roberton & Langendorfer 1982).

Exploration

Most studies of exploration have concerned themselves with how children investigate novelty in the physical (rather than the social) environment. Some basic concepts stem from the work of Hutt (1970a, b). She observed how preschool children approached, explored and later played with a novel toy, this being a rectangular metal box with lights, buzzers, counters and levers. She reported that more girls failed to approach and explore the novel toy, and that boys were subsequently more likely to use the toy for inventive or creative play.

These results were only partly replicated by Rabinowitz *et al.* (1975). These authors used a board with a picture of a clown driving a train engine, as the novel object. It too was equipped with buzzers and buttons (the clown's eyes) and levers. The four-year-old children in this study showed no sex differences in approach and exploration; however boys did play with the novel object for longer.

These two studies are open to the criticism that the novel toy had, in each case, more intrinsic interest to boys. McLoyd and Ratner (1983) attempted to control for this, by using three alternate novel objects, a car panel, a house panel, or a coloured panel, fitting on a large rectangular box with levers and the other usual manipulanda. An independent sample of 3–5-year-old preschoolers confirmed verbally that the car panel was preferred by boys, and the house panel by girls, while the coloured panel was sex-neutral. In the main study, in which another sample of children were observed, there were no sex differences in approach or exploration, and very few in play behaviour.

A much more naturalistic study of exploratory behaviour was reported by Henderson, Charlesworth and Gamradt (1982). They observed a large number of 3–8-year-olds in a 'Touch and See' room of a natural history museum. A few sex differences were found, with boys walking more and making more area changes, whereas girls sat and knelt more frequently. Nevertheless, the authors comment that 'sex did not appear to be as important a factor in response to the novel environment as companion and age differences' (p. 97).

Rather few studies have been made of social exploration in the age range we are concerned with. Doyle, Connolly and Rivest (1980) examined children in one-hour play sessions with a familiar or unfamiliar classmate. Only eight boys and eight girls were observed. Girls were described as showing more positive affect to unfamiliar as well as familiar playmates, though there was little difference in social participation, or the cognitive level of play. Berman and Goodman (1984) observed how boys and girls reacted in a playroom with a toddler aged between eight and nineteen months. There were no sex differences in the behaviour of preschool children (2–5 years), but with the older children (5–7 years) girls interacted with the baby much more than did the boys.

Choice of toys and activities

Observational studies of sex differences in toy and activity choices have often been carried out in nursery and playgroup settings. Typically, any one study observes children in one preschool institution, and comes up with a number of statistically significant sex differences. Another study will replicate some but not all of these findings; a test of significance only allows us to generalize to similar subjects in the same setting, so lack of generalizability of results may have many explanations, alluded to at the beginning of this section.

For example, Connor and Serbin (1977) devised a behaviourally based activity preference scale on observations of fourteen girls and twelve boys in one nursery class. 'Male' items were: airplane, balls, blocks, cube puzzle, large motor, lincoln logs/tinker toys/cooties, trucks, and wagon. 'Female' items were: crayons, doll, bed/cradle/stroller, dollhouse, dolls, kitchen, musical instruments, painting, record player, sewing board, telephone. These were differences significant at the 0.20 level on one-tailed tests, a very lenient criterion.

Fagot (1977a) collected data on 106 boys and 101 girls from fifteen classes in four different nursery schools. Summing all the data, the significant sex-preferred behaviours were, for boys: transportation toys, building blocks, carpentry/hammer/saw, and outdoor sandbox/mud play; for girls: art activities, play in kitchen, play with dolls, and dress-up.

Smith and Connolly (1980) collected data on two different classes of twenty-four children (each twelve boys and twelve girls) in a preschool playgroup. They only reported sex differences which were found to be significant, independently, for both classes. The only consistent differences for activities were that girls played more with the doll, and the rocking-boat.

In a study in the home environment of thirty-nine children aged 2–7 years (Giddings & Halverson 1981), the following sex differences were obtained: boys played more with vehicles, and watched more television; girls played more with dolls and in domestic roles. Another study of 165 children aged three and four years (Davie *et al.* 1984) found that boys preferred transportation toys and ball play, girls dressing up and domestic roles.

Despite variations, there is clearly some consistency in the finding that boys prefer transportation toys and block play, and that girls prefer dolls and domestic play. These and other trends tend to agree with adult stereotypes of sex-appropriate activities for children (Connor and Serbin 1977). However, those children who strongly choose sex-appropriate toys in preschool are not necessarily those who score highly on other measures of sex-role identity, based on home choice, or on parents' or teachers' ratings (Brush & Goldberg 1978).

Another aspect of activities is the degree of adult involvement with children. Carpenter and Huston-Stein (1980) looked at this in five preschool classrooms. They distinguished activities highly structured by teacher feedback or availability of adult models, from low structure activities. Independent of sex, children showed more compliance and less novel behaviour in high-structure activities than in low-structure activities; but girls spent more time in the former, boys in the latter.

Fantasy play

Fantasy, pretend and sociodramatic play is a common activity in the 3–6-year age range. According to some studies, boys engage in more fantasy play than girls at preschool. Sanders and Harper (1976) report such a difference for both solitary and interactive fantasy play, though girls did score higher for co-operative role-playing, for example playing 'house'. Smith and Connolly (1980) found no sex differences in the frequency of fantasy play, however, while Brindley *et al.* (1973) observed more in girls. The lack of consistency between these and other studies (see Fein 1981) is probably due to the definitions of fantasy used, the types of equipment and space available, the role of adults and teachers, and other environmental factors.

A more consistent finding is that boys and girls differ in the themes they adopt for fantasy and sociodramatic episodes. According to Brooks-Gunn and Matthews (1979), girls more often adopt relational roles (such as parent–child, husband–wife) in domestic type episodes such as 'cooking' or 'feeding baby'. Boys engage in a wider variety of episodes, such as 'taking a trip', or 'firework displays'. Other studies also find girls preferring domestic roles, and boys preferring fantastic roles or roles involving gross motor activity, such as monsters or spacemen (Fein 1981). Indeed, much of urban children's pretend play seems to reflect their knowledge of adult roles in a stereotyped way; the female role is the domestic one which they are familiar with from the home and also from books and other mass media (see Chapter 10); while the male role is relatively unknown from personal experience, and is derived largely from television or other media sources.

Rough-and-tumble, and aggression

Rough-and-tumble refers to play fighting, wrestling and chasing. The great majority of observational studies, in a number of cultures, have found this to be more frequent in boys (see Humphreys & Smith 1984). The difference may be greater for play fighting and wrestling, than chasing (Smith & Connolly 1972). Rough-and-tumble will be reviewed in detail later, in the context of an illustration of possible mechanisms producing sex differences.

Aggression also appears to be a characteristically male activity from early childhood on, and the review by Maccoby and Jacklin (1974) confirmed this. Some aspects of their review, notably the onset of the sex difference in the preschool years, and the postulation of a biological predisposition to these differences, disputed by Tieger (1980). Maccoby and Jacklin (1980) replied to these criticisms, using a meta-analysis of thirty-two studies on children six years or younger. Parke and Slaby (1983) also provide a thorough review. Another recent meta-analysis is of a total of 143 studies (Hyde 1984). This review suggests (contrary to Tieger 1980) that sex differences in aggression are larger in preschoolers than in college students. Hyde also found that sex differences, while quite consistent, were not all that large; they tended to be larger in naturalistic, observational studies, and smaller in more recent studies.

The kind of aggression being observed may well be an important consideration. Smith and Connolly (1980) found consistent sex differences for harassment (hostility deliberately directed at a person), but not for specific hostility (property/territory disputes). Another distinction is between physical and verbal aggression. By and large, boys are reported to be more aggressive both physically and verbally (Maccoby and Jacklin 1980), but there are exceptions (Archer & Westeman 1981).

Children's peer groups

A very commonly observed aspect of children's peer groups is that same-sex partners are more often chosen for activities or nominated as friends, from the preschool period through to adolescence. LaFreniere, Strayer and Gauthier (1984) observed affiliative activity in three groups of day care children at each of five age levels from seventeen months to six years. Same-sex choices were not more frequent than chance in the youngest age group (seventeen months), but they were evident by twenty-seven months and tended to increase with age, with about two-thirds of same-sex choices in four- and five-year-olds. Similar findings came from Smith and Connolly's (1980) study of three- and four-year-olds in playgroups, and many other studies (see Hartup 1983).

Some reports suggest that boys congregate in larger groups than girls do (Hartup 1983); but a large study in Israel, of 408 children in six kindergartens and six first grade classes (five- and six-year-olds) found no significant sex difference in group size (Hertz-Lazarowitz *et al*. 1981). However in a study of 181 fifth grade children (ten- and eleven-year-olds) in the United States, Lever (1976, 1978) found boys playing in larger groups, both from self-report and from observation. Quite likely, this sex difference increases with age as team games become more prevalent.

The amount and quality of interaction may also vary depending on the composition of children's groups. Most studies have looked at dyads. Langlois, Gottman and Seay (1973) found that five-year-olds engaged in more social interaction in same-sex than in opposite-sex pairs. At three years, though, boys were more sociable with girls than with boys. Jacklin and Maccoby (1978) by contrast reported that three-year-olds engaged in more social behaviour with same-sex partners, irrespective of sex. A possibly relevant difference is that the children were acquainted in the former study, but unacquainted in the latter.

Games in older children

Children tend to move from the constructive play, rough-and-tumble and fantasy play of the preschool and infant school, to more organized and publicly rule-governed games by the middle school years. Segregation of playground activities by sex is very marked at this period.

Based on report data from 5–11-year-old American children, Seagoe (1970) concluded that 'boys engage in play requiring more complex interpersonal interaction earlier and emphasise it more at all ages. Girls play with friends as much as boys do, but their play is more often of either an informal-individual or a competitive nature' (p. 143). Similar conclusions were reached by Lever (1976, 1978), on the basis of diary and observational data on ten- and eleven-year-olds. She reported that boys played outdoors more, in more age-heterogenous groups, and in more competitive team games (Lever 1976). Using measures such as role differentiation, interdependence, and number and specificity of rules, boys' games were more complex than those of girls (Lever 1978). Boys' games (such as football) were characterized by team spirit, leading roles, and face-to-face competition. Girls' games (such as jumprope) were characterized by less explicit goals, and indirect competition of an individual nature.

Explanations for sex differences

Despite some variations and inconsistencies, a fairly clear pattern of sex differences in children's social development and play is evident. These are best documented for urban children in the United States and UK; but some of these differences, for example in aggression, rough-and-tumble, and domestic role-playing, are well attested cross-culturally (Barry, Bacon & Child 1959; Whiting & Edwards 1973). The documenting of these differences does not, of course, imply that they are desirable, or inevitable.

In looking for explanations of these differences, we can examine what might be their immediate causation, and also what might be the longer-term historical or evolutionary explanations, which invoke some function of the behaviour. These can be thought of as corresponding to the questions 'how do sex differences develop?', and 'why do sex differences develop?'. The answers given to both sets of questions tend to vary between environmentalist and nativist-type explanations of various kinds; though some form of interactionist model (proposed by Archer & Lloyd 1982, for the causation of sex differences) seems the most promising general approach.

Causal mechanisms

A variety of immediate mechanisms probably interact with each other in bringing about sex differences. See Huston (1983) for a fuller review, and Block (1983) for a review of environmental factors.

Hormonal influences

The most direct link of biological sex to possible behavioural differences is via the effects of levels of sex hormones (produced by the gonads). For example, it has been argued that sex hormones can affect brain development, at the prenatal stage. An often-cited study by Money and Erhardt (1972) reported that girls who were exposed to a higher than usual level of androgen during the mother's pregnancy were more likely to be tomboyish, and less likely to play with girls and like feminine clothes, than matched controls. Erhardt and Meyer-Bahlberg (1981) conclude from this and similar studies that intense physical energy expenditure and rough-and-tumble play 'seem to be an essential aspect of psychosocial development and it appears to be influenced by sex steroid variations before birth' (p. 1313). However it is difficult, if not impossible, to separate out the possible effects of hormones on behaviour, from the effects of the parent's knowledge of the hormonal abnormalities, and the possible effect of the child's awareness of any physical abnormality on self-concept and behaviour. Indeed, children with hormonal abnormalities but without any physical abnormalities do not seem to show sex-inappropriate play interests (Hines 1982).

Behavioural compatibility

The tendency for young children to choose same-sex partners may, in part, be due to preferences of boys and girls for different activities. Thus, it could be that girls (for example) tend to like domestic play, and coming together through this, then tend to play together and make friends. This hypothesis was supported by Eisenberg, Tryon and Cameron (1984), in a study of four-year-olds in three preschool classes. They tried to distinguish whether the choice of activity influenced subsequent partner choice, or whether partner choice influenced subsequent activity choice. The evidence favoured the former alternative; 'most of the time, the child was not with a peer when he or she approached a toy, and the toy subjects approached were seldom possessed by another peer' (p. 1049). If the child chose a sex-appropriate toy, he or she was then more likely to be joined by a same-sex peer.

As these authors point out, this finding does not rule out the possibility that children who happen to choose sex-appropriate toys also happen to be friendly with same-sex partners for other reasons. However a causal relationship is also supported by data from questioning children themselves. In the Goldman and Goldman (1982) study of 5–15-year-olds, children were asked why they would choose to be a boy/girl (the great majority chose their own sex), and why they would choose a same-sex friend (as most did at least up to eleven years). The majority of reasons in each case were to do with activities and recreations (rather than with feelings, temperament, or social pressure, for example). 'I like jogging, climbing, rugby, soccer, games not normally played by girls' (eleven-year-old boy). 'I do recorder lessons and boys can't really do that. They'd think it cissy' (seven-year-old girl). By these ages, awareness of sex-appropriate behaviour is obviously strongly involved with any influence of behavioural compatibility on friendship choice.

Differential reinforcement

Children may be rewarded for sex-appropriate behaviour and punished for sex-inappropriate behaviour, by parents, teachers, and siblings or peers. There is evidence for each of these occurring.

In one study of three- and five-year-olds (Langlois & Downs 1980), the reactions of mothers, fathers and peers to sex-typed play behaviour were observed. With minor variations, all tended to reinforce sex-appropriate choices. However in the school setting there has been some evidence that feminine-type behaviours are preferred for both sexes. Fagot and Patterson (1969) found that teachers in two nursery classes reinforced both boys and girls for feminine-type behaviour, such as quiet play, more than for masculine-type behaviour. This has not been wholly confirmed by later work. In a similar study in three Dutch preschools, Fagot (1977b) found that teachers reinforced both boys and girls more for sex-appropriate behaviours. In her study of 207 children from fifteen different classes, Fagot (1977a) found that teachers and peers both criticized boys for engaging in stereotypic feminine behaviours, such as doll or kitchen play; but that girls who engaged in stereotyped masculine behaviours were not given negative feedback by peers, and only rarely by teachers. One factor which may contribute to these discrepancies was found by Fagot (1978); observations of six experienced and eight inexperienced preschool teachers showed that experienced teachers interacted with both boys and girls when they were engaged in feminine-preferred activities, whereas inexperienced teachers allowed themselves to be guided more by the children, and thus interacted more with boys when they engaged in masculine-preferred activities.

Lamb and Roopnarine (1979), and Lamb, Easterbrooks and Holden (1980), each studying one nursery class, found evidence that peers not only reinforce sex-appropriate play and punish sex-inappropriate play, but that this also affects the child's behaviour. Reinforcements tended to prolong the activity, and punishments to shorten it; especially if reinforcements were for sex-appropriate behaviour, and punishments for sex-inappropriate behaviour.

A detailed study by Fagot (1985) brings home very forcefully the importance of integrating reinforcement theory with other factors. Observing forty children aged twenty-one to twenty-five months in playgroups, Fagot recorded the reinforcement of behaviour by teachers and peers, and the child's reaction. From previous work, male-preferred activities were taken as: rough-and-tumble, transportation toys, large blocks and carpentry play; female-preferred activities as: doll play, dress up, art activities and dance.

Fagot found that teachers responded positively to female-preferred activities about twice as often as to male-preferred activities, irrespective of whether a boy or girl was involved. This impartiality as to the child's sex was not found in the children themselves. Girls responded positively to other girls about twice as often as to boys, irrespective of activity. Boys responded positively to other boys more than twice as often as to girls, unless the boys were in female-preferred activities. The pattern of reinforcement was thus gender-typed by recipient and activity.

Furthermore, the effectiveness of reinforcement also varied according to who was reinforcing, and what was reinforced. Using continuation of an activity as the criterion, it emerged that girls were influenced by other girls and by teachers, but less by boys. Boys were influenced by other boys, but less by girls or by teachers; boys were not influenced at all by girls or teachers if they were engaged in male-preferred activities.

These children were sufficiently young that they would be unlikely to have achieved gender identity. Thus, the effects of reinforcement seem to be filtered through the effects of behavioural compatibility, and/or an implicit, non-verbal response to gender not identified by the usual verbal tests of gender awareness.

In considering the implications of all these studies, it should be noted that the terms 'reinforcer' and 'punisher' are used in a very broad sense. For example, in Lamb, Easterbrooks and Holden (1980) the term 'reinforcer' includes 'observe' and 'join play', as well as 'praise'; while 'punisher' includes 'abandon play' as well as 'criticize'. Thus, these studies largely assume that peer presence (or absence) is a reinforcer (or punisher). Any intrinsic motivation or pleasure in engaging in certain activities by one sex would tend to bring about extrinsic 'reinforcement' through presence of same-sex peers in play. Thus, Fagot's (1985) finding that boys reinforce other boys more than girls, except when the boys are in female-preferred activities, could be reinterpreted as: boys join in play with other boys, but not if they are playing with dolls or other female-preferred activities. The results of these studies are thus not so different from what would be expected on the basis of behavioural compatibility.

Cognitive awareness of gender identity and sex-role conventions

It is clearly likely that a child's growing gender awareness will actually affect his or her behaviour. This could be by awareness of own and others' gender leading to observation and imitation of same-sex models; and by awareness of sex-appropriate behaviour in activities directly constraining own choices; Maccoby and Jacklin (1974) term these processes 'self-socialization', since they are social processes not depending on external reinforcement.

Weinraub *et al.* (1984) found a correlation between gender identity in two- and three-year-olds, and their degree of observed sex-typed toy preference. Similarly, the achievement of gender stability in preschoolers was related to gender-stereotyped choices by Eaton (1983). However, in a study of 5–8-year-olds, Marcus and Overton (1978) did not find a relationship between gender constancy, and sex-stereotyped choice of games or activities. One hypothesis (Eaton 1983) is that children who have achieved gender stability, but not constancy (typically, 5–7-year-olds) will be particularly likely to stay with sex-appropriate choices; this is because, at their current level of reasoning, a non-appropriate choice of activity, or dress, would threaten their own gender identity. Eaton (1983) cites the example of a four-year-old boy who refused to go to the girls' washroom, saying 'I don't want to be a girl'. Once gender constancy is achieved, however, cross-sex activities would be less threatening.

This argument supposes that children aware of their own gender identity are also aware of which toys or activities are sex-typed. Against this, Perry, White and Perry (1984) found that the acquisition of sex-role stereotypes about toys lagged well behind that of sex-role preferences for such toys, in 2–5-year-olds; and Eisenberg, Murray and Hite (1982) found that three- and four-year-olds seldom gave sex-role oriented reasons as to why they had chosen a certain toy, even though they did give such reasons more often to explain toy choices of other children.

Damon (1977) interviewed children about their awareness of sex-role conventions, such as sex-typed activities. He suggests a series of levels.

At level 0 (up to about four years) ideas are confused and children tend to follow their own desires. At level 1 (around five and six years) children are aware of conventions and tend to regard them as binding. At level 2 (around six or seven years) some awareness of exceptions to rules develops. At level 3 (around eight or nine years) the child has some understanding of why sex-linked rules and conventions exist, while a more mature conception of this (level 4) is achieved in adolescence. This analysis (like that of Eaton 1983) suggests that by five and six years, children would be especially resistant to engaging in cross-sex behaviours because of their level of conception of gender. Before this age, as the mixed research results indicate, the causal influence of children's gender awareness of behaviour is not well established.

The content of children's conceptions of gender identity and sex-role conventions will be influenced by observation of same- and opposite-sex models. Parents, teachers, siblings and peers can influence behaviour by modelling sex-appropriate choices which a child may imitate. The mass media also predominantly portray sex-typed behaviour and activities in boys and girls (see Chapter 10). The degree of stereotyping in children's books, for example, was found to affect sex-typed toy choice in preschool children, at least in the short term (Ashton 1983). Once gender identity is acquired, all these influences could magnify sex differences in behaviour, both by observation and imitation, and by deliberate choice of sex-appropriate activities (self-socialization), even if the causal role of these influences earlier in development is still under question.

Functional explanations

Historical and evolutionary models look for the origin of sex differences, and of postulated causal mechanisms, in more long-term circumstances: for example, the nature of sex roles in urban or capitalist society, or the selective pressures which acted in our evolutionary history.

Evolutionary explanations generally postulate some continuity of human sex differences with sex differences in our primate and mammalian ancestors, modulated by the particular selection pressures acting in hominid evolution. For example, Harper and Sanders Huie (1978) develop such an argument, based on the sexual dimorphism found in primates regarding physical size and strength, and hence (it is argued) in need for aggressive capability; and on the division of labour in the hunting and gathering way of life in later hominids and present-day hunter-gatherer societies. Thus, preferences of boys for outdoor play, play-fighting, gross motor activity and team competition are related ultimately to the hunting role of our male ancestors, and the predisposition of girls for care-giving roles and more solitary and sedentary activities, to the gathering and child-care roles of our female ancestors.

Parker and Gibson (1979) have developed a model in which language and intelligence developed through hominid evolution, primarily as adaptations for complex feeding strategies, including extractive foraging with tools. They postulate that aimed throwing of missiles was an important component of hunting. Given the division of labour just discussed, it would be expected that boys would engage in more aimed throwing than girls, and would be better at this. Parker (1984) sees sex differences in agonistic exercise games generally as being (in an evolutionary context) adaptive for later adult behaviour; "like many other sex differences, these differences in play-fighting are ultimately caused by sexual selection for male ability to compete by fighting or intimidating rivals" (p. 284). Similar theories are characteristic of the sociobiological approach to human nature (e.g. Daly & Wilson 1978; Wilson 1978).

These evolutionary explanations do presuppose that some of the immediate causal mechanisms producing sex differences are linked ultimately to genetic differences between males and females. Hormonal influences are an obvious candidate, and indeed are explicitly invoked by Harper and Sanders-Huie (1978). Nevertheless evolutionary theories are quite compatible with interactionist models which postulate a variety of causal mechanisms, including immediate environmental ones. For example, Wilson (1978) argues that:

> Modest genetic differences exist between the sexes; the behavioral genes interact with virtually all existing environments to create a noticeable divergence in early psychological development; and the divergence is almost always widened in later psychological development by cultural sanctions and training. Societies can probably cancel the modest genetic differences entirely by careful planning and training, but the convergence will require a conscious decision based on fuller and more exact knowledge than is now available. (p. 129).

Evolutionary explanations would seem nonetheless to be incompatible with a view that sex differences are purely cultural, that is that any sex difference would be equally easy to socialize, given a supportive ideology and social structure. They are thus discordant with a widely held approach (e.g. Archer & Lloyd 1982; Mead 1949) that it is only the classification of gender that is biologically determined, but not to any extent the behavioural content of these gender classifications.

The view of these last-named authors is that the ultimate explanation for sex differences in childhood is mainly or entirely due to the social structure, and thus historical and not biological factors. Similarly Lever (1978), asking what produces the distinct game patterns of boys and girls, argues that 'the answer is mainly historical and cultural' (p. 480). She points to the influence of recently prevailing social beliefs in the masculine nature of sport and the physiological inferiority of females, on the encouragement of, and provision of resources for, boys' and girls' games. She also argues that the strong emphasis on boys' team games is a relatively recent historical phenomenon (which may be changing yet again, Parker 1984).

Anthropological research suggests that socialization pressures do vary with type of society. Pressure for girls to help in domestic tasks, and for boys to range further from home helping in tasks such as cattle herding, seem to be greater in settled agricultural or pastoral communities than in hunter-gatherer societies (Barry, Bacon & Child 1959; Draper 1975). Divale and Harris (1976) argue that a particular phase in the social evolution of such settled, band level societies, in which resource (protein) scarcity was prevalent, is the historical origin of the 'male supremacist complex', evidenced in male dominance and warfare. Other anthropologists and historians (Engels 1942; Shorter 1975) have pointed to the modern nuclear family, linked to the market economy and the rise of capitalism, as reinforcing the role of women in child care and domesticity, and the role of men in external positions of power, competition and economic provision. These theorists would then see childhood sex differences as due to socialization pressures producing conformity to adult and societal standards.

A general model relating cultural practices (including sex roles) via child-rearing procedures, to maintenance systems (economy and social structure), and hence back to ecology, was proposed by Whiting and Child (see LeVine (1973) for an updated discussion). Indeed, the recognition that ecology and social structure influences gender roles via socialization processes can be argued to be compatible with evolutionary theories. As Weitz (1977) points out, 'most economic theories are ultimately based on what we can only call biological factors', such as female pregnancy and child care, and perhaps male aggression. Equally, evolutionary explanations are clearly insufficient by themselves; a sociobiological account such as Wilson's (1978) cannot by itself explain why we might make 'a conscious decision' to 'cancel the modest genetic differences', for example (see quote from Wilson [1978] above).

An illustration of an interactionist model

An interactionist model, in the sense of Archer and Lloyd (1982), implies a continuing interplay between the child and the environment, with no overriding control of development from within the organism or from the environment.

Sex differences in rough-and-tumble play are taken as an example for illustration. It is a reliably sex-typed behaviour, and there is considerable evidence that there are hormonal influences at the prenatal stage. The activity features prominently in children's and adult's stereotypes of sex-appropriate behaviour; and fathers (more than mothers) engage in rough-and-tumble more with boys (than girls) by the second year. However differential reinforcement by parents, in the sense of praise or discouragement, probably does not occur until later in development (see Humphreys and Smith, 1984, for a review).

Figure 6.1 illustrates some likely factors involved in sex differences in rough-and-tumble, as it may occur in two-year-old children, before they become very aware of their own gender identity, and of the sex-typed nature of rough-and-tumble. The effect of prenatal hormones is

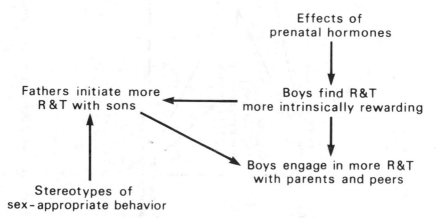

Figure 6.1 Sex differences in rough-and-tumble play (R&T) at around two years of age: likely influences

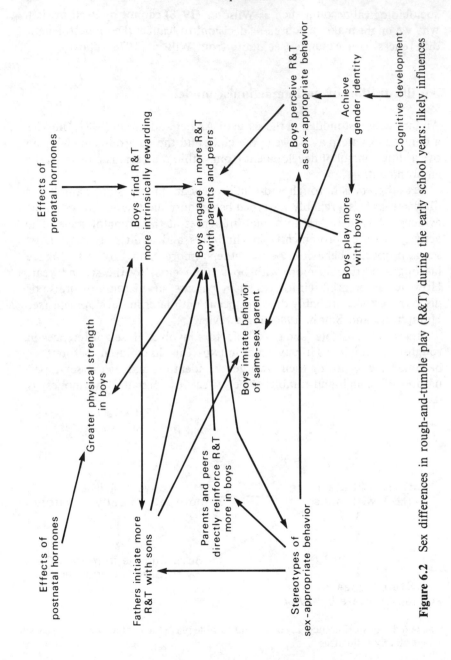

Figure 6.2 Sex differences in rough-and-tumble play (R&T) during the early school years: likely influences

postulated, though a sex difference could be sustained by the influence of stereotypes acting on parents in initiating rough-and-tumble play overtures with boys and girls. It is postulated that differential reinforcement is not acting directly at this age, though it could be added if appropriate evidence were found.

Figure 6.2 illustrates a more complex interplay of factors likely to be involved in children a few years older. Two major new factors are introduced. First, it is assumed that, at least by ages five or six, the child's awareness of gender identity will lead to imitation of same-sex models and preference for same-sex partners; and that awareness of sex-appropriate behaviour will also directly influence sex differences in rough-and-tumble. Second, the effects of direct reinforcement (for example parents and teachers discouraging girls from rough-and-tumble) are included. A feedback between participation in rough-and-tumble, and physical strength (which increases more in boys in the school years) is also postulated.

These are not meant as formal models, since they are speculative and no doubt incomplete. Other factors are doubtless involved. (For example, if girls prefer to stay closer to teachers, this in itself could lead them into other activities than rough-and-tumble). The objective is simply to illustrate the multi-causational nature of this, and no doubt many other, sex differences as they develop through childhood. The illustrations could of course be adapted, with suitable omissions and inclusions, to apply to sex differences in other behaviours or activities. Only some immediate causal factors are suggested. Possible historical/evolutionary factors involved are left for the reader to surmise.

Acknowledgements

John Archer, Helen Cowie and Charlie Lewis made helpful comments on an earlier draft of this manuscript.

References

Archer, J. & Lloyd, B. (1982) *Sex and gender*. Harmondsworth: Penguin.
Archer, J. & Westeman, K. (1981) Sex differences in the aggressive behaviour of school children. *British Journal of Social and Clinical Psychology*, *20*, 31–36.
Ashton, E. (1983) Measures of play behavior: the influence of sex-role stereotyped children's books. *Sex Roles*, *9*, 43–47.

Barry, H. A., Child, I. L. & Bacon, M. K. (1959) The relation of child training to subsistence economy. *American Anthropologist, 61,* 51–63.

Berman, P. W. & Goodman, V. (1984) Age and sex differences in children's responses to babies: effects of adults' caretaking requests and instructions. *Child Development, 55,* 1071–1077.

• Block, J. H. (1983) Differential premises arising from differential socialization of the sexes: some conjectures. *Child Development, 54,* 1335–1354.

Brindley, C., Clarke, P., Hutt, C., Robinson, I. & Wethli, E. (1973) Sex differences in the activities and social interactions of nursery school children. *In* R. P. Michael & J. H. Crook (eds) *Comparative ecology and behaviour of primates.* London: Academic Press.

Brooks-Gunn, J. & Matthews, W. S. (1979) *He and she: How children develop their sex-role identity.* Englewood Cliffs, NJ: Prentice-Hall.

Brush, L. R. & Goldberg, W. A. (1978) The intercorrelation of measures of sex-role identity. *Journal of Child Psychology and Psychiatry, 19,* 43–48.

Carpenter, C. J. & Huston-Stein, A. (1980) Activity structure and sex-typed behavior in preschool children. *Child Development, 51,* 862–872.

Connor, J. M. & Serbin, L. A. (1977) Behaviorally-based masculine- and feminine-activity-preference scales for preschoolers: correlates with other classroom behaviors and cognitive tests. *Child Development, 48,* 1411–1416.

Daly, M. & Wilson, M. (1978) *Sex, evolution and behavior.* North Scituate, Mass.: Duxbury.

Damon, W. (1977) *The Social World of the Child.* San Francisco: Jossey-Bass.

Davie, C. E., Hutt, S. J., Vincent, E. & Mason, M. (1984) *The young child at home.* Windsor: NFER-Nelson.

Divale, W. T. & Harris, M. (1976) Population, warfare, and the male supremacist complex. *American Anthropologist, 78,* 521–538.

Doyle, A., Connolly, J. & Rivest, L. (1980). The effect of playmate familiarity on the social interactions of young children. *Child Development, 51,* 217–223.

Draper, P. (1975) Cultural pressure on sex differences. *American Ethnologist, 2,* 602–616.

Eaton, W. O. (1983) Gender understanding and sex-role stereotyping in preschoolers: implications for caregivers. *Child Care Quarterly, 12,* 28–35.

Eaton, W. O. & Keats, J. G. (1982) Peer presence, stress, and sex differences in the motor activity levels of preschoolers. *Developmental Psychology, 18,* 534–540.

Eisenberg, N., Murray, E. & Hite, T. (1982) Children's reasoning regarding sex-typed toy choices. *Child Development, 53,* 81–86.

Eisenberg, N., Tryon, K. & Cameron, D. (1984) The relation of preschoolers' peer interaction to their sex-typed toy choices. *Child Development, 55,* 1044–1050.

Engels, F. (1942, orig. 1884) *The origin of the family, private property, and the state.* New York: International Publishers.

Erhardt, A. A. & Meyer-Bahlberg, H. F. L. (1981) Effects of prenatal sex hormones on gender-related behavior. *Science, 221,* 1312–1318.

Fagot, B. I. (1977a) Consequences of moderate cross-gender behavior in preschool children. *Child Development, 48,* 902–907.

Fagot, B. I. (1977b) Teachers' reinforcement of sex-preferred behaviours in Dutch preschools. *Psychological Reports, 41,* 1249–1250.

Fagot, B. I. (1978) Reinforcing contingencies for sex-role behaviours: effect of experience with children. *Child Development, 49,* 30–36.

Fagot, B. I. (1985) Beyond the reinforcement principle: another step toward understanding sex role development. *Developmental Psychology,* in press.

Fagot, B. I. & Patterson, G. R. (1969) An in vivo analysis of reinforcing contingencies for sex-role behaviors in the preschool child. *Developmental Psychology, 1,* 563–568.

Fein, G. G. (1981) Pretend play in childhood: an integrative review. *Child Development, 52,* 1095–1118.

Feiring, C. & Lewis, M. (1980) Temperament: sex differences and stability in vigor, activity, and persistence in the first three years of life. *Journal of Genetic Psychology, 136,* 65–75.

Giddings, M. & Halverson, C. F. (1981) Young children's use of toys in home environments. *Family Relations, 30,* 69–74.

Goldman, R. & Goldman, J. (1982) *Children's sexual thinking.* London: Routledge & Kegan Paul.

Halverson, L. E., Roberton, M. A. & Langendorfer, S. (1982) Development of the overarm throw: movement and ball velocity changes by seventh grade. *Research Quarterly for Exercise and Sport, 53,* 198–205.

Harper, L. V. & Sanders, K. M. (1975) Preschool children's use of space: sex differences in outdoor play. *Developmental Psychology, 11,* 119.

Harper, L. V. & Sanders Huie, K. (1978) The development of sex differences in human behavior: cultural impositions, or a convergence of evolved response-tendencies and cultural adaptations? *In* G. M. Burghardt & M. Bekoff (eds) *The development of behaviour: comparative and evolutionary aspects.* New York and London: Garland STPM Press, pp. 297–318.

Hartley, D. (1981). Infant-school children's perception of the behaviour of same- and opposite-sex classmates. *British Journal of Social Psychology, 20,* 141–143.

Hartup, W. W. (1983). Peer relationships. *In* P. H. Mussen & E. M. Hetherington (eds) *Handbook of child psychology*: vol. 4 *Socialisation, personality and social development,* 4th edn. New York and Chichester: John Wiley.

Henderson, B. B., Charlesworth, W. R. & Gamradt, J. (1982) Children's exploratory behavior in a novel field setting. *Ethology and Sociology, 3,* 93–99.

Hertz-Lazarowitz, R., Feitelson, D., Zahavi, S. & Hartup, W. W. (1981) Social interaction and social organization of Israeli five- to seven-year-olds. *International Journal of Behavioral Development, 4,* 143–155.

Hines, M. (1982) Prenatal gonadal hormones and sex differences in human behavior. *Psychological Bulletin, 92,* 56–80.

Humphreys, A. P. & Smith, P. K. (1984) Rough-and-tumble in preschool and playground. *In* P. K. Smith (ed.) *Play in animals and humans.* Oxford: Basil Blackwell, pp. 241–266.

Huston, A. C. (1983) Sex-typing. *In* P. H. Mussen & E. M. Hetherington (eds) *Handbook of child psychology*; vol 4 *Socialisation, personality and social development.* New York and Chichester: John Wiley.

Hutt, C. (1970a) Curiosity in young children. *Science Journal*, *6*, 68–71.

Hutt, C. (1970b) Specific and diversive exploration. *In* H. Reese & L. Lipsitt (eds) *Advances in child development and behavior*, vol. 5. New York: Academic Press.

Hyde, J. S. (1984) How large are gender differences in aggression? A development, meta-analysis. *Developmental Psychology*, *20*, 722–736.

Jacklin, C. N. & Maccoby, E. E. (1978) Social behavior at thirty-three months in same-sex and mixed-sex dyads. *Child Development*, *49*, 557–569.

Kuhn, D., Nash, S. C. & Brucken, L. (1978) Sex role concepts of two- and three-year-olds. *Child Development*, *49*, 445–451.

LaFreniere, P., Strayer, F. F. & Gauthier, R. (1984) The emergence of same-sex affiliative preferences among preschool peers: a development/ethological perspective. *Child Development*, *55*, 1958–1965.

Lamb, M. E., Easterbrooks, M. A. & Holden, G. W. (1980) Reinforcement and punishment among preschoolers: characteristics, effects, and correlates. *Child Development*, *51*, 1230–1236.

Lamb, M. E. & Roopnarine, J. L. (1979) Peer influences on sex-role development in preschoolers. *Child Development*, *50*, 1219–1222.

Langlois, J. H. & Downs, A. C. (1980) Mothers, fathers, and peers as socialization agents of sex-typed play behaviors in young children. *Child Development*, *51*, 1217–1247.

Langlois, J. H., Gottman, N. W. & Seay, B. (1973) The influence of sex of peer on the social behavior of preschool children. *Developmental Psychology*, *8*, 93–98.

Lever, J. (1976). Sex difference in the games children play. *Social Problems*, *23*, 478–487.

Lever, J. (1978) Sex differences in the complexity of children's play and games. *American Sociological Review*, *43*, 471–483.

LeVine, R. A. (1973) *Culture, behavior and personality*. Chicago: Aldine.

Liss, M. B. (1983) *Social and cognitive skills: sex roles and children's play*. New York: Academic Press.

Maccoby, E. E. and Jacklin, C. N. (1974) *The psychology of sex differences*. Stanford, Calif.: Stanford University Press.

Maccoby, E. E. & Jacklin, C. N. (1980) Sex differences in aggression: a rejoinder and reprise. *Child Development*, *51*, 964–980.

McLoyd, V. C. & Ratner, H. H. (1983) The effects of sex and toy characteristics on exploration in preschool children. *Journal of Genetic Psychology*, *142*, 213–244.

Marcus, D. E. & Overton, W. F. (1978) The development of cognitive gender constancy and sex-role preferences. *Child Development*, *49*, 434–444.

Mead, M. (1949) *Male and female*. New York: Morrow.

Melson, G. F. (1977) Sex differences in use of indoor space by preschool children. *Perceptual and Motor Skills*, *44*, 207–213.

Money, J. & Erhardt, A. A. (1972) *Man and woman, boy and girl*. Baltimore: Johns Hopkins University Press.

Parke, R. D. & Slaby, R. G. (1983) The development of aggression. *In* P. H. Mussen & E. M. Hetherington (eds) *Handbook of child psychology*: vol. 4.

Socialisation, personality and social development, 4th edn. New York and Chichester: John Wiley.

Parker, S. T. (1984). Playing for keeps: an evolutionary perspective on human games. *In* P. K. Smith (ed.) *Play in animals and humans*. Oxford: Basil Blackwell, pp. 271–293.

Parker. S. T. & Gibson, K. R. (1979) A developmental model for the evolution of language and intelligence in early hominids. *Behavioral and Brain Sciences*, *2*, 367–408.

Perry, D. G., White, A. J. & Perry, L. C. (1984) Does early sex typing result from children's attempts to match their behavior to sex role stereotypes? *Child Development*, *55*, 2114–2121.

Rabinowitz, F. M., Moely, B. E., Finkel, N. & McClinton, S. (1975) The effects of toy novelty and social interaction on the exploratory behavior of preschool children. *Child Development*, *46*, 286–289.

Sanders, K. M. & Harper, L. V. (1976) Free-play fantasy behavior in preschool children: relations among gender, age, season and location. *Child Development*, *47*, 1182–1185.

Seagoe, M. V. (1970) An instrument for the analysis of children's play as an index of degree of socialization. *Journal of School Psychology*, *8*, 139–144.

Shorter, E. (1975). *The making of the modern family*. New York: Basic Books.

Slaby, R. G. & Frey, K. S. (1975) Development of gender constancy and selective attention to same-sex models. *Child Development*, *46*, 849–856.

Smith, P. K. & Connolly, K. (1972) Patterns of play and social interaction in preschool children. *In* N. Blurton Jones (ed.) *Ethological studies of child behaviour*. Cambridge: Cambridge University Press.

Smith, P. K. & Connolly, K. J. (1980) *The ecology of preschool behaviour*. Cambridge: Cambridge University Press.

Smith, P. K. & Hagan, T. (1980) Effects of deprivation on exercise play in nursery school children. *Animal Behaviour*, *28*, 922–928.

Thompson, S. K. (1975) Gender labels and early sex-role development. *Child Development*, *46*, 339–347.

Tieger, T. (1980) On the biological basis of sex differences in aggression. *Child Development*, *51*, 943–963.

Weinraub, M., Clemens, L. P., Sockloff, A., Ethridge, T., Gracely, E. & Myers, B. (1984) The development of sex role stereotypes in the third year: relationships to gender labeling, gender identity, sex-typed toy preference, and family characteristics. *Child Development*, *55*, 1493–1503.

Weitz, S. (1977) *Sex roles: biological, psychological and social foundations*. New York: Oxford University Press.

Whiting, B. & Edwards, C. P. (1973) A cross-cultural analysis of sex differences in the behavior of children aged three through 11. *Journal of Social Psychology*, *91*, 171–188.

Williams, J. E., Bennett, S. M. & Best, D. L. (1975) Awareness and expression of sex stereotypes in young children. *Developmental Psychology*, *11*, 635–642.

Wilson, E. O. (1978) *On human nature*. Cambridge, Mass: Harvard University Press.

CHAPTER SEVEN Family and Sex Roles in Middle Childhood

John and Elizabeth Newson

Introduction

One could be forgiven for thinking that, to research psychologists, children become invisible as they pass through middle childhood, earning definition only in so far as they make up a primary school population. We once provocatively (we hoped) set as an examination question '"Middle childhood is of no interest to the developmental psychologist" – discuss'; not one person attempted it. Perhaps the rot set in when Freud chose to use the somewhat dismissive term 'latency period'; certainly the explosion of research interest in early development, as psychologists have discovered the willingness of mothers (mainly) to welcome them into their homes and even bring their babies and toddlers into university laboratories, has done little to redress the balance. The phrase 'yawning gap' is apposite for the way many developmentalists still see the years between preschool and adolescence, so far as the child's development within the family environment is concerned.

Yet what goes on in the family setting is likely to involve more powerful forces than can possibly be exerted elsewhere, if only because the family is individual-oriented in a way that cannot be tolerated within the necessarily group-oriented structures of larger institutions (Newson 1978). Evidence has long been building up to show that, far from presenting a *tabula rasa* as passive reflectants of environmental pressures, children contribute actively to their own socialization; and this has highlighted *negotiation* (whether verbal, non-verbal or pre-verbal, explicit or implicit) as paramount in the socialization process. Negotiation becomes inevitable when parents and children have an intimate knowledge of each other as individuals with a shared history of needs and demands; the longer the history persists (and the more inescapable this joint knowledge), the more complex the negotiative web and the accommodations which derive from it (Newson 1976; Newson, Richardson & Scaife 1978). Greater communicative ability and increased influence from the outside world will both contribute to this complexity; so that we can expect socialization to enter a phase of qualitative reconstruction during the middle years of childhood, rather than merely consolidating or lying fallow. Partly as a result of the closer impingement of the outside world, issues such as sex role, which might have been bypassed earlier on, inevitably come to be more clearly spelled out at this stage.

The data base for this discussion is a longitudinal study of 700 children growing up in Nottingham through the 1960s and 1970s. With the exclusion of single-parent, immigrant-parent and handicapped children (all of which groups were the subjects of separate studies), the children formed a social-class-stratified but otherwise random sample. The sample of 700 included at least 100 children in each of five social classes, based on the Registrar General's classification (father's occupation modified by mother's occupation or qualifications) as follows: classes I and II combined (professional and managerial); class III white collar; class III manual (skilled); class IV (semi-skilled); class V (unskilled). For shorthand purposes, the first two groups (non-manual) are designated middle-class, while the last three groups (manual) are designated working-class. Most of the information derives from semi-structured interviews lasting around three hours with the children's mothers (and some fathers) at the age-stages of one year, four years, seven years, eleven years and sixteen years (and the study is continuing into the second generation). In presenting this discussion of parental attitudes and practices relevant to sex roles in middle childhood, we will therefore choose to take seven and eleven years as our defining boundaries for this period; but the longitudinal nature of the work allows us to give the discussion further perspective by glancing at data obtained at four and sixteen years and beyond. Obviously the strength of such data is that it was obtained contemporaneously with each age, and is uncontaminated by knowledge of what was to come; only now can we add the long-term perspective.

In planning the study as we did, we were anxious not to prejudge what might be important variables in leading parents to 'choose' one child-rearing practice or another; on the other hand, we needed to make it possible to allow data to fall in natural lines of cleavage and to make reliable statements about what we found. At a time when social class was often glibly described as 'no longer existing', it was with some tentativeness that we built into the design the possibility of comparing children by class, including dividing class III in a way which, at that time, the Registrar General was not doing; the study was not seen by us then as an investigation into class inequalities (one of its chief claims to importance as time went on), and we felt on much firmer ground as we prepared to analyse the data by sex of child. We should emphasize at this point, however, that while social class proved from the start of the child's life (for example, mother's age at the time of conception) to be a major and continuing issue, sex was a much less salient variable than class in the early years; and though, during middle childhood in fact, it became an increasingly important variable, it never became as pervasively powerful a factor as social class in deciding the constraints and possibilities of children's lives.

This is not to say that parents were ignoring the child's sex in the early years. There were times, even at one year, when sex affiliation was commonly seen by parents as determining their own behaviour. For instance, mothers frequently gave as a reason for picking up a baby boy quickly when he cried after being put down, 'You have to with boys, don't you, cause he might get a rupture'. However, when we actually analysed the speed with which mothers would pick up their crying babies, there was no difference between their responses to boys and to girls; 'a rupture' just gave a good physical excuse for 'indulgence' of boys, and mothers did without the excuse when it came to girls (Newson 1963).

Similarly, folk beliefs about what small children are like suggest that girls might be more likely to have imaginary companions whose existence they communicated to their mothers, and that boys are more difficult to train not to wet the bed; neither of these areas showed significant sex differences at four years, nor were there differences in prevalence of bed-time comfort habits. When it comes to parents' own behaviour, many mothers and fathers accompany their descriptions of smacking four-year-old boys with the comment, 'Well, you have to with a boy, don't you?' However, analysis of frequency of smacking at four in terms of several variables, shows a fairly complex association with social class, an association of high-frequency smacking with overcrowded housing (class held constant), but only a minor association with sex, shown in a slight tendency ($p < .03$) for girls to be smacked 'seldom' (less than once a week) and not shown in other categories (Newson 1968). This was the more surprising since we know boys to be more prone to the kind of 'trouble' characterized by impetuous inquisitiveness and failure to check with the adult (such as we see repeatedly, for instance, in sex differences for accidental poisoning statistics at every stage of the preschool period) (Department of Prices and Consumer Protection 1976).

Chaperonage

By four socialization had acquired an urgency for parents in that they were conscious that they would soon have to present their child to the more public world of school, and for a large part of the day would be unable to cover up for his or her inadequacies; yet the child's contact with the world outside was still under their control, in that they could bodily remove her from neighbourhood situations if they wished. By seven the child to a far greater extent begins to belong to the wider culture, and parents know that new loyalties and temptations will increasingly draw him/her away. It is at this stage that they are repeatedly forced to set the benefits of independence against its dangers, and it is perhaps in these areas that parents most consciously begin to treat girls and boys differently. In looking at the area of 'chaperonage' first, we would emphasize that no part of child-rearing can be insulated from the rest, so that these salient areas inevitably become linked within a very broad framework.

What we called the 'chaperonage factor' was defined as:

> the extent to which children in their ordinary everyday experience come under the supervision of their parents (or a parental delegate), either by remaining within the immediate parental orbit, or by acceding to certain conditions (in particular, staying within boundaries and keeping the parent precisely informed) when they move beyond that orbit. (Newson 1976, p. 99).

A higher degree of chaperonage is associated with higher social class; but there is a class/sex interaction and, unusually, the sex of the child operates more powerfully than class, girls being consistently more closely chaperoned than boys. The 'index of chaperonage' at seven years was in fact derived from contributory data on a number of topics, most of which themselves showed highly significant sex differences. Table 7.1 shows sex and class differences firstly in mean scores on the chaperonage index as such, and secondly on those contributors to the index which showed sex differences at a significance level of $p < 0.001$. The other measures contributing to the index (whether there was a rule forbidding the child to 'play out' after school, without reporting home first; whether there was an adult at home on the child's return from school; whether the child's friends played at his house; whether there were strict geographical boundaries laid down for the child) all showed sex differences in the same direction but at a lower level of significance, except the last which showed

no significant sex difference. In addition, information which did not contribute to this index but which seems relevant was derived from the
mothers' descriptions of their children's general personality: 67 per cent
of the boys were described unequivocally as 'outdoor children' (i.e. not
even partly 'indoor'), compared with 52 per cent of girls so described
(p < .001).

The results in Table 7.1 (together with circumstantial data given in the
original report but which there is no space for here) confirm that 'by the
age of seven, and in a whole variety of ways, the daily experience of little
boys in terms of where they are allowed to go, how they spend their time
and to what extent they are kept under adult surveillance is already
markedly different from that of little girls! (Newson 1976, p. 100). It
may help to point out that the difference in mean index scores is of a
similar order to the difference in height between men and women, which
most would agree is a 'marked difference'. If this was difficult for us to
show at four years, it must be remembered that at that age supervision
is almost total anyway, so that there is little leeway for treating boys and
girls differently in this respect.

The implications of girls leading more protected and sheltered lives
than boys must undoubtedly be important in social developmental terms,
since children who are kept under closer and more continuous surveillance by adults inevitably come under consistently greater pressure to
conform with adult standards and values. There are likely to be other
consequences also; for instance, traffic accident statistics show a
sex/class factor (until eleven years) very complementary to our 'fetched
from school' figures, the ratio of boys' to girls' traffic accidents at seven
being 2 : 1 (Howarth, Routledge & Repetto-Wright 1974). Between seven
and eleven years, 21 percent of girls and 35 percent of boys in our own
sample suffered some accident which needed out-patient treatment
(p < .001).

By eleven years, 86 percent of mothers said they were inclined to worry
when their children were 'off out' , but this rose to 92 percent for girls'
mothers and fell to 80 per cent for boys' (p < .001). The major worry
concerned possible attack, traffic coming second as a main cause of
anxiety. In both, there are sex differences: 21 percent of boys' mothers,
compared with 14 percent of girls' mothers were most worried by fears
of traffic (p < .02); whereas 66 percent of girls' mothers worried about
attack, especially sexual molestation, compared with 42 percent of boys'
mothers (p < .001). These anxieties are reflected in the index of chaperonage which we applied to eleven-year-olds. Clearly it is not feasible to

Table 7.1 Boys' and girls' mean scores on the 'chaperonage' index at seven years together with sex differences shown on data contributing (positively or negatively) to that index

	Social class					Overall population
	I&II	IIIwc	IIIman	IV	V	
Chaperonage index mean score						
boys	9.6	9.2	9.1	8.6	8.4	9.0
girls	10.6	10.3	10.3	10.0	9.2	10.2
Significance: class trend p < .01; sex differences p < .001						
	%	%	%	%	%	%
Children who 'play or roam around in the street'						
boys	75	78	83	75	89	81
girls	54	59	70	73	77	67
Significance: class trend p < .001; sex differences p < .001						
Children who 'often can't be found when wanted'						
boys	13	12	16	28	25	18
girls	5	4	7	4	10	6
Significance: class trend p < .01; sex differences p < .001						
Mothers who have firm rule that child gives prior notice of destination						
boys	72	70	70	64	65	69
girls	83	81	89	80	67	84
Significance: class trend not significant; sex differences p < .001						
Children who are fetched from school						
boys	22	21	13	7	16	15
girls	45	20	29	28	26	30
Significance: class trend p < .01; sex differences p < .001						

Source: condensed from Newson 1976
Note: In this and the next table, significance of social class differences is given in relation to boys' and girls' data combined. For the chaperonage index, the statistical test for class trend was derived from the class × sex analysis of variance. For the remaining sections the percentage differences between classes were subjected to a chi-squared trend test. All the class × sex interactions in this table were routinely analysed, but none proved to be statistically significant. Note also that 'overall population' figures are weighted to show findings relevant to a true random population (given the exclusions above-mentioned), rather than to a class-stratified population.

derive such an index from the same questions as were asked at seven; parents accept that eleven-year-olds *must* be more geographically mobile than seven-year-olds, if only because secondary schools cast a wider net than primary schools. The child is also more capable of breaking without detection whatever geographical 'rules' might be imposed at eleven. We therefore based the index at eleven on whether the child used buses for leisure journeys on his own, only to get to school or not at all; whether he went into the city centre on his own; whether he went into the city centre on his own; whether he would make journeys to the other side of the city alone, with a same-age child, or only with an older person; and whether his maximum journey time on his own was less than half an hour, around that time or substantially longer. This gives us an eight point score range; if we now define as 'low scorers' the least-chaperoned 30 percent of all children and as 'high scorers' the most chaperoned 30 percent, we find that boys are more likely than girls to score 'low' by $36:22$ percent ($p < .001$), while girls are more likely than boys to score 'high' by $36:24$ percent ($p < .01$). The position in terms of social class is different at eleven, in the sense that many of the more culturally creative opportunities now open to children are community-based, taking place in organized groups; at this point, middle-class parents seem to relax their restrictions on mobility, despite their expressed anxieties, because they now find the advantages convincing. Class differences are in fact negligible for low scorers on chaperonage, and for high scorers the position is actually reversed, high chaperonage increasing as we move down the scale ($p < 0.01$). In this context, the persistence of sex differences is particularly interesting.

Friendships and activities

Patterns of friendship, in so far as these too show sex differences, may well be linked with patterns of chaperonage. Mothers are not wholly and invariably welcoming to the idea of having their children's friends in to play, and their doubts are often expressed in terms of 'a crowd of children wrecking your furniture'. The fact that the children who manage to have a friend in most frequently at seven are girls ($p < .01$) may have something to do with the finding that by eleven rather more girls than boys prefer to play with a special friend rather than being 'one of a crowd'. Girls may also learn to be more selective as a result of their mothers' attitudes; although at eleven sex does not affect which children's mothers are 'unhappy' about one or more of their friendships (33 percent of the sample), mothers of girls are more likely to criticize their undesirable friends (42 percent, compared with 22 percent for boys, $p < 0.001$); does this reflect greater amenability in girls to their mothers in general and to verbal persuasion in particular?

Given that the entire sample had spent its primary school years in mixed schools it is especially interesting that at eleven, despite increased mobility in and beyond the neighbourhood, almost all 'special friends' were the same sex as the child: 65 percent of mothers could name their child's single 'best friend', 64 per cent being the same sex. We had found convincing reasons for this among seven-year-olds, in terms of preferred play patterns – girls had preferred the kind of 'pretend' play in which a plot was played out at length and complementary roles sustained, demanding a higher level of linguistic competence than boys' 'pretend' play which was less complementary, less verbally sustained and more competitive or even duplicative in terms of role – so that it was intriguing to find like-sex preference lasting well beyond the peak period for pretend play. It may be that children's interests continue to sustain this although for a different reason. For instance, boys at eleven are far more likely than girls to have active sports interests *in addition* to those followed at school or in organized associations – 57 percent compared with 24 percent ($p < .001$) – and these are likely to be pursued with a crowd of other boys; whereas girls are more involved than boys with dancing lessons, and with less team-based sports such as skating and horseriding. Girls in fact have a much greater variety of 'miscellaneous hobbies' (categorized as such *because* of their variety): 46 percent of girls compared with 25 percent of boys had non-sport hobbies (collections not counted here).

Most of the children seemed happy in their 'best friendships', but 14 percent of those who had single best friends sometimes 'got upset' about them (as distinct from just quarrelling), and girls were rather more prone to 'upset' than boys (19 percent compared with 11 percent, $p < .01$). The identification of same-sex children as the 'best friend' might of course partly derive from the mother's perception of what is appropriate as a 'best friendship'; but a difference between 1 percent and 64 percent can hardly be wholly attributed to distorted perception of the real situation, and must at least be supported by children's overt behaviour. Obviously we have to ask whether this persistent identification of boys with boys and girls with girls is induced into children, explicitly and implicitly, by the attitudes of parents and teachers. Would it, indeed, be possible to create a situation in which the interests and attitudes of primary school children, and hence their friendship patterns, were *not* polarized according to sex?

Polarization in interests is not, of course, the same thing as sexual latency; it can hardly be suggested, for instance, that later sexual activity is wholly dependent on shared interests other than joint interest in sexual activity itself. In some ways, in fact, boys and girls may differ more sharply in adolescence as far as non-sexual interests are concerned; but cross-sex relationships then tend to become compelling because of the intense motive force of sexuality, which does not, as in ordinary friendship, need joint interests to sustain it, at least in the short term.

Nonetheless, sex differences in interests between seven and eleven may be not only maintained by a sexual latency which makes contact between the sexes unrewarding, but also encouraged by adults – simply because adults are conscious of the power of sexual motivation and have opinions about when it 'ought' to be activated. That is, children's care-givers may reinforce the idea that little boys and girls are not sexually attracted to each other before puberty, out of their own fear that, if this belief were not maintained, children might engage in sexual activity too prematurely. Some parents do in fact touch on such ideas when *in a joking manner* they talk about 'his girl-friend' or 'her little boy-friend' rather than simply using 'friend' as they would for a same-sex child. It is perhaps significant that working-class parents are much more likely to make this kind of facetious innuendo *and* that they are also the group most likely to take active measures, including punishment, against children showing sexual interest in each other (Newson 1968 (especially), 1976).

The majority of our sample were pre-pubertal at eleven (94 percent of girls were pre-menstrual); but, since both the growth spurt preceding puberty and the changes of puberty itself arrive earlier for girls than boys, we might have expected sex differences both in the degree of psychological change generally, and in the amount of cross-sex interest shown at eleven. Obviously, in either case we are talking about phenomena observable by the mother; however, mothers are probably the best source available for such observations. On the basis of the question 'Would you say that N has changed a lot since she/he was seven?', 40 percent of the children were thought hardly to have changed at all, 30 percent to have changed somewhat, and 30 percent to have changed a great deal during middle childhood; slightly more change was observed further down the social scale, but there were no sex differences.

Discussion of cross-sex interests was introduced (in addition to questions about non-specific friendship patterns) by asking: 'Has the question of girl-friends/boy-friends come up at all yet – I mean, is there anyone N feels a bit romantic about?' Asked in this way, sex-role stereotyping would predict greater 'romantic' interest from girls; however, 20 percent of girls and 22 percent of boys have some kind of romantic attachment that the mother knows about. Half the girls' attachments and three-quarters of the boys' attachments are reciprocated by the child named.

In so far as parental expectations are generally believed to have some effect on children's behaviour (and nowhere more than in sex-role matters), it seemed relevant to ask mothers when they were expecting active 'romantic interest' to start. 23 percent were expecting this by eleven (not necessarily those whose children had started), and, as in actuality, there were no sex differences; 39 percent (including these) expected it at thirteen or before, and again there were no sex differences; in fact, the only group which stands out as exceptional in expectations is class V mothers of boys, 21 percent of whom, rather oddly, expect such interests to be delayed until after sixteen (13 percent of the sample as a whole expect such a delay).

Alongside this data should be set the whole question of how parents approach information-giving on sexual matters, even though there is not space to do this topic justice here; complete discussions will be found in Newson (1968 and in press). In summary, willingness to give sexual information is heavily class-biased, such discussion being avoided until an increasingly later age as one moves down the social class scale; but in learning about reproduction (where a baby comes from – how it gets out – how it got in), there is little difference for boys and girls. However, there are two topics of sex information where mothers see an element of 'warning', and in both of these girls at eleven are better informed (by their mothers) than boys: menstruation and sexual molestation. More than three-quarters of the girls in our sample 'knew about' menstruation by eleven, compared with only 21 percent of boys; 42 percent of boys were considered too young to tell at this age, even if the subject were to come up, and well over half of this group's mothers were deliberately hiding tampons and sanitary towels from boys in order to avoid being embarrassed by their questions. We have already mentioned molestation as the major anxiety affecting mothers when their children were 'off out', and it is usual for parents to warn their children about 'strangers'; this of course raises very complex issues (Newson 1976, and in press), and we wanted to know how explicit these warnings might be. We therefore asked, 'Have you explained *why* it can be dangerous to go off with someone or get in someone's car? ... Would you explain anything about sexual danger, or do you think it's better not to mention that?' There were neither class nor sex differences among the 17 percent of children with whom this had already been discussed; but among the 48 percent of mothers who did not intend to mention it, there was a class trend (fewer avoiding the topic further up the scale) which was entirely produced by the unwillingness of working-class mothers, especially the unskilled group, to discuss this with their boys: 43 percent of class V mothers (no different from mothers of other classes) would avoid the topic with girls, compared with 70 percent with boys.

The interviews elicited many detailed accounts of what mothers had said in discussion with their eleven-year-olds, which we have quoted at length elsewhere (Newson, in press) but have no room for here. At the end, however, we could hardly say that we had done much more than scratch the surface:

> The question remains, of course, how far the way in which children learn about sexual matters may have a lasting effect upon them for good or ill. There is much anecdotal evidence to suggest that it is not easy to shed early inculcations of disgust or guilt; but do we really know even this, let alone the protective effects of more sensitive introductions? All that is certain is that mothers generally think this is a significant area of communication, whether or not they shy away from it. The difficulties of addressing such an enquiry would be daunting; nonetheless, since this is likely to be one of those areas in which the more impersonal school contribution cannot quite compensate, the answers would surely be worth having.

Communication

There are other findings which throw additional light on communication between parents and children and how it may be affected by the sex of the child. At both seven and eleven we attempted to investigate the 'sharing, caring' aspects of the relationship with mother and father respectively, and at seven we found this particularly difficult, perhaps because of the more nurturant element at seven; for instance, we asked mothers to judge which parent the child seemed closer to, and although they were able to answer this question, neither sex differences nor class differences emerged more than negligibly. Rather, we noted:

> a tendency for children to turn to the opposite-sexed parent to express dependency or to solicit indulgence, and to the like-sexed to enjoy more

grownup companionship on an equal level, sometimes with a spice of almost conspiratorial adventure for both the pair. By and large, this schema (seemed) to hold true independent of male or female traits regarded as characteristic of fatherly or motherly roles. (Newson 1976, p. 268).

At eleven we investigated the amount of talking that went on between mother-child and father-child pairs separately as well as together, asked about the topics discussed, and also probed shared activities in parent-child couples. Gender polarization turns out to be of particular interest at this stage. 56 percent of all children share some specific regular activity with their mother; (there are no class differences, but 71 percent of girls do this, compared with 42 percent of boys (p < .001); 53 percent of children share an activity with their father, and this time there is a clear class trend showing a decrease lower down the scale; in each class, more boys do so than girls (boys 63 percent overall, girls 44 percent, p < .001).

Looking at range and depth of conversations between parent-child pairs, we find children of both sexes rather dependent on their mothers for conversation, particularly for 'serious' conversation. The class differences are the more salient here, showing a massive trend away from conversation of any sort at the lower end of the scale: 'serious conversation with mother' drops from 62 percent in class I and II to only 14 percent in class V, and a quarter of working-class eleven-years-olds do not even have much casual conversation with their mothers, on mothers' own report. However, boys are for once at a linguistic advantage over girls by virtue of their fathers making more effort to talk to them: 40 percent of middle-class fathers have serious conversations with their sons, compared with 29 percent with their daughters; but at the lower end of the scale this difference only holds true for casual conversations.

It is possible, however, to come much closer to the whole picture of communication between mother and son compared with mother and daughter; and this we did by deriving an 'index of communication' from mothers' accounts of thirteen different topics. These included offers of advice when upset over friendships, knowledge of the child's opinions and fears, helping with homework, show of affection, coaxing and reasoning with the child when he was angry, offering of information on intimate topics and valuing the child for rapport and companionship rather than other things, as well as the 'conversation' measures already mentioned; it also included (as negative quantities) such 'anti-communication' measures as deliberate withholding of information and teasing that went beyond playfulness (full discussion of this index will be found in Newson (in press)).

Table 7.2 High and low scorers on the index of communication between mother and child at eleven years

	Social class					Overall population
	I&II	IIIwc	IIIman	IV	V	
	%	%	%	%	%	%
High scorers (9 or more)						
boys	51	39	18	31	10	27
girls	54	49	36	47	26	41
both	52	44	27	39	18	34

Significance: class trend p < .001; middle class vs working class p < .001; boys vs girls p < .001

	I&II	IIIwc	IIIman	IV	V	Overall
Low scorers (6 or less)						
boys	23	35	52	42	70	46
girls	14	16	32	31	39	28
both	19	26	42	36	55	37

Significance: class trend p < .001; middle class vs working class p < .001; boys vs girls p < .001

Table 7.2 shows major class and sex differences in range and depth of children's communication with their mothers. 'High' and 'low' scores are defined as those scores which delimit the top and bottom thirds (approximately) of the sample. It can be seen that the sparseness of boys' communication with their mothers is much too great to be compensated for by their slightly higher level of conversation with their fathers. The class interaction makes this sex difference considerably more marked for working-class children.

The index of communication to some extent replaced the indices of child-centredness which we devised for four-year-olds and seven-year-olds (Newson 1968, 1976), but which were no longer so appropriate at eleven. Those indices were also heavily class biased, but did not show the substantial sex differences that we find here. Communication, like child-centredness, reflects the mother's willingness to take the child seriously as a person rather than possession: both include a respect for the child's rights to information, the right not to lose dignity through unkind teasing, the right to be valued as someone worth both talking to and listening to. To this extent, the communication index measures quite directly the messages the child receives which identify him or her as a person of worth and considerability. Because such messages are reiterated through every part of the day-to-day contact between mother and child, even small class/sex differences must be important for the whole child-rearing pattern. The divisive nature of class difference is beyond doubt; but here we are also seeing sex differences, especially in relation to class V children, in an area of experience which may well contribute to eventual personality or achievement outcomes. And in fact this is found to be so: looking ahead, children who attained a criminal record before the age of twenty had significantly lower scores on mother/child communication at eleven (Newson, in press).

Although sex differences were not found in child-centredness at seven and we had no communication index as such for that age, one combination of findings at seven foreshadows our suggestion that girls may be taken more seriously by their mothers. We asked both about the child's ambitions for herself and about the mother's ambitions for her: not just in education, but on 'what you would like her to do when she's grownup'. Mothers found this a somewhat amusing question for its very prematurity; but it also had the advantage that at seven the child's school progress is not yet determined, so that mothers' ambitions were not wholly coloured by actual achievement. Overall, as one might expect, mothers were looking beyond their present social status for their children; but girls are in fact consistently favoured over boys, in terms of professional ambitions held for them by their mothers, throughout the working class — in particular, four times as many girls as boys in the skilled group and three times as many in the unskilled group (Newson 1977). When we actually look for the reason for this, we find it in the specific occupations mentioned by mothers; and, ironically, it comes directly out of sex-role stereotyping. Teaching and nursing are seen as highly desirable occupations for girls in every class; whereas teaching is mentioned a quarter as often for boys, and nursing not at all. Working-class mothers are naturally familiar in daily life with the teaching and nursing professions; if they do not see these as men's jobs, they tend to choose for boys the more skilled or less dangerous types of manual work.

The correspondence between mother's and child's ambitions is equally interesting: it is much higher between girls and their mothers than between boys and their mothers. This is partly because children of seven often hold ambitions which are in some sense romantically inspired, and romance is not necessarily about unreality. For instance, although there were a few children hoping to be astronauts, the favourite boys' choice in every class except class V (where it was also popular but tied) was policeman; but very few mothers found this acceptable. Nursing was easily top choice for girls, followed by teaching. Thus boys' romantic ambitions were discounted by their mothers, whereas girls' were taken seriously and backed up by mothers' own hopes. Whether this willing conformity to sex-role stereotype is to be deplored is a moot point. At the time we commented:

> if mothers and daughters both tended to believe that going into service as a kitchen-maid was the most appropriate ambition for girls, we might indeed regard such sex-typing as destructive. In so far as mother and daughter are at this stage mutually supportive in *professional* ambitions, however, one might see girls as advantaged over the boys by virtue of this stereotype. This is likely to be more true of working-class girls, for whom teaching or nursing qualifications will be a step up, than for middle-class girls, for whom such a stereotyping may remove choices that they might otherwise have considered (Newson 1977)

The long-term view

We have mentioned poor mother–child communication at eleven as a sex-differentiated factor which is associated with the outcome in later life of criminal record before the age of twenty; but there are other indices distinguishing boys and girls in middle childhood which are closely linked with outcomes, and to which we should briefly refer. Chaperonage at seven, already discussed, is one of a number of factors linked with verbal reasoning scores at eleven years, more highly chaperoned children scoring higher *within class* ($p < .001$ – Newson 1977): so too is home–school concordance at seven, in which high scorers are more likely to be girls ($p < .01$ – Newson (1977)). We have not had space here to discuss punishment and its outcomes; at seven, frequency of smacking (with the hand) was higher with boys than with girls ($p < .001$ – Newson 1976), while at eleven both smacking frequency and use of implement were greater with boys ($p < .001$ in each case – Newson, in press)), and mothers of boys were also more likely to score high on an index of their commitment to formal corporal punishment: each of these measures proved to be predictive of the child scoring high on an index of being 'troublesome' (on mother's report) at the age of sixteen, and also was associated with criminal record by the age of twenty ($p < .001$ in each case – Newson 1976).

In many ways, then, girls' experience of child-rearing is different from boys in terms that might, and apparently do, affect their 'ways of being' in later life; in particular, their experience supports the continued verbal superiority of girls which is so generally found that it had to be allowed for when educational selection at eleven plus was normal policy. Chaperonage fosters verbal interaction with adults; information-giving on intimate topics demands lengthy verbal explanations; less smacking predicates alternative disciplinary strategies, which are inevitably more verbal. At first sight, it might indeed seem that sex differences are created by differential parental treatment.

It is not as simple as that, however. Talking to parents over the entire socialization period, it is very evident that a major element in child-rearing for almost all parents is *responsiveness* to the child they have, for good or ill. A recurrent theme has been the modification of intended parental behaviour to meet individual personalities and individual situations; the blue-print parents have for child-rearing when they first start has been many times redrawn (and redrawn differently for their different children) by the time the child reaches adulthood. Given this degree of adaptation (and we are not saying that adaptive behaviour is necessarily constructive or helpful for the child), it is not credible that differential treatment is imposed upon unwilling recipients. Colin Rogers' argument (Chapter 8) that teachers' expectations of boys and girls are partly formed and maintained by the original behaviour of the two sexes, and that expectations can only affect pupils if pupils respond to them, is equally true for parents and their children: and we would suggest that inbuilt sex-linked orientations in children provide a hospitable environment for parental treatment which becomes and remains increasingly differentiated because it can do no other if it is to respond to the child as he/she is.

What these orientations consist of is another matter. Elsewhere (Newson, Richardson & Scaife 1978) we have somewhat tentatively suggested (following Erikson) a basic genetic difference that epitomizes girls as 'person-oriented' and boys as 'thing-oriented'. In the light of the socialization process *as a whole*, such a schema perhaps makes more sense than most attempts to list fragmented sex differences; for it explains not only the initial impetus for a series of cultural forces, but how these can build up, sustain and perpetuate the massive and durable complexity that characterizes sex roles in later life. It is in these terms that the discussion seems likely to progress most constructively.

158   *Part II Developmental Issues*

References

Department of Prices and Consumer Protection (1976) *Child Poisoning from Household Products.* London: HMSO.

Howarth, C. I., Routledge, D. A. & Repetto-Wright, R. (1974) An analysis of road accidents involving child pedestrians. *Ergonomics, 17 (3),* 319–330.

Newson, Elizabeth (1978) Unreasonable care: the establishment of selfhood. *In* G. Vessey *Human values.* Sussex: Harvester Press (and New Jersey: Humanities Press), pp. 1–26.

Newson, John and Elizabeth (1963) *Infant care in an urban community.* London: Allen & Unwin (and Harmondsworth: Penguin under title *Patterns of . . .*).

Newson, John and Elizabeth (1968) *Four years old in an urban community.* London: Allen & Unwin (and Harmondsworth: Penguin).

Newson, John and Elizabeth (1976) *Seven years old in the home environment.* London: Allen & and Unwin (and Harmondsworth: Penguin).

Newson, John and Elizabeth (1977) *Perspectives on school at seven years old.* London: Allen & Unwin.

Newson, John and Elizabeth (in press) *Transition into adolescence.*

Newson, J. and E., Richardson, D. & Scaife, J. (1978) Perspectives in sex-role stereotyping. *In* J. Chetwynd and O. Hartnett (eds) *The sex role system.* London: Routledge & Kegan Paul.

CHAPTER EIGHT   Sex Roles in Education
Colin Rogers

Throughout this book, the nature and effects of sex roles are documented with respect to a number of different areas of human activity. It would be naive to assume that schools can be isolated from these general effects. Patterns of behaviour that are typical of each sex are not likely to be dropped at the school gates, to be picked up again only at 3.30 p.m. on the way home. Schools are a part of society and the boys and girls, men and women within them are subject to the same general influences on their behaviour there as elsewhere.

Within a general consideration of the psychology of sex roles, an examination of sex roles at school is important for two main reasons. First, school occupies much of a young person's life. What happens there may have a profound influence on their behaviour in later life. Second, the educational process itself may be affected by the ways in which sex roles spell out different patterns of behaviour for each sex. This has implications for the ways in which children perform academically.

The concern of this chapter will be to investigate the nature of sex roles as they affect behaviour in school classrooms, with particular reference to the ways in which these roles may exert an influence upon the academic attainments of each sex. The chapter will begin with an outline of the nature of the differences between the sexes in terms of academic attainment. It will then go on to examine the ways in which teachers and pupils interact with each other within the classroom, and the ways in which the expectations of teachers for certain patterns of performance might have a bearing on the final levels of attainment of each sex. The attention will then switch from the teacher to the pupil, through an examination of the pupils' reactions to teacher behaviour. Recent work in attribution theory will be used here in formulating a general framework for the analysis of pupil reactions to the experience of school, followed by a more specific analysis of sex differences in these processes. A concluding section will draw attention to some of the major implications of this work for the development of an understanding of sex roles in school.

The pattern of attainment

The Department of Education and Science provides regular information concerning the performance of children in public examinations, frequently categorizing the data by pupil sex. The interested reader will be able to obtain fuller details by examining the Statistics of Education published annually with summary updates provided by the Statistical Bulletins. The summary provided here is taken from Statistical Bulletin 11/84 (1984) and provides information of pupils who left school during the year 1982–3.

Some 765,000 pupils left schools in England during this period. Overall, some 27 percent of these school leavers intended to go on to pursue some form of full-time further education. The corresponding percentages for boys and girls were 23 percent and 32 percent respectively. While a greater proportion of the girls were going on to some form of further education, the pattern is different if the proportions are calculated separately for different types of further education. For example, 8.5 percent of boy school leavers were going on to degree courses while the corresponding figure for the girls was only 6.5 percent. Teacher training courses reveal a different pattern again. The percentage of boys going on to such courses was 0.1 percent compared to 0.6 percent of the girls. Recent years have seen considerable reductions in the availability of teacher training places. In 1971/2 the proportions of boys and girls going on to such courses were 1.3 percent and 5.0 percent respectively. The proportional drop has been greatest amongst the boys but in terms of absolute numbers it is clearly girl school leavers who have been most affected by the reduction in these places.

Closer examination of the available data reveals subtler differences. For example, the proportions of the boys and girls attempting A-level examinations were very similar. Of the boys leaving, 19.6 percent had attempted A-levels, the corresponding figure for the girls being 19.2 percent. These attempts resulted in 17.4 percent of the boys leaving school with at least one A-level pass compared with 16.9 percent of the girls. The gap widens when one looks separately at the figures for those obtaining three or more A-level passes; here the percentage of boy leavers was 10.3 percent while that for the girls was only 8.8 percent. The last figure is one of the few which demonstrates a simple 'advantage' for boys in terms of qualifications obtained, as long as the subject being taken is not specified. At O-level, girls tend to do rather better. For example, 11.4 percent of girls left school with five or more higher grade

O-level passes (GCE grades A, B, C or CSE grade 1), but with no A-levels, compared with 9.2 percent of the boys. However, when one does take the subject to be taken into account the picture begins to look very different. The figures will only be given for O-level here in order to avoid spending too much time on this. The patterns at O-level are important because, given the nature of the present English examination system in practice, what happens here will have a determining effect on a great deal that follows.

The pattern of differences is much as would be expected (which in itself tends to suggest that sex roles might be involved). A higher percentage of girls than boys leave with higher grade passes in subjects such as English (girls 45 percent, boys 34 percent) and French (girls 19 percent, boys 11 percent), whereas the opposite is the case in subjects such as maths (girls 27 percent, boys 32 percent) and physics (girls 8 percent, boys 22 percent). The difference is not simply one of arts versus science, for a higher percentage of girls obtain higher grade passes in biology (girls 20 percent, boys 13 percent). The biggest differences are in subjects such as craft and design (girls 3 percent, boys 18 percent) and domestic and commercial studies (girls 17 percent, boys 3 percent). The differences at A-level follow the same pattern. While the percentages leaving with passes in each subject are lower at A- than at O-level, the magnitude of the difference between the sexes is greater.

It is not necessary for present purposes to go into these figures in any greater detail. Two general conclusions can be drawn. First, while girls could not be said to be disadvantaged with respect to the total number of them that go on to take any kind of further education after school, they do not do as well at gaining access to degree courses. Second, while again they do not fail to gain qualifications at school, there is a strong tendency for the pattern of qualifications that they do obtain to be sex-typed. The same point applies equally well to the boys, of course, only it should be noted that the subjects in which boys gain the higher percentages of qualifications are also those that are typically rated as being the most difficult by pupils of both sexes, for instance physics and maths (Duckworth & Entwistle 1974). In short, it is perhaps not unfair to characterize the available data as showing that girls and boys do equally well at school as long as one ignores the difficulty (and possibly by implication also the prestige) of their areas of attainment; boys' successes are gained in the more difficult areas.

These differences in attainment are of considerable concern at present. Much of this concern is due to the belief that the subjects in which girls participate less often (and do less well in) are becoming increasingly important (Eddowes 1983; Harding 1983; Kelly, Whyte & Smail 1984). Furthermore, authors such as Byrne (1975) and, more recently, Deem (1984) have argued that co-education, now the dominant form of school organization, tends to amplify, rather than reduce these differences.

Teacher expectations and pupil gender

It can readily be established that teachers believe boys and girls to be different from each other in a variety of different ways, and at all age levels represented within the school system. Many of these beliefs reflect those held in society as a whole, with girls expected to be quieter, neater, better behaved, more co-operative and easier to control (Byrne 1975; Delamont 1980; Stanworth 1983). However, a more substantial and educationally significant claim can be made, namely that the sex-typed beliefs that teachers hold about pupils will exert a causal influence upon pupils' levels of academic performance.

The research of Rosenthal and Jacobson (1968) is generally credited with establishing the 'expectancy effect' as a topic of major concern in educational research. By giving teachers expectations for above average gains for arbitrarily specified pupils at the beginning of a school year, Rosenthal and Jacobson claimed to be able to show that the pupils who had been expected to gain actually did so. While they had not observed the teachers in action in the classroom, they suggested that the style of interaction which developed between pupil and teacher would be altered by the expectation. This would not necessarily be something that would happen as the result of any deliberate strategy adopted by the teacher. Indeed the researchers claim that most teachers were unable to remember the names of the pupils identified to them at the start of the experimental period by the end of that school year.

While this classic piece of research has been extensively criticized (e.g Elashoff & Snow 1971; Jensen 1969) for a variety of reasons including technical deficiencies, recent reviews of the research generated by this study have concluded that the effect has been well enough established (Blease 1983; Braun 1976; Brophy 1983; Rogers 1982). This not to say that teacher expectations will always have causal influences upon the performance level of pupils. Indeed, the conclusion reached by Rogers (1982) was that such effects will be relatively rare. The full reasoning behind this conclusion cannot be detailed here, but essentially the claim is made that the process by which teachers' expectations might actually come to influence pupils' performance is a long and complex one. Like any process, if only requires a breakdown to occur at one point and the effect will not occur.

In the case of the teacher expectancy process some of the more important steps will include the following: the teacher will have to form some impression of the child; this impression will need to give rise to expectations for future levels of performance; the behaviour of the teacher will have to vary as a function of the expectations he or she holds for individual pupils; any one pupil will have to notice, in some way, these differences in teacher behaviour and react by behaving in an appropriate manner so that so their final performance comes to be more like that expected by the teacher. Finally it must be noted that if an expectancy effect is to operate, that is if the teacher's expectations are to exercise an influence upon the pupils' behaviour, then the expectations held in the first place by the teacher must be in some way inaccurate. A full account of the operation of this entire process is beyond the scope of this chapter, and so a more selective review of the available evidence will be undertaken. The focus of attention will be on the nature of teacher expectations towards pupils as a function of the pupils' sex, differences in the behaviour of teachers towards boys and girls and the nature of pupils' reactions to these differences.

Sex as a basis for teacher expectations

The literature on teacher expectations and their effects has given only scant regard to the problem of defining expectations. This matter will be briefly discussed here before going on to look at the evidence concerning sex as a basis for expectations, as it is believed that such discussion is particularly relevant to the concerns of this chapter.

Impressions and expectations are not the same thing. While one could not expect anything of another person without having some minimal impression of them, having an impression does not imply the holding of an expectation. To expect something of an individual requires knowledge of the situation in which they are to be operating as well as knowledge of the individual. Teachers will generally be well-informed about the former: they will know the demands of the classroom setting as well as anybody, and be able to anticipate the responses of given individuals to it. Their knowledge of the individual child may be less adequate: if teachers are using inaccurate information in this respect, then they could form erroneous expectations.

Expectations themselves, however, can differ. Rogers (1982) draws attention to the difference between probabilistic and prescriptive expectations. The former can be regarded as a weaker type of expectation that is perhaps less likely to give rise to expectancy *effects*. Here the holder of the expectation is simply stating that he or she believes something is likely to happen; there is no suggestion that it ought to. To expect a friend to be quiet at a party because he or she is believed to be shy is not to say that he or she *ought* to be quiet. Prescriptive expectations are likely to be stronger in their effects. Here the expectation takes on something of the force of a moral imperative. The headteacher who tells the assembled new pupils that this is a school that expects high standards of behaviour and work is not simply saying that it is likely that these new pupils will conform to this pattern, it is clearly being implied that they should.

The distinction between probabilistic and prescriptive expectations is an important one as far as an understanding of teacher expectations and their possible effects is concerned. It is clearly the prescriptive expectations that are more likely to become self-fulfilling prophecies. It is here that processes are likely to be set up, not necessarily deliberately, to ensure that other people do conform to one's expectations for them. A somewhat similar point is made by Blease (1983) when he argues that it will be expectations that are shared by a network of individuals within the same social setting that will be more likely to produce expectancy effects. If all teachers hold very similar expectations for a given pupil, that pupil is more likely to come to conform to the expectations than if the expectation is only held by a single teacher.

On both accounts (the prescriptiveness of an expectation and the degree to which any expectation is likely to be held by most people in any given setting) it seems very reasonable to suggest that expectations based on pupil gender are going to be important. As will be made clear elsewhere in this book, sex roles do carry a prescriptive element. People who clearly fail to conform to the pattern of behaviour considered appropriate to their sex will quickly find their behaviour being sanctioned. Similarly, teachers will hold broadly comparable views concerning the types of behaviour that are likely to be exhibited by children as a function of the child's sex. Delamont (1980) suggests, indeed, that teachers as a group are likely to be somewhat more conservative in their definition of sex-appropriate behaviour than are other sections of the population.

She also points out that society as a whole, and perhaps particularly the news media, will be quick to react in a possibly hostile manner should teachers begin to suggest alternatives to the accepted definitions of sex-appropriate behaviour.

Perhaps not surprisingly therefore, one of the earlier studies of the effects of teacher expectations identified pupil sex as an important factor. Palardy (1969) assessed the attitudes of teachers of primary school aged children with respect to the assumed ease with which boys and girls would learn to read. He found that teachers who held the common belief that girls will learn to read more readily than boys had pupils in their class some six months later who reflected that pattern. The girls had higher reading attainment scores than the boys. Where this attitude was not held, that is where the teachers had professed that boys and girls would learn to read with equal facility, the sex differences in attainment were not found. The pupils in the sample had been matched in terms of 'reading readiness' at the beginning of the study.

However, not all of the research has demonstrated such clear-cut results. In a meta-analysis of a large number of studies concerned with factors that might inform teachers' expectations for pupil performance, Dusek and Joseph (1983) come to the conclusion that the sex of a pupil is not a relevant factor. Individual studies, of course, support this view. Adams and Cohen (1976) find that among a series of items of information presented to teachers about pupils, the sex of pupils had very little effect on what the teachers came to expect from those pupils.

Dusek and Joseph employ another distinction between types of expectations that is now fairly common in the literature, that between academic and social expectations (see also Crano & Mellon 1978; Rogers 1982). The labels are fairly self-explanatory, and the lack of impact of gender on expectations noted by Dusek and Joseph is stronger in connection with academic expectations. Teachers' expectations for a pupil's classroom behaviour are somewhat more likely to be based on gender than are expectations that are directly concerned with academic performance, but the relationship is still not a strong one. Their analysis also shows, however, that sex-role behaviour is a stronger influence on teacher expectations than gender itself. An important study here is that of Bernard (1979). Bernard found that teachers would expect higher levels of intelligence, independence and logic from pupils described as possessing typically masculine characteristics. Pupils with patterns of behaviour that were more typically feminine were judged to be likely to have greater difficulty with future study and to be less suited to the study of physics. It should be remembered that these judgements related to sex-role behaviour and not to sex itself. It should also be noted that Dusek and Joseph (1983) concluded that the available evidence does no more than suggest that sex-role behaviour might influence teacher expectations.

In some respects, this research tells us more about the problems inherent in the literature on teacher expectancies than it does about the expectancies themselves. The studies reviewed by Dusek and Joseph (1983) typically do not involve the expectations held by teachers of their actual pupils. In an attempt to gain experimental rigour researchers have provided teachers with information concerning hypothetical pupils. In this way it is possible to claim that the effects of the particular information provided have been isolated from any other items of information that might have been available to the teacher in the real classroom. Dusek and Joseph, however, claim that the effects of gender, and perhaps particularly sex-role behaviour, may appear to be greater if tested within the context of the real classroom.

The evidence available from classroom-based research tends to support this view. It is important to point out that this research has not been carried out with the explicit intention of testing claims concerning the nature and effect of teacher expectations.

Differences in the treatment of boys and girls can be documented from an early age. For example, Adams and Passman (1979) found that for preschool children greater adult attention was forthcoming for the achievements of boys than was the case for girls. It will be demonstrated later how these differences are reflected in the reactions to success and failure of preschool boys and girls. At the primary age level, Entwisle and Baker (1983) demontrate how the expectations of parents are differentiated according to their children's sex. This difference however, interacted with social class, so that while middle-class parents expected girls to be better at reading and boys at mathematics, working-class parents expected girls to be better than boys at both.

Differences related to social class were also picked up in an observational study reported by Clarricoates (1980). Observing the interactions of teachers and pupils in four primary schools, serving catchment areas ranging from an inner-city district to a very small rural community, she documents a wide range of differences in the ways in which boys and girls are treated by teachers. These forms of gender differentiation were most obvious in the inner-city school, but are to be found in all types of school. Teachers were least tolerant of boys who demonstrated behaviour that might be considered effeminate and were more tolerant of aggression when it was displayed by boys. This applied both to physical and verbal forms of aggressive behaviour.

Sex was also used by teachers as a way of dividing pupils into groups for managerial purposes even though the activities in question had no particular sex specific basis. So boys and girls would leave and enter the class separately, collect their milk separately and so on. From the teachers' point of view, such forms of sex differentiation may have no particular significance. A primary school class is likely to be better managed and controlled if various activities are carried out by the pupils in subgroups rather than en masse, and dividing the pupils by sex is an obvious and easy way of doing this. Neither the teacher, nor the pupils will need to exert much effort to recall which pupil is supposed to be in which group.

Clarricoates (1980) points out that the teachers themselves claimed not to treat the pupils differently. This suggests that if the gender-based expectations of teachers are assessed in a relatively abstract manner (as was the case in the studies reviewed by Dusek and Joseph (1983) differences may well not appear. In practice however, the differences may be quite apparent.

A similar point can be made at the secondary level. Spender (1982) concludes from a review of a number of pieces of research that pupil differentiation by gender on the part of teachers is so pervasive that the teachers and pupils themselves become adapted to it. This is so, she claims, to the extent that if boys receive less than two-thirds of teacher attention, then both boy and girl pupils and the teachers will assume that the girls are being given more than their fair share. This is not because teachers believe that it is appropriate to give boys more attention than girls (they would typically refute any such suggestion). Rather the normative background is so biased in favour of the boys that departures from it produce contrast effects leading to the overestimation of the attention now being given to girls. A number of studies come to broadly similar conclusions (see e.g. Byrne 1975; Kelly 1981; Kelly, Whyte & Smail 1984; Spender & Sarah 1980; Stanworth 1983; Sutherland 1981).

The sex differences in attention and treatment are likely to be more pronounced in some curriculum areas than others. Reports on behalf of the Schools Council by Eddowes (1983) and Harding (1983) document the difference in mathematics and science respectively while Kelly (1981) and Kelly, Whyte and Smail (1984) provide futher evidence concerning the differences in the science area and the difficulties likely to be encountered in trying to implement changes.

While space does not permit a detailed review of this literature, the overall picture that emerges is that from initial entry to school (and indeed prior to this as well), boys and girls will receive quite different types of treatment and will therefore have quite different educational experiences. Boys receive more teacher attention and, particularly at the primary level, the greater part of this extra attention will be disciplinary in nature. By the time of entry into secondary school these differences have been accepted by all concerned as being entirely normal, to the extent that they will often go unnoticed by teacher and pupil alike. Differences in attention are perhaps most likely to be found at the secondary level in those areas of the curriculum that are traditionally regarded as masculine (mathematics, science and technology). If we are to arrive at an understanding of the ways in which these differences might give rise to differences in pupil performance, we need to have a framework in which to assess the pupil reaction. The remainder of this chapter will be concerned with this aspect of the overall process.

Pupils' reactions to classroom events

The paradox involved in a consideration of sex differences in school is that the apparently favourable environment in which girls spend their primary years gives way to a situation in which, at the secondary level, girls are apparently less confident and less willing to undertake difficult tasks. The boys, who are regarded at the primary level as being more troublesome and as having styles of behaviour that are less conducive to successful school-based learning, are the ones who at the secondary level emerge with the greater degree of success in the more difficult areas of study.

One potentially fruitful approach to the study of the processes involved in this transitional development is provided by attribution theory. Numerous introductory texts are available for the reader new to this material (Ames & Ames 1984; Kelley & Micheala 1980; Shaver 1975; Weiner 1979). Attention will be given here to attempts to use attribution theory concepts to explain achievement-related behaviour. The origins of the theory lie in the work of Weiner (1974, 1979, 1980, 1984), but the reader should be aware of the existence of somewhat different approaches (Covington 1984; Covington & Beery 1976; Covington & Omelich 1979). The basic claims are essentially simple, and rest on the assumption that individuals are motivated to explain significant events by attributing them to causes. In the case of achievement-related behaviour (that is behavioural instances where it is possible to succeed or fail) the event to be explained will be the success or failure itself. While many individual causes may be used by many individuals, Weiner's claim is that these causes can be classified in terms of a few simple dimensions. Included in these dimensions are two that have received the lion's share of research attention to date (although as Weiner (1979) himself makes clear, there are other dimensions available that may prove to be equally if not more important in the longer term).

The first of these concerns the stability of the perceived cause. Ability, for example, would be a stable cause of success (or the lack of ability a stable cause of failure) as ability itself is not seen to vary within one individual over time. Effort, however, is unstable, as this is a cause that will be seen to vary over time. The second dimension concerns the location of the perceived cause. Causes can be either internal, to be seen as residing within oneself (both the two causes, ability and effort, referred to above, would be of this type) or they can be seen as being located outside of oneself (examples here would be the perceived difficulty of the task or the amount of luck that one had experienced). Any particular perceived cause, therefore, can be located on the two-by-two array produced by these two dimensions.

Weiner's theory is concerned with examining the processes involved in determining the particular judgement that any individual might make in any given case, and with the consequences of the making of that judgement. A simple example at this point should help to make the rudiments of the approach clear. If certain individuals typically make attributions to a lack of ability for their failures (that is they explain their failures by concluding that they failed due to a lack of ability) then they will be likely to expect further failure. Their lack of ability is seen as a stable feature and will therefore continue to depress performance. Given this analysis, it would be perfectly rational for them to conclude that any further expenditure of effort on this task would be pointless. Such a conclusion, if put into practice, would be likely to prove to be self-fulfilling, as reductions in effort will generally lead to reductions in the quality of performance. Had these individuals instead attributed failure to lack of effort, the prognosis would have been different. As effort is seen to be unstable, there would be no good reason to suppose that future success was not possible. Individuals who typically attributed their successes to ability but failures to lack of effort would increasingly come to see themselves as being capable of relatively high levels of performance. On the contrary, individuals who typically attributed success to effort but failure to lack of ability, would increasingly come to see themselves as people who could only succeed through the application of effort under circumstances in which high levels of ability were not called for. In adults, ability generally tends to be seen as a fixed capacity that sets a clear ceiling on performance levels (Nicholls 1984).

The relevance of this to the present discussion is simple; it has been claimed that girls (and women) will be more likely to display the second, and less adaptive 'attributional style' than will boys (or men).

Sex differences in attributional style

These differences can be identified at preschool age. Löchel (1983) reports that in a sample of boys and girls aged between four and five years, a number of sex-typed differences in attributional patterns for success and failure could be identified. Löchel further claims that these differences indicate that girls are likely to use a less adaptive style. For example, they were less likely to claim that success indicated that they possessed relatively high levels of ability, while boys were more likely to use self-defensive attributions for their failures. One particularly important finding here is that even at this age the 'sex appropriateness' of the task interacted with the more general findings. Girls, for example, were particularly likely to attribute failure to a lack of relevant ability if the failure occurred on a 'masculine' task. (In this study the masculinity or femininity of a task was defined both in terms of typical differences between the sexes in quality of performance, and in terms of the degree to which each sex would indicate a preference for a particular task.)

Several other studies (Horner 1972; and the work of Dweck and her colleagues, e.g Dweck *et al.* (1978)) have demonstrated similar patterns of differences across a range of different age groups and tasks. Deaux (1976) has provided one general systematization of these results. Her claim is that the important factor is the degree to which a particular success or failure might have been expected on the grounds of sex-typing. Success on a task considered to be appropriate to one's sex is more likely to be attributed to a stable causal factor than one that would not have been so anticipated. As attributions to stable factors enhance the degree to which more of the same will be anticipated, such a pattern will lead to an ever-increasing expectation that success is more likely in cases where the task in hand is considered to be appropriate to oneself.

An important study that attempts to link the development of these general differences between the sexes in terms of attributional style with the pattern of early school experience outlined above, has been reported by Dweck *et al.* (1978). The findings of this study are strongly suggestive of a connection between the apparently more favourable environment of the primary schoolgirl and the older schoolgirl's less adaptive attributional patterns. The research shows that the greater attention received by the boys in class is primarily due to the greater amount of disciplinary actions that are directed against them. Even criticisms of boys' work are often directed to aspects such as the neatness of presentation rather than to the quality of the work itself. While this may make the classroom environment appear to be more hostile to the boy than to the girl, it also has the effect, argues Dweck, of enabling the boy to accept teacher criticism *without* assuming that this indicates a lack of ability on his part. Whilst the girls experiences an overall lower level of criticism, a higher proportion of the criticism that they do receive is directed at the actual quality of the work they have done. It therefore becomes much more difficult for the girl to avoid concluding that teacher criticism implies a lack of ability on her part.

Dweck has further developed her case by demonstrating that boys and girls respond differently to feedback indicating that they have failed, but that these different reactions depend crucially on who has delivered the feedback (Dweck & Bush 1976). Boys will show a more positive reaction to failure feedback originating from an adult that will girls (that is the boys will be more likely to respond by attempting to improve). The opposite is the case if the failure feedback is delivered by a peer. In other words, when the feedback comes from an adult, girls are more likely to assume that this implies a lack of ability on their part and therefore assume that success is likely to be beyond them. The finding that these differences are reversed when the source of the feedback changes from adult to peer suggests that the differences are specific products of particular interactional patterns, which further implies that changing the interactional patterns might change the nature of the performance outcomes.

This view, that patterns of attributions are the product of particular situational factors, is supported by further research suggesting that different situations can produce different attributional patterns and that existing attributional styles can be modified. For example, Ames (1984) and Nicholls (1984) provide evidence to support the claim that competitive situations will produce different patterns of attributions to those produced under co-operative conditions. They would also claim that in many respects the patterns produced under co-operative conditions are more likely to promote high levels of intrinsic motivation. Further, studies by Andrews and Debus (1978), DeCharms (1976, 1984) and Dweck (1985) all illustrate that in various ways it is possible to change less adaptive attributional styles into more adaptive ones.

Conclusion

An attributional analysis of classroom interactions and their consequences is still in its infancy, but signs of progress can be detected (Rogers 1982, in press). The significance of this approach for the study of sex roles in education is that it provides a theoretical basis for linking together a variety of observations concerning the ways in which boys and girls behave (and are treated in school) with the development of particular approaches to work on the part of the pupils. The provision of such a theoretical basis is important, for it would appear to be the case that some of the links between classroom events and developing attitudes are not immediately apparent.

A further important consequence of the adoption of an attributional basis for the analysis of classroom events is the emphasis that will be placed upon the contribution of the pupils themselves in establishing the nature of sex roles in education. As stated in the introduction to this chapter, pupils will not leave sex-typed patterns of behaviour behind them at the school gates. However, these established patterns of behaviour are not in themselves the whole story. School provides for the pupil a new range of experiences and challenges from which will be generated new patterns of behaviour and new attitudes and motivational styles. These new styles are, however, generated and not just passively acquired. Pupils and teachers interact together to produce the particular set of behaviours and attitudes that characterizes each sex within school. If we wish to acquire an understanding of the ways in which teachers influence pupils, with respect to sex roles, it will not be sufficient to analyse the beliefs of teachers (or indeed of pupils) alone. Sex roles in education are produced by the process of schooling, and it is this process that we must attend to if our understanding is to grow.

References

Adams, G. & Cohen, A. (1976) An examination of cumulative folder information used by teachers in making differential judgements of children's abilities. *The Alberta Journal of Educational Research, 22,* 216–225.

Adams, R. E. & Passman, R. H. (1979) Sex differences in the interaction of adults and pre-school chidren. *Psychological Reports, 44,* 115–118.

Ames, C. (1984). Competitive, cooperative and individualistic goal structures: a cognitive-motivational analysis. In R. Ames & C. Ames *Research on motivation in education.* vol. 1 *Student motivation.* London: Academic Press.

Ames, R. & Ames, C. (1984) *Research on motivation in education:* vol. 1 *Student motivation.* London: Academic Press.

Andrews, G. R. & Debus, R. L. (1978) Persistence and the causal perception of failure: modifying cognitive attributions. *Journal of Educational Psychology, 70,* 154–166.

Bernard, M. (1979) Does sex-role behaviour influence the way teachers evaluate students? *Journal of Educational Psychology,* 71, 553–562.

Blease, D. (1983) Teacher expectations and the self-fulfilling prophecy. *Educational Studies, 9,* 123–130.

Braun, C. (1976) Teacher expectation: socio-psychological dynamics. *Review of Educational Research, 46,* 185–213.

Brophy, J. E. (1983) Research on the self-fulfilling prophecy and teacher expectations. *Journal of Educational Psychology, 75,* 613–661.

Byrne, E. (1975) *Women and education.* London: Tavistock.

Clarricoates, K. (1980) The importance of being Ernest ... Emma ... Tom ... Jane: the perception and categorisation of gender conformity and gender deviation in primary schools. *In:* R. Deem (ed.) *Schooling for Women's Work.* London: Routledge & Kegan Paul.

Covington, M. V. (1984) The motive for self-worth. *In* R. Ames & C. Ames *Research on motivation in education:* vol. 1 *Student motivation.* London: Academic Press.

Covington, M. V. & Beery, R. (1976) *Self-worth and school learning.* New York: Holt, Rinehart & Winston.

Covington, M. V. & Omelich, C. L. (1979) Are causal attributions causal? A path analysis of the cognitive model of achievement motivation. *Journal of Personality and Social Psychology, 37,* 1487–1504.

Crano, W. D. & Mellon, D. M. (1978) Causal influence of teachers' expectations on children's academic performance: a cross-lagged panel analysis. *Journal of Educational Psychology, 70,* 39–49.

Deaux, K. (1976) Sex: a perspective on the attribution process. *In* J. Harvey, W. J. Ickes & R. F. Kidd *New directions in attribution research,* vol.1, Hillsdale, NJ: Erlbaum.

DeCharms, R. (1976) *Enhancing motivation: change in the classroom.* New York: Irvington.

DeCharms, R. (1984) Motivation enhancement in educational settings. *In* R. Ames & C. Ames *Research on motivation in education:* vol. 1 *Student motivation.* London: Academic Press.

Deem, R. (ed.) (1984) *Co-education reconsidered*. Milton Keynes: Open University Press.

Delamont, S. (1980) *Sex roles and the school*. London: Methuen.

Department of Education and Science (1984) *English school leavers 1982–83*, Statistical Bulletin, 11/84.

Duckworth, D. & Entwistle, N. J. (1974) Attitudes to school subjects: a repertory grid technique. *British Journal of Educational Psychology*, 44, 76–78.

Dusek, J. B. & Joseph, G. (1983) The bases of teacher expectancies: a meta-analysis. *Journal of Educational Psychology*, 75, 327–346.

Dweck, C. S. (1975) The role of expectations and attributions in the alleviation of learned helplessness. *Journal of Personality and Social Psychology, 31*, 674–685.

Dweck, C. S. & Bush, E. S. (1976) Sex differences in learned helplessness: I, Differential debilitation with peer and adult evaluators. *Developmental Psychology, 12*, 147–156.

Dweck, C. S., Davidson, W., Nelson, S. & Enna, B. (1978) Sex differences in learned helplessness: II. The contingencies of evaluative feedback in the classroom; III. An experimental analysis. *Developmental Psychology, 14*, 268–276.

Eddowes, M. (1983). *Humble pi: the mathematics education of girls*. York: Longman for Schools Council.

Elashoff, J.D. & Snow, R. E. (eds) (1971) *Pygmalion reconsidered*. Worthington, Ohio: Charles A. Jones.

Entwisle, D. R. & Baker, D. P. (1983) Gender and young children's expectations for performance in arithmetic. *Developmental Psychology, 19*, 200–209.

Harding, J. (1983) *Switched off: the science education of girls*. York: Longman for Schools Council.

Horner, M. S. (1972) Towards an understanding of achievement-related conflicts in women. *Journal of Social Issues, 28*, 157–175.

Jensen, A. (1969). Review of *Pygmalion in the classroom,* by Rosenthal and Jacobson. *Scientific American, 51*, 44a–45a.

Kelly, A. (1981) *The missing half: girls and science education*. Manchester: Manchester University Press.

Kelly, A., Whyte, J. & Smail, B. (1984) *Girls into science and technology: final report*. GIST, University of Manchester.

Kelley, H. H. and Michaela, J. L. (1980) Attribution theory and research. *Annual Review of Psychology, 31*, 457–502.

Löchel, E. (1983) Sex differences in achievement motivation. *In* J. Jaspars, F. D. Fincham & M. Hewstone, *Attribution theory and research: conceptual, developmental and social dimensions*. London: Academic Press.

Nicholls, J. G. (1984) Conceptions of ability and achievement motivation. *In*: R. Ames & C. Ames *Research on motivation in education*: vol. 1 *Student motivation*. London: Academic Press.

Palardy, J. (1969) What teachers believe – what children achieve. *Elementary School Journal, 69*, 370–374.

Rogers, C. (1982) Impressions and attributions within the classroom. *In* C. Antaki & C. Brewin (eds) *The applications of attribution theory to clinical and educational practice*. New York: Academic Press.

Rogers, C. (1982) *A social psychology of schooling*. London: Routledge & Kegan Paul.

Rogers, C. (in press) Attributing for success and failure in the classroom. *In* A. Desforges & C. Desforges *Psychology and primary schooling*. Brighton: Falmer Press.

Rosenthal, R. & Jacobson, L. (1968) *Pygmalion in the classroom*. New York: Holt, Rinehart & Winston.

Shaver, K. G. (1975) *An introduction to attribution processes* Cambridge, Mass.: Winthrop.

Spender, D. (1982) *Invisible women: the schooling scandal*. London: Writers and Readers Publishing Cooperative.

Spender, D. & Sarah, E. (1980) *Learning to lose*. London: The Women's Press.

Stanworth, M. (1983) *Gender and schooling*. London: Hutchinson.

Sutherland, M. (1981) *Sex bias in education*. Oxford: Blackwell.

Weiner, B. (1974) *Achievement motivation and attribution theory*. Morristown, N.J.: General Learning Press.

Weiner, B. (1979) A theory of motivation for some classroom experiences. *Journal of Educational Psychology*, *71*, 3–25.

Weiner, B. (1980) *Human motivation*. New York: Holt, Rinehart & Winston.

Weiner, B. (1984) Principles for a theory of student motivation. *In* R. Ames & C. Ames *Research on motivation in education*: vol 1 *Student motivation*. London: Academic Press.

CHAPTER NINE Sex Roles in Adolescence
Clive R. Hollin

The principal difficulty with the topic of adolescence is the lack of a satisfactory definition of the term. Perusal of several basic texts (Adelson 1980; Muuss 1962; Rogers 1972) reveals a variety of approaches to adolescence. It can simply be defined in terms of chronological age; or as a time of physiological change; or as a period when certain moral and cognitive developmental stages are reached. Psychological thought on adolescence follows a number of approaches; psychodynamic theory (e.g. Freud 1966) psychophysiological theory (e.g. Peterson & Taylor 1980), and social learning theory (e.g. McCandless 1970) have all been utilized to explain adolescence. However, looking at the historical picture (Aries 1962; Elder 1980; Muncie 1984) it is clear that adolescence, indeed childhood, is not the sole province of psychological inquiry. Adolescents are a relatively recently created social group, the product of an affluent mid-eighteenth-century society where a falling infant mortality rate, a corresponding growing population, and the need for a smaller workforce, resulted in a surplus of young people. Alongside a number of legal and educational changes, this newly formed social group was gradually absorbed into the economy so that now the adolescent or 'teenage' market is an integral part of the Western financial system. In any theory of adolescence it is therefore evident that sociological factors must be included (see Gillis 1974). Thus Muncie (1984) has expressed concern about:

> The many attempts of psychologists to 'discover' the distinguishing features of adolescence. 'Identity confusion', 'schizoid characteristics', 'ego experimentation', 'psychological disequilibrium', 'a second period of negativism' and 'ideological instability' are just a few of the bewildering array of concepts that have been invented to pin down new and disturbing aspects of this stage of life. (p. 46)

Whilst psychological theorizing may well be more confusing than explanatory, the fact remains that there is a time in human development when particular biological changes occur. These pubertal changes take place between the age of ten and seventeen years for the majority of the population, with males typically two years behind females (Peterson &

Taylor 1980). I have therefore pragmatically chosen age to define adolescence here, only considering studies which have sampled a population between ten and seventeen years of age. Finally, in structuring this chapter I have borrowed from the A: B: C model familiar in behavioural theory (Skinner 1953). If the *B*ehaviour is taken to be the sex roles, then the *A*ntecedent conditions are those which nurture their development, and finally there are the *C*onsequences which result from their presence. To follow this model we begin with the Antecedent or setting conditions for the development of sex roles in adolescence.

The development of sex roles in adolescence

Contemporary theory strongly holds that gender identity is formed in the first years of life (see Maccoby & Jacklin 1974); from that early stage of being designated as 'male' or 'female' we act appropriately, and reap the due rewards and punishments. Thus the distal antecedents for sex roles can be traced back to childhood: discussion of early sex-role development and socialization is presented in Part 2 of this book and in a number of recent publications (Archer 1984; Archer & Lloyd 1982; Best *et al*. 1977; Kuhn, Nash, & Bruchan 1978; Pitcher & Schultz 1983; Wittig 1983). When adolescence is reached, a considerable amount of sex-role development has already taken place; but a number of writers suggest that 'late childhood' or 'early adolescence' heralds a new phase in sex-role development and therefore these proximal antecedents merit attention.

Pleck (1975) took the theoretical position that in early adolescence there is a 'developmental phase of traditional masculinity-femininity development' (p. 173). That is, it is suggested that during this developmental stage, adolescents are learning the rules of sex-role differentiation, and trying to make themselves and others conform to these perceived roles. Whilst this is a developmental advance, during this stage adolescents are rigid in their beliefs about gender appropriate rules, and are intolerant of deviations from the norm. Following this stage Pleck (1975) suggests that adolescents mature to a stage of 'psychological androgyny in accordance with their inner needs and temperaments' (p. 172). Ullian (1976) provided some support for this vew: it was found that at ten years of age rigid beliefs about masculinity and femininity are apparent, but by 14–16 years of age a more flexible belief system exists.

However, Archer and Lloyd (1982) were critical of this interpretation of the results, suggesting that they could be seen in terms of a series of gradual rather than discrete stages.

Emmerich and Shepard (1982) compared the interest preferences of males and females during late childhood (mean age 10.7 years), early adolescence (mean age 13.8 years), and late adolescence (mean age 16.7 years). Although the age trends were complex, and varied according to sex, race, cognitive maturity, and socioeconomic class, some clear differences in sex-differentiated preferences between groups were found. For some items (e.g. being a doctor) there was a clear bias (towards males) in late childhood which neutralized during adolescence. However, on other items (e.g. being a nurse) the bias (towards females) was consistent over all age groups. Emmerich and Shepard (1982) tentatively suggest that the age differences reflect sex-role developmental changes after late childhood; but, as they note, there may have been differences between groups *prior* to the study. Thus, whilst there is some support for the stage theory, the evidence is not conclusive.

Lerner, Sorell and Brackney (1981) offered a different theoretical view from that of Pleck: they suggested that rather than proceeding through fixed developmental stages, sex roles should be considered as 'reciprocally and plastically related to changing sociocultural and historical circumstances' (p. 721). In other words, we should look to changing environmental demands rather than phases of personal development for explanations of sex-role functioning in adolescence (also see Abrahams, Feldman & Nash 1978). Lerner, Sorell and Brackney interpret their own experimental findings with young adults in this light, but as a whole experimental evidence is limited. Lamke (1982a) tested both views on the basis of their respective predictions for levels of self-esteem in early adolescence (mean age 13.7 years). The findings supported the predictions made by the environmental model, calling into question the validity of the developmental stage model. Other studies have demonstrated the importance of environmental influences in the formation of sex roles. Television is one potent source of social influence and its effects on sex-role development are increasingly being studied (Jeffries-Fox & Jeffries-Fox 1981). A longitudinal study of adolescents by Morgan (1982) suggested that television has a causal influence on sex-role stereotypes for females, whilst for males this effect is only slight. Whether this is due to sex differences in development during adolescence, or reflects the content of the television programmes, or both, brings us back to the initial theoretical debate.

The family is an environment in which much learning takes place, and a number of studies have considered the role of the family in relation to sex roles. Rollins and White (1982) reviewed the evidence and concluded that the relationship between mothers' and daughters' sex-role attitudes would be influenced by the type of family environment. To test this hypothesis they examined the sex-role attitudes of mothers and daughters in families where the mother was permanently at home, or employed because of economic necessity, or employed from career choice. Sex-role attitudes were measured for the areas of marriage, children and careers. Significant correlations were found between mothers' and daughters' attitudes for all three areas regardless of family types (the only exception being for attitudes towards children in the 'career' families). A between-groups comparison of mothers' attitudes revealed that similar, more traditional, attitudes were held by the non-working and 'economic' working groups; the 'career' group held significantly less traditional attitudes. A similar between-groups analysis for the daughters' attitudes revealed an identical pattern of results. It is, however, unfortunate that fathers' attitudes were not also measured, as without this information the exact process of sex-role attitude formation cannot be judged.

Hertsgaard and Light (1984) tested the perceptions of 500 adolescent females of both their mothers and fathers. The females rated their mothers as significantly higher on femininity and fathers higher on masculinity (using the Personal Attributes Questionnaire (Spence, Helmreich & Stapp 1974)). The greatest differences were in rating mothers as more emotional and more aware of the feelings of others; and fathers as more independent, better able to cope with pressure, and feeling superior. Hertsgaard and Light (1984) conclude that adolescent girls perceive their parents as possessing stereotypical masculine and feminine traits. Thus, *if* sex roles are based on the same-sex parent they will mirror traditional values although, as Rollins and White (1982) demonstrated, this will be modified by the circumstances of the parents. More research addressing male as well as female perceptions is needed to add to our understanding of sex-role acquisition.

In summary, despite the history of research (Mussen 1961) it would be unwise to dismiss either 'stage' or 'environmental' theories at present. Indeed, the debate as to the relative importance of 'inner' cognitive process and 'outer' environmental events in determining human behaviour is not confined to the study of sex roles but is central to the whole of psychology. It can be speculated, however, that an interaction between the two views will eventually prove most productive. This may mean that physical and psychological changes at adolescence will modify sex roles, perhaps differently for males and females. However, exactly which aspects of learning are changed will depend on current social perspectives. The next section seeks to examine the content of sex-role stereotypes in adolescents.

Sex roles in adolescence

Some investigators have used sex role inventories to assess adolescent personality characteristics: Rudy's (1968) study is in this tradition. A sample of 120 male and female fourteen- and fifteen-year-olds completed a battery of scales, rating the desirability of attributes such as 'aggressive', 'proud', and 'stern'. It was found that the male subjects rated the 'masculine' attributes as significantly more desirable than the females' ratings of the 'feminine' attributes. However, there was no significant difference in the male and female subjects' ratings of the desirability of opposite sex attributes. Rudy suggests that this pattern of results reflects the social pressures, particularly for young males, to adopt stereotyped sex-role traits.

Whilst research of this type has led to greater sophistication in psychological assessment, it tells us little about what *behaviour*, rather than personality traits or personal values, is expected of males and females according to the stereotypes.

A number of attempts have been made to look for this type of information. Morgan (1982) used a five-item true-false scale of sex-role stereotypes which contained items such as 'By nature, women are happiest when they are making a home and caring for children'. Emmerich and Shepard (1982) used two types of scale: the first asked about preferences for interests and activities and the second for interpersonal qualities such as kindness and conformity. With an adolescent population they found that sex-stereotyped preferences were stronger among males than females on items concerned with fixing bikes and cars, playing rough team sports, becoming a nurse or a doctor, and doing well in science or mathematics. With the 'male' and 'female' interpersonal qualities no evidence of sex-role stereotyping was found.

Whilst there are several small-scale studies of the type noted above, a major investigation has been reported by Tittle (1981) and the results of this will be discussed in detail. Adolescents' beliefs about sex roles were examined in two ways. They were questioned about overall male and

Table 9.1 Mean responsibility ratings for family activities

	Sex of adolescent[a]	
Activity	*Female*	*Male*
Clean the house	2.7	2.5
Managing family money	3.2	3.4
Repairing household appliances	3.7	3.9
Mowing the lawn	3.7	4.1
Taking out garbage	3.4	3.6
Washing family car	3.4	3.7
Taking children to doctor	2.8	2.9
Earning salary to support family	3.4	3.8
Deciding when car needs tune-up	3.8	4.0
Teaching children sports	3.3	3.8
Fixing a broken lamp	3.7	3.9
Deciding to move to another city	3.1	3.2
Deciding to buy a large item (e.g. colour TV, washing machine)	3.0	3.1

Source: Adapted from Tittle (1981)
[a]n = 600

female responsibility for activities within a family with children; and about what percentage of responsibility the husband and wife should accept for three important family responsibilities. Firstly, the adolescents rated twenty activities on a scale from one to five, from 'Only a Woman's Responsibility' to 'Only a Man's Responsibility' (a rating of three indicates 'Could be either Person's Responsibility'). Significant sex differences were found on thirteen of the twenty-two items; these are shown in Table 9.1 along with the mean ratings for each sex. From Table 9.1 it is noticeable that in almost every case it is the females who give the less stereotyped response.

Secondly, the adolescents were asked to assign a 'percentage responsibility' for three major family activities. A clear pattern emerged: over the whole sample earning money was deemed the man's responsibility, keeping house was the woman's and caring for children was more equally divided (see Table 9.2). The only sex difference in these judgements was for earning money, with significantly more males (72.3 percent) than females (63.4 percent) assigning this as being a husband's responsibility.

Tittle (1981) summarizes her findings as follows: 'Overall, the attitudes towards sex roles still exhibit many of the traditional views of the appropriate roles for females and males in the family setting. These attitudes

Table 9.2   Mean percentage responsibilities for family activities

Activity	Percentage responsibility		
	Husband	*Wife*	*Other*
Earning money	67.8	32.1	—
Keeping house	34.8	63.6	1.9
Caring for children	43.4	55.3	1.2

Source: Adapted from Tittle (1981)

are found to be more conservative for adolescent males than adolescent females' (p. 245). This latter comment echoes an emerging trend in sex-role research (Archer 1984; Der-Karabetian & Smith 1977; Emmerich & Shepard 1982; Kriedberg, Butcher & White 1978).

In summary, there are several lines of related research. These concern the personal characteristics of masculinity, femininity, or androgyny; beliefs about the appropriate personal qualities of other males and females; and beliefs about what domestic and social activities are gender appropriate. Whilst not thoroughly researched, it seems that in adolescence all these aspects are relatively firmly fixed, especially so for males as regards stereotyping for activities.

The consequences of sex roles in adolescence

Sex-role stereotyping in adolescence has two direct consequences – on future adult development and on other aspects of adolescent functioning. Sex roles in adulthood are considered in Part 3 of this book and so we will concentrate here on the latter aspect. The range of variables studied in relation to sex roles is wide, covering a variety of individual and social factors (see Archer & Lloyd 1982; Hartnett, Boden & Fuller 1979; Lloyd & Archer 1976; Maccoby & Jacklin 1974): I have drawn them together here under the categories of psychological, behavioural and psychopathological consequences of sex roles in adolescence.

Psychological consequences

Expectations for family life   Bernard (1976) suggested that sex roles influence adolescent expectations for future marriage and children.

Table 9.3 Values associated with marriage and parenthood

Marriage values	
Female preferred	Financial security
	Emotional support
	Prestige
Male preferred	A normal life
	Your own home
	A feeling of leadership
Parenthood values	
Female preferred	Variety
	Friendship
	A chance to express love
Male preferred	Respect of others
	A stable marriage
	A tie to the future

Source: Adapted from Tittle (1981)

Support for his suggestion came from a study by Wrigley and Stokes (1977) which found the predicted correlation between sex-role ideology and expected number of children. Similarly Tittle (1981) asked adolescents at what age they expected to finish their education, marry, and have children. Whilst there was no sex difference in anticipated age at completing education, males expected to marry at a significantly later age than females (25.8 and 24.2 years). In keeping with this difference, males anticipated their first child at 27.2 years of age, compared with 26.1 years for females; and the second child was anticipated at 29.1 and 28.2 years for males and females respectively. Along with these differences, there were also significant sex differences in the values associated with marriage and parenthood. These are summarized in Table 9.3.

Thus it appears that adolescent females are ready to marry at an earlier age for reasons of support and security, whilst males wish to wait a little longer to establish their own territory, command the respect of others, and lead the family. The traditional stereotypes of the accommodating female and the dominant male appear from this to be alive and well.

Expectations of success and failure   Horner (1972, 1974) suggested that
in early life females acquire a 'motive to avoid success'. Central to this
thesis is the assumption that success is a male goal, and thus for females
success produces an approach-avoidance conflict. Success is desirable for
its associated rewards of achievement, finance, and so on; but is to be
avoided as it may lead to 'unfemininity' and social and sexual rejection.
This hypothesis has generated a great deal of research, and it is now
thought that the 'motive to avoid success' is both important and complex
(see Ward 1979).

Fear of success in adolescents was investigated by Viaene (1979) who
advanced the hypothesis that if success is not compatible with a feminine
sex role, then individuals high in femininity who achieve success will
attribute it to external causes such as luck or fate. Conversely, individuals with a masculine sex-role orientation will be more likely to
attribute success to their own ability. Female and male adolescents completed an experimental task (anagram solving) which could be
manipulated to produce success or failure. They also completed the Bem
Sex Role Inventory (BSRI) and a measure of locus of control (Rotter
1966). The results indicated that masculinity was positively associated
with success in terms of personal ability in three of the four study groups,
whilst femininity was only weakly associated with explanations relying on
personal ability. The findings for sex role identity were not strong, unlike
those for sex differences: males explained their performance in terms of
task difficulty, whilst females blamed lack of ability for failure. Viaene
(1979) comments that: 'It would seem that the degree of sex typing . . .
can hardly be considered a crucial factor in explaining sex differences in
causal attributions' (p. 132). These results fail to support those of many
previous studies: but this may well be because an adolescent rather than
an adult population was employed. O'Connell and Perez (1982) found
a *greater* fear of success in sixteen-year-olds than in twenty-year-olds,
but no sex differences were immediately apparent amongst these subjects. However, they also found that when the success or failure was
looked at in terms of being gender appropriate or inappropriate the
pattern of results then fitted the theoretical predictions.

The importance of whether the fear of success is for one's own sex or
for the opposite sex was emphasized in a study by Weinreich-Haste
(1984). Male and female adolescents (aged fifteen years) were given
stories to read and their task was to continue the story. The experimental
manipulation was whether the character in the story was working in a
sex-appropriate field – trainee nursing or trainee engineer. It was found

that in continuing the story the boys were more likely to predict failure, the girls more likely to predict success. Whilst fear of success was influenced by whether the stimulus was sex-appropriate, and also by whether the adolescent's mother was employed – introducing a new variable – no clear support for the fear of success hypothesis was found.

Clearly Horner's ideas may require some modification for adolescents, and it seems important that experimental studies must carefully consider the type of task employed. Additionally, it may be that fear of success changes over time, and Weinreich-Haste (1984) acknowledges this: 'Possibly there has been considerably more change in sex-role norms for girls, permitting them to succeed and to work in sex-inappropriate fields. As yet, boys may not fail or work in sex-inappropriate fields' (p. 262). It remains for future research to test this hypothesis.

Self-perception The way in which each of us constructs our self-image, or self-concept, is one of the fundamental questions philosphers and psychologists have considered for generations. Self-perception has been studied extensively in adolescents (e.g. Zigler & Child 1973) but it is only recently that it has been looked at in conjunction with sex roles. The aspect of self-perception which has received most attention in this line of research is *self-esteem* – our perception of our own worth and value.

Connell and Johnson (1970) found that adolescent males with high masculinity had greater self-esteem than low masculinity males and high femininity females. However, in females sex-role identification was not related to self-esteem. Connell and Johnson (1970) suggest that the masculine role may have a reward value greater than the feminine role, regardless of whether the role is adopted by a male or female. Spence and Helmreich (1978) found however that both masculinity and femininity showed a positive relationship to high levels of self-esteem for males and females. Wells (1980), using the original BSRI (Bem 1974) found that a masculine sex-role orientation was predictive of self-esteem for female adolescents; however, neither masculine nor feminine sex-role orientation was associated with self-esteem in male adolescents. Lamke (1982a) found that for both males and females, masculinity is related to high levels of self-esteem. Lamke (1982b) suggested that the discrepant results of Wells may have been due to the use of the original BSRI, since superseded by the improved short BSRI (Bem 1981). Using the short BSRI, Lamke (1982b) found that for both male and female adolescents a masculine sex-role orientation was predictive of high self-esteem.

Additionally, there was an indication of a relationship between femininity and self-esteem in the male adolescents. Massad (cited in Rust & McCraw 1984) found a similar pattern of results to Lamke. In male adolescents high masculinity was associated with high self-esteem; among female adolescents both high masculinity and high femininity were associated with high self-esteem. In agreement with the majority of previous studies, Rust and McCraw (1984) found that high levels of masculine sex-role orientation were associated with high levels of self-esteem for both male and female adolescents. High levels of femininity were related to significantly lower self-esteem in males but not females; at finding at variance with Lamke (1982b).

The general pattern of results for adolescents is similar to that found for older age groups (Silvern & Ryan 1979; Spence, Helmreich & Stapp 1975), suggesting that once formed the self-image remains stable, at least for self-esteem. The confusion over the pattern for the interaction between sex, sex-role identity, and self-esteem remains unresolved. The different findings may reflect the use of different inventories across studies, or cultural, racial, or socioeconomic differences between subject groups.

Whilst masculinity and androgyny appear to be related to high self-esteem, it would be erroneous to conclude that women with low masculinity are less well adjusted. Nielsen and Edwards' (1982) review and empirical evidence found: 'No difference in positive self-concept for women who perceived their feminine roles as liberal, those who saw their roles as traditional, and those who had a neutral orientation' (p. 547). This study was not conducted with adolescents, so until research is conducted the overall relationship between sex-role orientation, overall self-concept and psychological adjustment remains unclear.

Behavioural consequences

Career choice Sex differences in career aspirations and choice have been the subject of a great deal of empirical research (see Archer & Lloyd 1982; Marini 1978; Tittle 1981). The *processes* involved in determining career choice in relation to sex cover a wide range of social, political and economic forces (Oppenheimer 1975), whilst *values* about career choice are transmitted through familial processes (Berson 1979; Gettys & Cann 1981; Maccoby & Jacklin 1974; Peterson *et al.* 1982). Certain educational subjects have acquired a 'masculine' image, and others a 'feminine' image (Weinreich-Haste 1979), with corresponding examination performances from males and females (Murphy 1979). Indeed, the sex-typing of occupational choice has reached a level at which suggestions have been made for counselling to modify the aspirations of young women (Kenkel & Gage 1983).

Sex roles and career choice in adolescence has received considerably less attention than sex differences and career choice. Feather and Said (1983) carried out a study of sex, sex-role identity, ideal and realistic occupational choice, and rating of occupational choice for male dominance and status in a sample of Australian adolescents. A sex difference consistent with previous research (Helmreich, Spence & Holahan 1979) was found which was particularly strong for males: the males selected occupations perceived as male-dominated, whereas females made choices of 'feminine' occupations. The results for sex-role identity were not so pronounced. There was some indication that both feminine and masculine males were relatively more interested in occupations of higher male dominance, but the sex-role scores were only weakly related to the other dependent measures. Feather and Said (1983) suggest that this weak effect is consistent with other findings (e.g. Spence & Helmreich 1978, 1979; Wertheim, Widom & Wortzel 1978) and that it illustrates the theoretical point that 'sex role expectations and attitudes should be distinguished from the effects of instrumental and expressive personality traits when occupational choices are considered' (p. 113).

Delinquency The traditional view within criminology is that females are less delinquent than males (see Rutter & Giller 1983). However, recent trends in criminal activity, including adults as well as adolescents, indicate a shift to greater female involvement in some types of crime (see Norland & Shover 1977). Given the perception of law-breaking as a 'masculine' activity, the inference has been drawn that the increase in female criminal activity reflects a change in sex-role orientation in the female population (Jensen & Eve 1976; Weis 1976; Widom 1981). Indeed, there is considerable debate over the proposition that women's liberation is causally linked to crime, and violent crime in particular (Adler 1975; Smart 1977). In a well-argued discussion, Norland and Shover (1977) pointed out the theoretical flaws in such arguments, and also noted the absence of any empirical data. Since then McCord and Otten (1983) have conducted a large self-report survey, over a wide age range, and could find no support for the view that pro-feminist attitudes contributed to criminality. In a similar self-report study with young adults (mean age 18.8 years), however, Cullen, Golden and Cullen (1979) did find some support for the hypothesis of a relationship between sex-role and delinquency. They note: 'Independent of gender, male traits appear to contribute to delinquent involvement' (p. 308).

The empirical evidence with adolescent delinquents is limited. Mannarino and Marsh (1978) carried out the first experimental study with delinquent girls aged between thirteen and seventeen years. They compared a non-delinquent control group with a delinquent group in which the females were convicted for promiscuity or illicit sexual behaviour, and a second delinquent group where the offences – arson, theft, assault – were deemed 'anti-social'. The three groups completed the Gough Femininity Scale (Gough 1952) on which a high score indicates greater 'psychological femininity'. Whilst the 'sex' delinquents and non-delinquent controls scored very similarly on the scale, the 'anti-social' delinquents scored significantly lower than both other experimental groups. Mannarino and Marsh (1978) suggested that the 'overly masculine sex role of the anti-social delinquents' (p. 648) contributed towards their delinquency. There is a question mark over this assertion: the Gough scale specifically assesses *femininity*, and therefore it is a questionable assumption that low femininity is equivalent to masculinity. It would be more accurate to say that Mannarino and Marsh (1978) found low feminine sex-role orientation in anti-social delinquents. Thornton and James (1979) surveyed a sample of 978 male and female 13–19-year-olds on a range of variables including self-reported delinquency and the Masculine Gender Role Scale. As expected, they found a greater incidence of delinquency amongst the males. However, across the whole population, no relationship was found between level of delinquency and degree of masculinity. This finding is at odds with that of Mannarino and Marsh (1978), although this is probably explained by the different scales used in the two studies. As a whole, however, the evidence is extremely limited for young offenders.

Sexual behaviour   One of the stereotypes about adolescence, perhaps in keeping with the physiological changes taking place, is that it is a time of sexual awakening. Some adolescents do experience sexual activity, and Cvetkovich *et al.* (1978) investigated sex-role identity and sexual experience in a sample of American adolescents (aged 16–17 years). They found that sexually experienced female adolescents held more traditional views of the female role than non-experienced females, suggesting that 'The actives seemed to be liberal but not liberated' (p. 232). This finding, they further suggest, may indicate that some adolescent females use sexual activity to facilitate the process of identifying their sex-role and sexual identity.

A view advanced by a number of writers (e.g. Ausubel 1954; McCandless 1970) is that adolescent males approach relationships with a physical orientation, whilst females take an affectional orientation. McCabe and Collins (1979) suggested that for contemporary females this may not now be the case; individuals may vary in their approach to dating depending upon their sex-role orientation. Three Australian subject groups, aged 16–17 years, 19–20 years, and 24–25 years, completed the BSRI and a scale measuring 'dating orientation'. A clear relationship between sex-role identity and dating orientation emerged in the youngest age group: 'Irrespective of their biological sex, feminine adolescents do not generally desire as much sexual involvement as masculine or androgynous adolescents' (p. 419). Whilst adolescent males show a greater wish for physical involvement than females, this sex difference diminishes with age: the females show an increasing wish for physical involvement as age increases. Regardless of sex, age, or sex-role identity, the desire for more affection increased as commitment to a relationship grew. This casts doubts over the 'physical males' and 'affectional females' stereotype: initially males may have a greater desire than females for physical involvement, with the difference diminishing over time, but it appears that both sexes begin dating with an affectional orientation. McCabe and Collins (1979) add the caveat that their study was conducted with 'better-educated middle-class adolescents' and so the results may not generalize to other socioeconomic groups.

This point is reinforced by a second study by McCabe (1982), in which a much larger sample aged from sixteen to twenty-five years (n = 2,001) from varied backgrounds completed the same measures as in the 1979 study. A number of results of the previous study were replicated (although the data were not analysed according to age): those with masculine and androgynous sex-role identity wanted greater physical involvement than those with a feminine sex-role identity; males desired more physical intimacy than females (and were more permissive); and there was a strong effect of 'dating experience' so that both the desire and experience of intimacy was higher in both sexes at the later stages of dating. However, it was with regard to desire for affection that different findings emerged. Those with a feminine sex-role orientation expressed a greater wish for affection than those with a masculine sex role. Similarly, females expressed a greater wish for affection than males. On the basis of the improved sampling, McCabe (1982) is inclined to accept the latter study as stronger support for the view that the desire for affection is a feminine trait, so individuals with a feminine sex role will want a higher level of affection.

However, as McCabe (1982) did not analyse the data according to age, it is unknown whether all the findings would apply specifically to adolescents. So, with the additional proviso that both studies were conducted in Australia where cultural norms may be different to Britain, it does seem to be the case that adolescents approach their first relationships with expectations built on conventional stereotypes. It is heartening – or perhaps disheartening, depending on your point of view – that these notions are quickly modified with experience. This is an area ripe for more research, particularly regarding the link with social class noted by McCabe and Collins (1979).

Psychopathology

As with career choice there is a considerable body of research into sex differences in psychopathology (see Archer & Lloyd 1982; Maccoby & Jacklin 1974). Similarly, there is a large literature on psychopathology in adolescence (e.g. Evans 1982; Weiner 1982), which describes a number of sex differences in types of adolescent psychopathology. However, to the best of my knowledge, there is no research which has specifically addressed the influence of sex roles in adolescent psychopathology. This may well be a potentially fruitful field for research, especially in areas such as eating disorders where there is thought to be an aetiological relationship between the disorder, pubertal physiological changes and sexual identity (Garfinkel & Garner 1982).

Research into sex-role identity and personal adjustment has not, as yet, considered specific adolescent psychopathologies but has concentrated upon constructs such as 'personal adjustment' and 'psychological health'. This line of investigation is well-founded for older populations (Orlofsky & Windle 1978; Selva & Dusek 1984; Small, Teagno & Selz 1980), although it is only more recently that adolescent populations have been studied. Keyes and Coleman (1983) hypothesized that during adolescence females are confronted with societal pressure to subdue the 'masculine' traits of independence and achievement in favour of more acceptable 'feminine' traits such as submissiveness (Douvan 1979). Thus the adolescent female, especially if high achieving, is plunged into a position of conflict not experienced by the male adolescent. This sex-role conflict, it is suggested, may be manifested by an increase in psychological stress. Keyes and Coleman (1983) set out to test whether adolescent females experienced more conflict and problems with personal adjustment than male adolescents; and whether adolescents experiencing sex-role conflict show less optimal personal adjustment. Subjects completed the Texas Social Behaviour Inventory (TSBI) (Helmreich, Stapp & Ervin 1974) as a measure of personal adjustment; the General Health Questionnaire (GHQ) (Goldberg 1972); 'real', 'ideal', and 'society expects' ratings on the PAQ; and note of educational ambition was also made. Differences between the three ratings on the PAQ were used to gauge sex-role conflict.

The results failed to show any sex differences on personal adjustment, although there were some differences in sex-role conflict. Overall, females appeared to experience more conflict over sex roles, particularly on masculine PAQ items; however, there was also evidence of male conflict on some PAQ ratings. No relationship was evident between high academic ambition and personal adjustment for either sex. There was, however, considerable support for the proposition that sex-role conflict would be related to personal adjustment. Adolescents of both sexes who reported the highest levels of sex-role conflict also showed the lowest levels of self-esteem and the highest levels of physical and psychological malaise. This study therefore illustrates that both sexes experience sex-role conflict and that this conflict is related to personal adjustment. In a further study of the relationship between gender stereotypes and personal adjustment Keyes (1984) found that, using both the TSBI and GHQ, androgynous adolescents showed the lowest levels of malaise. The highest malaise scores were found in male and female adolescents characterized as feminine in sex-role orientation, with the effect being strongest in the males. Overall, however, whilst the first steps have been taken, knowledge is limited. It remains for future research to determine the exact qualitative nature of the relationship between sex-role conflict and adjustment, with respect to both specific psychopathologies and the future development of adolescents experiencing the conflict.

Conclusion

Throughout this chapter the comment has repeatedly been made that very little is understood about sex roles in adolescence. This reflects, I suggest, the relative recency of the growth of interest in sex roles, and the large number of variables which may be associated with them. There is a very real danger that what little knowledge we possess may be applied prematurely. The call has gone out, and programmes have been designed, to change 'unsuitable ' sex-roles: in an area where understanding is so limited this strategy is fraught with obvious danger, perhaps especially so with children and adolescents. A great deal more empirically based knowledge about the antecedents and consequences of sex-role development in adolescence is required before attempts at change are even considered.

References

Abrahams, B., Feldman, S. S. & Nash, S. C. (1978) Sex role self-concept and sex role attitudes: enduring personality characteristics or adaptions to changing life situations? *Developmental Psychology, 14*, 393–400.

Adelson, J. (ed.) (1980) *Handbook of adolescent psychology.* New York: John Wiley.

Adler, R. (1975) *Sisters in crime: the rise of the new female criminal.* New York: McGraw-Hill.

Archer, J. (1984) Gender roles as developmental pathways. *British Journal of Social Psychology, 23*, 245–256.

Archer, J. & Lloyd, B. (1982) *Sex and gender.* Harmondsworth: Penguin.

Aries, P. (1962) *Centuries of childhood.* London: Jonathan Cape.

Ausubel, D. P. (1954) *Theory and problems of adolescent development.* New York: Grune & Stratton.

Bem, S. L. (1974) The measurement of psychological androgny. *Journal of Consulting and Clinical Psychology, 42*, 155–162.

Bem, S. L. (1981) *Bem sex-role inventory professional manual.* Palo Alto, California: Consulting Psychologists Press.

Bernard, J. (1976) Change and stability in sex-role norms and behaviour. *Journal of Social Issues, 32*, 207–233.

Berson, J. S. (1979) Perceived costs of combining career and family roles: the influence of early family history on adult role decisions. *In* O. Hartnett, G. Boden & M. Fuller (eds) *Women: sex-role stereotyping.* London: Tavistock Publications.

Best, D. L., Williams, J. E., Cloud, J. M., Davis, S. W., Robertson, L. S., Edwards, J. R., Giles, H. & Fowles, J. (1977) Development of sex-trait stereotypes among young children in the United States, England, and Ireland. *Child Development, 48*, 1375–1384.

Connell, D. M. & Johnson, J. E. (1970) Relationship between sex-role identification and self-esteem in early adolescence. *Developmental Psychology*, *3*, 268.

Cullen, F. T., Golden, K. M. & Cullen, J. B. (1979) Sex and delinquency: partial test of the masculinity hypothesis. *Criminology*, *17*, 301–310.

Cvetkovich, B. G., Grote, B., Lieberman, E. J. & Miller, W. (1978). Sex role development and teenage fertility-related behaviour. *Adolescence*, *13*, 231–236.

Der-Karabetian, A. & Smith A. J. (1977) Sex-role stereotyping in the United States: is it changing? *Sex Roles*, *3*, 193–198.

Douvan, E. (1979) Sex role learning. *In* J. Coleman (ed.) *The school years*. London: Methuen.

Elder, G. H. (1980) Adolescence in historical perspective. *In* J. Adelson (ed.) *Handbook of adolescent psychology*. New York: John Wiley.

Emmerich, W. & Shepard, K. (1982) Development of sex-differentiated preferences during late childhood and adolescence. *Developmental Psychology*, *18*, 406–417.

Evans, J. (1982) *Adolescent and pre-adolescent psychiatry*. London: Academic Press.

Feather, N. T. & Said, J. A. (1983) Preference for occupations in relation to masculinity, femininity, and gender. *British Journal of Social Psychology*, *22*, 113–127.

Freud, A. (1966) Instinctual anxiety during puberty. *The writings of Anna Freud; the ego and the mechanisms of defence*, revised edn. New York: International Universities Press.

Garfinkel, P. E. & Garner, D.M. (1982) *Anorexia nervosa: a multidimensional approach*. New York: Brunner/Mazel.

Gettys, L. D. & Cann, A. (1981) Children's perceptions of occupational stereotypes. *Sex Roles*, *7*, 301–308.

Gillis, J. R. (1974) *Youth and history*. London: Academic Press.

Goldberg, D. P. (1972) *The detection of psychiatric illness by questionnaire: a technique for the identification and detection of non-psychotic illness*. Institute of Psychiatry, Maudsley Monographs, No. 21. London: Oxford University Press.

Gough, H. (1952) *The adjective check list*. Palo Alto, California: Consulting Psychologists Press.

Hartnett, O., Boden, G. & Fuller, M. (1979) *Women: sex-role stereotyping*. London: Tavistock Publications.

Helmreich, R. L., Spence, J. T. & Holahan, C. K. (1979) Psychological androgyny and sex role flexibility: a test of two hypotheses. *Journal of Personality and Social Psychology*, *37*, 1631–1644.

Helmreich, R., Stapp, J. & Ervin, C. (1974) The Texas Social Behaviour Inventory (TSBI): an objective measure of self-esteem or social competence. *JSAS Catalogue of Selected Documents in Psychology*, *4*, 79.

Hertsgaard, D. & Light, H. (1984) Adolescent females' perceived parental sex-role attributes. *Psychological Reports*, *55*, 253–254.

Horner, M. S. (1972) Motive to avoid success and changing aspirations of women. *In* J. Bardwick (ed.) *Readings on the psychology of women*. New York: Harper & Row.

Horner, M. S. (1974) The measurement and behavioural implications of fear of success in women. *In* J. Atkinson & J. Raynor (eds) *Motivation and achievement.* New York: John Wiley.

Jeffries-Fox, S. & Jeffries-Fox, B. (1981) Gender differences in socialisation through television to occupational roles: an exploratory approach. *Journal of Early Adolescence, 1*, 293–302.

Jensen, G. & Eve, R. (1976) Sex differences in delinquency: an examination of popular sociological explanations. *Criminology, 34*, 427–448.

Kenkel, W. F. & Gage, B. A. (1983) The restricted and gender-typed occupational aspirations of young women: can they be modified? *Family Relations, 32*, 129–138.

Keyes, S. (1984) Gender stereotypes and personal adjustment: employing the PAQ, TSBI and GHQ with sample of British adolescents. *British Journal of Social Psychology, 23*, 173–180.

Keyes, S. & Coleman, J. (1983) Sex-role conflicts and personal adjustment: a study of British adolescents. *Journal of Youth and Adolescence, 12*, 443–459.

Kriedberg, G., Butcher, A. L. & White, K. M. (1978) Vocational role choice in second- and sixth-grade children. *Sex Roles, 4*, 175–181.

Kuhn, D., Nash, S. C. & Bruchan, L. (1978) Sex-roles concepts of two- and three-year-olds. *Child Development, 49*, 445–451.

Lamke, L. K. (1982a) The impact of sex-role orientation on self-esteem in early adolescence. *Child Development, 53*, 1530–1535.

Lamke, L. K. (1982b) Adjustment and sex-role orientation in adolescence. *Journal of Youth and Adolescence, 11*, 247–259.

Lerner, R. M., Sorrell, G. T. & Brackney, B. W. (1981) Sex differences in self-concept and self-esteem of late adolescents: a time-lag analysis. *Sex Roles, 7*, 709–722.

Lloyd, B. B. & Archer, J. (eds.) (1976) *Exploring sex differences.* London: Academic Press.

McCabe, M. P. (1982) The influence of sex and sex role on the dating attitudes and behaviors of Australian youth. *Journal of Adolescent Health Care, 3*, 29–36.

McCabe, M. P. & Collins, J. K. (1979) Sex role and dating orientation. *Journal of Youth and Adolescence, 8*, 407–425.

McCandless, B. R. (1970) *Adolescents: behaviour and development.* Hinsdale, Illinois: Dryden Press.

McCord, J. & Otten, L. (1983) A consideration of sex roles and motivations for crime. *Criminal Justice and Behaviour, 10*, 3–12.

Maccoby, E. E. & Jacklin, C. N. (1974) *The psychology of sex differences.* Stanford: Stanford University Press.

Mannarino, A. & Marsh, M. (1978) The relationship between sex role identification and juvenile delinquency in adolescent girls. *Adolescence, 13*, 643–652.

Marini, M. M. (1978) Sex differences in the determination of adolescent aspirations: a review of research. *Sex Roles, 4*, 723–753.

Morgan, M. (1982) Television and adolescents' sex role stereotypes: a longitudinal study. *Personality and Social Psychology, 43*, 947–955.

Muncie, J. (1984) *'The trouble with kids today': youth and crime in post-war Britain.* London: Hutchinson.

Murphy, R. J. L. (1979) Sex differences in examination performance: do these reflect differences in ability or sex-role stereotypes? *In* O. Hartnett, G. Boden & M. Fuller (eds) *Women: sex-role stereotyping*. London: Tavistock Publications.

Mussen, P. (1961) Some antecedents and consequents of masculine sex-typing an adolescent boys. *Psychological Monographs: General and Applied*, *75*, Whole No. 506.

Muuss, R. E. (1962) *Theories of adolescence*. New York: Random House.

Nielsen, E. C. & Edwards, J. (1982) Perceived feminine role orientation and self-concept. *Human Relations*, *35*, 547–558.

Norland, S. & Shover, N. (1977) Gender roles and female criminality: some critical comments. *Criminology*, *15*, 87–104.

O'Connell, A. N. & Perez, S. (1982) Fear of success and causal attributions of success and failure in high school and college students. *Journal of Psychology*, *111*, 141–151.

Oppenheimer, V. K. (1975) The sex-labeling of jobs. *In* M. T.S. Mednick, S. S. Tangi & L. W. Hoffman (eds.) *Women and achievement: social and motivational analyses*. New York: Halsted Press.

Orlofsky, J. L. & Windle, M. T. (1978) Sex-role orientation, behavioural adaptability and personal adjustment. *Sex Roles*, *4*, 801–811.

Peterson, A. C. & Taylor, B. (1980) The biological approach to adolescence. *In* J. Adelson (ed.) *Handbook of adolescent psychology*. New York: John Wiley.

Peterson, G. W., Rollins, B. C., Thomas, D. L. & Heaps, L. K. (1982) Social placements of adolescents: sex-role influence on family decisions regarding the careers of youth. *Journal of Marriage and the Family*, *44*, 647–658.

Pitcher, E. G. & Schultz, L. H. (1983) *Boys and girls at play: the development of sex roles*. New York: Praeger.

Pleck, J. H. (1975) Masculinity-femininity: current and alternative paradigms. *Sex Roles*, *1*, 161–177.

Rogers, D. (1972) *The psychology of adolescence*. New York: Appleton-Century-Crofts.

Rollins, J. & White, P. N. (1982) The relationship between mothers' and daughters' sex-role attributes and self concepts in three types of family environment. *Sex Roles*, *8*, 1141–1155.

Rotter, J. B. (1966) Generalised expectancies for internal versus external control of reinforcement. *Psychological Monographs*, *80*, Whole No. 609.

Rudy, A. J. (1968) Sex-role perceptions in early adolescence. *Adolescence*, *3*, 453–470.

Rust, J. O. & McCraw, A. (1984) Influence of masculinity femininity on adolescent self-esteem and peer acceptance. *Adolescence*, *14*, 359–366.

Rutter, M. & Giller, H. (1983) *Juvenile delinquency: trends and perspectives*. Harmondsworth: Penguin.

Selva, P. D. & Dusek, J. B. (1984) Sex role orientation and resolution of Eriksonian crises during the late adolescent years. *Journal of Personality and Social Psychology*, *57*, 204–212.

Silvern, L. E. & Ryan, V. L. (1979) Self-rated adjustment and sex-typing on the Bem Sex Role Inventory: is masculinity the primary predictor of adjustment? *Sex Roles*, *5*, 739–763.

Skinner, B. F. (1953) *Science and human behaviour*. London: Collier-Macmillan.

Small, A., Teagno, L. & Selz, K. (1980) The relationship of sex role to physical and psychological health. *Journal of Youth and Adolescence, 9*, 305–314.

Smart, C. (1977) *Women, crime and criminology: a feminist critique*. Boston: Routledge & Kegan Paul.

Spence, J. & Helmreich, H. (1978) *Masculinity and femininity: their psychological dimensions, correlates, and antecedents*. Austin: University of Texas Press.

Spence, J. & Helmreich, R. (1979) Comparison of masculine and feminine personality attributes and sex-role attitudes across age groups. *Developmental Psychology, 15*, 583–584.

Spence, J., Helmreich, R. & Stapp, J. (1974) The Personal Attributes Questionnaire: a measure of sex role stereotypes and masculinity-femininity. *JSAS Catalogue of Selected Documents in Psychology, 4*, 43.

Spence, J., Helmreich, R. & Stapp, J. (1975) Ratings of self and peers on sex role attributions and their relation to self-esteem and conceptions of masculinity and femininity. *Journal of Personality and Social Psychology, 32*, 29–39.

Thornton, W. E. & James, J. (1979) Masculinity and delinquency revisited. *British Journal of Criminology, 19*, 225–241.

Tittle, C. K. (1981) *Careers and family: sex roles and adolescent life plans*. Beverly Hills: Sage Publications.

Ullian, D. Z. (1976) The development of conceptions of masculinity and femininity. In B. B. Lloyd & J. Archer (eds.) *Exploring sex differences*. London: Academic Press.

Viaene, N. (1979) Sex differences in explanations of success and failure. *In* O. Hartnett, G. Boden & M. Fuller (eds) *Women: sex-role stereotyping*. London: Tavistock Publications.

Ward, C. (1979) Is there a motive in women to avoid success? *In* O. Hartnett, G. Boden & M. Fuller (eds) *Women: sex role stereotyping*. London: Tavistock Publications.

Weiner, I. B. (1982) *Child and adolescent psychopathology*. New York: John Wiley.

Weinreich-Haste, H. (1979) What sex is science? *In* O. Hartnett, G. Boden & M. Fuller (eds) *Women: sex-role stereotyping*. London: Tavistock Publications.

Weinreich-Haste, H. (1984) Cynical boys, determined girls? Success and failure anxiety in British adolescents. *British Journal of Social Psychology, 23*, 257–263.

Weis, J. C. (1976) Liberation and crime: the invention of the new female criminal. *Crime and social justice, 6*, 17–27.

Wells, K. (1980). Gender-role identity and psychological adjustment in adolescence. *Journal of Youth and Adolescence, 9*, 59–73.

Wertheim, E. G., Widom, C. S. & Wortzel, L. H. (1978) Multivariate analysis of male and female professional career choice correlates. *Journal of Applied Psychology, 63*, 234–242.

Widom, C. S. (1981) Perspectives of female criminality: a critical examination of assumptions. *In* A. Morris & L. Gelsthorpe (eds) *Women and crime*. Cambridge: Institute of Criminology.

Wittig, M. A. (1983) Sex role development in early adolescence. *Theory into Practice*, *22*, 105–111.

Wrigley, A. P. & Stokes, C. S. (1977) Sex role ideology, selected life plans, and family size preferences: further evidence. *Journal of Comparative Family Studies*, *8*, 391–400.

Zigler, E. & Child, K. (1973) *Socialisation and personality development*. Reading, Mass.: Addison-Wesley.

PART III

SEX ROLES IN ADULTHOOD

CHAPTER TEN   Sex Roles and the Mass Media
Kevin Durkin

British television viewers have for over twenty years enjoyed a weekly programme called *Top of the Pops*, which is devoted to the current popular music. The format of the programme has remained relatively constant over the years, consisting of short presentations of 'live' or video recorded renditions of the latest hit records, interspersed with brief overviews of the rank-ordered sales achievements of the industry's stars. The programme is recorded in a studio complete with an audience of young people dancing to the music and, from time to time, the cameras pan the audience. When this happens, at least one camera is usually located very low, thus affording a generally upwards perspective on the legs and undergarments of the female participants.

Social scientists who have been studying the programme's enduring services to Western youth culture since its inception are aware that this particular camera technique was an innovation which coincided with the advent of the mini-skirt during the late 1960s. Presumably, the retention of the sub-ankle camera in the face of the fluctuating location of hemlines since that time owes a little to the perseverance of the accommodations made by the medium to the culture, and much to the optimism of the cameramen.

It is difficult to tell what contribution this aspect of *Top of the Pops* has made to the enormous popularity of the programme, which regularly attracts audiences of several millions. It is interesting to reflect, however, that this minor voyeurism has been a part of family life for a couple of decades, and hence part of the sociocultural contexts in which countless people have passed through their adolescence. It is also obvious to anyone familiar with the mass media that *Top of the Pops* is not unique in the perspective it favours on women's bodies. Many television programmes and films, most newspapers, and large numbers of magazines devote considerable attention to female thighs and breasts. The proverbial visitor from Mars would find much evidence that we attach great significance to these physical components of this subset of our species, and perhaps rather less to others.

Probing a little further, the Martian would discover that the other gender category on this dichotomized planet has a somewhat different relationship to the media. First he is portrayed in a wider range of contexts, with some emphasis upon physical properties and competence but much also upon his psychological suitability for mastering the environment. Second, the other gender actually does seem to have had more success in mastering the environment, and this is reflected in the predominance of males in running the media: for example, they control where the lens points during *Top of the Pops*. The Martian might wonder how all of this came about and how the system perpetuates itself and ensures that new members adapt satisfactorily to it.

Several contributors to this volume address questions concerned with the origins and continuities of the human sex-role system. This chapter will focus on just one feature of these complex processes, and that is the part played by the mass media in transmitting and encouraging particular conceptions of the sexes and their potentialities. It will begin by summarizing what we know of the content of the media with respect to sex roles and will then turn to the rather more difficult question that occurred to our Martian: how might this contribute to the functioning of the system in general? Finally, we will consider what happens when the content is changed, so that the media are used to promote portrayals of non-traditional male and female roles.

The portrayal of females and males in the mass media

The mass media present the sexes in markedly different ways. There are of course differences between the sexes, and certain types of media coverage, such as that favoured by the *Top of the Pops* cameramen, or the *Benny Hill Show*, reveal some of these with enthusiastic attention to detail. However, the overall concerns of the media rarely seem to be the provision of a veridical account of human beings and the actual distributions of their diverse properties. Instead, the media select certain categories of people and certain forms of behaviour for particular emphasis and derogate others by acknowledging them infrequently and/or unfavourably.

For example, although in most populations women slightly outnumber men, the mass media present radically different sex ratios. In most areas of television entertainment, males outnumber women by about 70:30 (Durkin 1985a). Men are more likely to be shown as stars (Dominick 1979) and they perform the vast majority of the voiceovers in commercials (McArthur & Resko 1975; Manstead & McCulloch 1981). Men form a higher proportion of the leading characters in films (Butler & Paisley 1980) and male characters and masculine themes dominate children's fictional literature (Braman 1977; Butler & Paisley 1980). In newspapers, 81 percent of photographs include men, 30 percent include women, and male figures are paramount in the front page, the inside news sections, the business sections and the sports sections (Miller 1975). Even the obituary columns devote more space to male demise (over 80 percent, according to Miller (1975). Readers of the present volume who are studying a discipline which is pursued by more females than males in most undergraduate settings, may find it especially interesting to reflect that psychology textbooks have been found to use more male examples and sources than either general population distributions or researchers' gender would predict (see Birk *et al.* 1974, cited in Butler & Paisley 1980, p. 124).

Numerical imbalance is a gross reflection of the differential values that the media attach to men and women, but there are many other indicators at varying levels of subtlety. A reasonably obvious one is the age distribution of males and females: in general women are shown in a quite narrow age band, up to about thirty years in much of television (Aronoff 1974), magazines and films (Butler & Paisley 1980), while the male age range extends much higher, and it is quite common to encounter older men in the media who enjoy prestige and attractiveness (Butler & Paisley 1980; Durkin, 1985a; Harris & Feinberg 1977). Correlated, unsurprisingly, with this factor is the widespread emphasis upon female physical attractiveness and the use of beautiful young women to support images of powerful men in films and TV (Butler & Paisley 1980; Durkin, 1985b) and to add sexual decoration, often irrelevent to the product, in advertisements in magazines and newspapers (Butler & Paisley 1980; Sexton & Haberman 1974).

Only slightly less noticeable to the untrained eye is the variation in occupational and social status accorded to males and females in fictional media. Men are more often shown employed in settings outside of the home and often in high-status and dynamic jobs, while women are cast in a narrow range of occupations, most commonly those of housewife, nurse, secretary and air stewardess (Butler & Paisley 1980; Durkin 1985a). In newspaper reports, women's marital status and hair colour are often mentioned, irrespective of the relevance of these data to the specific individuals involvement in the news item (Foreit *et al.* 1980). Many nonfictional media roles, such as quiz show presenters (Karpf 1980), weather forecasters (Durkin 1985c), and radio DJs (Karpf 1980) are presented predominantly or exclusively by men.

When the behaviour and settings of the males and females shown in the various media are analysed, yet more predictable differences emerge. Men are shown as more aggressive and autonomous (Gerbner 1972; Hodges, Brandt & Kline 1981) and more likely to be dominant over females than to be dominated by them (Lemon 1977). Females tend to be shown with superior nurturant and empathetic abilities (Harvey, Sprafkin & Rubinstein 1979). Parents and children perusing toy catalogues are likely to find that stereotypes are endorsed there by the depiction of child models playing with the toys traditionally deemed appropriate to their sex (Schwartz & Markham 1985), and even the background music of TV ads for toys have been found to vary in dramatic style according to sex typing of product (Welch *et al.* 1979).

The mass media are clearly rich in highly traditional sex-role stereotypes and they are evidently biased towards an overrepresentation of what we might loosely call a 'man's world'. However, with the possible exception of men's sex magazines, most media attend sometimes to issues of women's rights and feminism. There are several well-known popular books on feminist topics, there are a number of feminist novelists in the best selling lists, and feminist discussions or plays are occasionally broadcast on TV and radio. Yet although these minority expressions in the mass media may be explicitly committed to undermining the *status quo* and redressing the balance, there is unsystematic but persuasive evidence that the broader context of media representation provides strategies that promote the depiction of these as eccentric or lunatic fringe endeavours.

For example, feminist TV characters are sometimes given jargon-ridden scripts, making them easy prey for neighbouring media such as TV critics in newspapers (see Baehr 1980). Similarly, attention to women's issues can be 'ghettoized' in the press by allocation to particular pages or columns (Baehr 1980), and contentious positions voiced in discussion programmes can be 'neutralized' by subsuming them in the 'cosy, reassuring tone' of afternoon radio chat shows for women (Karpf 1980). When charges of sexism are raised against the media, they often respond by belittling the attack and trivializing the issues. In 1985 a complaint by a British Labour MP that a TV commercial for British Caledonian, in which male passengers sing about the charms of the airline's stewardesses, was sexist, led to much scorn within the media. Within a day the chat show host Terry Wogan led a string of the company's female cabin staff in uniform on to his programme to ask whether they felt the advertisement was demeaning to women. Needless to say, they did not. (Male cabin staff were not consulted at all about their exclusion from the advertisement.) Because TV commercials are ephemeral, and commonly acknowledged to bear only a fragile correspondence with reality, and because Mr Wogan's show is an early evening light entertainment slot, and because the pleasant-looking young women seemed perfectly happy with their 'fly me' image, it would involve access to either a feminist consciousness or a critical body of social science literature to resist the conclusion that the MP was getting heated up about a quite trivial issue. By the time *Top of the Pops* came on, one would imagine that many viewers would have forgotten the matter altogether.

To sum up, the media do not treat the sexes equally.They pay more attention to men and aggrandize those members of this sex who achieve economic, political or physical dominance over others. They underrepresent women (though within the sex they overrepresent high socioeconomic status), and they often reveal preoccupations with female sexual properties at the expense of other attributes. The mass media are vast and pluralistic enterprises, and do afford some space to occasional exceptions to these generalizations and to some dissenters, but their exceptionality itself reflects what are the dominant patterns – and it also seems that the media have ways of overwhelming irregularities.

The consequences

Most of the research to date on sex roles in the mass media has been concerned with content, and only a summary of this wide-ranging literature was attempted in the preceding section. The summary serves to indicate what is *transmitted* by the media, and this is an interesting topic in its own right. I have not dealt here with the question of *why* this content takes the form it does, partly because it seems obvious that the transmission reflects the characteristics and interests of those who control the machinery itself, but partly because the main contribution that psychologists can hope to make to this topic is to uncover the processes of *reception*. That is, our proper concern as a discipline is the question of how human beings discern, encode and respond to information available in their environments.

Unfortunately, with respect to sex roles in the mass media, these process issues turn out to be much more difficult and less immediately rewarding than the study of content. For this reason, there is more speculation than evidence available when we turn to the question of the consequences of using sex-stereotyped media and, still more problematically, much of the speculation is based upon atheoretical assumptions that do not easily find support in what psychologists know of human information acquisition and social behaviour.

For example, a frequent assertion in many feminist discussions of the topic is that the media 'condition' people to adopt particular views of the world, and this shapes them to behave in role-appropriate ways. While this is an understandable anxiety given the sheer volume of distortion inherent in the media that pervade our lives, it is not a very illuminating way of accounting for the complexities of human development. It can lead both to understatement of the phenomena requiring attention and to a metaphor of personal adjustment which is as demeaning of human subjects as the traditional stereotypes themselves. Hence, by assuming that the consequences of the media can be diagnosed as 'conditioning' we may fail to analyse the problem adequately and thus limit the prospects for 'cure'. After all, once people of either sex have been reduced to the conceptual status of arbitrarily shaped plastic, then the demand for and quality of methods to 'reshape' them scarcely appear profound or pressing concerns.

There are very difficult methodological and measurement problems involved in attempting to gauge the impact of the mass media upon people's social attitudes and behaviour. A fundamental difficulty is that so many media are integrated into our lives in so many ways, that any attempt to evaluate the functions of one of them is confounded by the co-occurrence of the others. As other contributors to this volume attest, there are many other sources of potential influence concerning sex role allocations, and these too co-occur with any media presence. Equally perplexing is the sheer breadth of the audience, people themselves, who exhibit such diversity in terms of demographic characteristics, social orientation and developmental status that it soon becomes apparent that it is naïve to think of the mass media as having an homogeneous 'effect' upon all of them.

Several researchers have attempted to measure the relationship between consumption of a particular mass medium and the strength of the individual's traditional sex-role beliefs. Most of these have been concerned with television viewers, including young children (Frueh & McGhee 1975), adolescents (Morgan 1982), and adults (Gunter & Wober

1982). None of these, or any other published study as far as I am aware, has found a strong, positive relationship between amount of viewing and sex-role beliefs. Indeed, Gunter and Wober (1982) found that on *some* measures heavy viewers of action-drama programmes had slightly more positive attitudes towards women than did light viewers. Some studies, such as that of Frueh and McGhee (1975), which report modest associations between viewing and traditional beliefs, are often cited as illustrations of TV 'effects' upon sex-role development, but correlational evidence can always be interpreted in a number of ways (the most obvious being that heavily sex-typed individuals might *choose* to watch more sex-stereotyped TV because it is consonant with their world views). More problematically still, there are measurement weaknesses in some of these studies and serious theoretical shortcomings (see Durkin, 1985b), for a more detailed discussion of the developmental literature). There are also several studies which report finding *no* statistical relationship between amount of viewing and sex-role beliefs (Durkin, 1985b, d).

Should the depressing complexity of the real world and the disappointing lack of evidence for the additive impact of mass media stereotypes lead us to assume that the media are not implicated in our sex-role systems, or that if they are, we will never have the research technology to enable us to analyse their functions? I think not. What these considerations do suggest is that if we are to improve our understanding of the relationships between media and people with respect to sex-role issues we need to develop more sophisticated theories and more ingenious approaches.

A starting point may well be to recognize that the processes at stake are *social* rather than *unidirectional* (cf. Durkin, 1985b). Curiously, many accounts of supposed external influences on social behaviour which purport to offer 'social' explanations of human development take a very one-sided (asocial) view of the transaction. In the present context, for example, the media are thought to 'teach' or 'condition' the passive subject, whose own contributions seem to be minimal. A richer perspective may be afforded if we consider what the media user him/herself brings to the engagement and how this interacts with the content of the media.

When we do this, we have to acknowlege that even the youngest media user is not cocooned and inactive, but is developing his or her understanding of the import of gender from very early in life as a social participant (Durkin, 1985b) and soon develops firm views about the significance and correlates of sex-role membership. In this context, it is unlikely that information is simply 'coming in' from the media to accumulate in the developing person's psyche, but rather that he or she will influence the input and will play an active part in determining how to react to it.

In fact, there is quite a lot of evidence that children do interpret sex-role images or themes in the media according to what they already know about sex roles. For example, as children's knowledge of gender constancy increases, they are more likely to attend selectively to same-sex figures on screen (Slaby & Frey 1975) and to take account of television messages that certain types of toy are sex-specific (Ruble, Balaban & Cooper 1981). Further, when 4–9-year-old children are questioned about sex-stereotyped television material, they show a ready ability to elaborate and embellish upon the scenarios in ways which indicate that they can relate it to their existing understanding (Durkin 1984). They can explain that hypothetical fathers not actually seen in a programme are out 'at work', while mothers not seen are 'washing the dishes', and they account for a range of televised male–female interactions in similar ways – by recourse to traditional scripts for sex-role behaviour. Older children reveal sex bias in their preferences for particular characters in stories, with boys in particular showing less favourability towards female than male characters (Connor & Serbin 1979) – a finding consistent with the stronger contraints upon cross-sex identification by males.

It seems that by imposing their pre-existing beliefs upon what they view, children may *use* the media to confirm or supplement their developing social knowledge. Adults probably do the same. For example, Lull, Mulac and Rosen (1983) found that high feminist sympathizers viewed substantially less television per day than low feminist sympathizers, but listened to more progressive rock programmes on the radio. It seems unlikely that this form of musical entertainment causes increased feminism, but quite plausible that people exercise some control over their media usage to select those aspects of content that are either compatible with, or least offensive to, their social perspectives.

This does not, of course, establish that we live in a balanced world in which individuals rigidly predetermine their own media exposures from a range of equally treated visions of possible social orders. Nor does it vindicate the media for their sexist practices. It does suggest, though, that the medium-audience relationship is interactive. This means that to understand the effects of the media we need to understand the social contexts in which they are used, and these are quite varied, as other contributors to this book demonstrate.

Placing the media in their social context acknowledges something of the complexity of the issues facing psychologists in this area, but does not in itself explain how the system functions. Unfortunately, because the bulk of research in this field has focused upon content, there are still remarkably few empirical investigations of reception (Durkin, 1985b). There is a pressing need for more experimental and field research and many issues have simply not been addressed yet. Rather than speculate about these, it may be helpful to consider one issue relating to the media–audience relationship that has received some attention, and that is the question of how effective are non-sexist and counter-stereotyped media images.

Changing representations of sex roles in the mass media

Overall, the sex-role stereotypes in the popular media are *not* being reduced drastically in the wake of the upsurge in the women's movement. Recent reviews find occasional modest changes through the 1970s (Butler & Paisley 1980; Durkin 1985a). However, in the popular media such topics as sex roles, women's rights and male and female career opportunities do command attention from time to time and even if these are not sufficiently common to register massively on content analyses, most people are likely to encounter some manifestation of the questioning of traditional sex roles. What effects might these elements in the mass media have upon the audience? I have already suggested above that the media may often be able to render these innocuous by packaging or trivializing them, and few tests have been conducted to investigate how these processes actually occur in everyday media use. But it is possible to learn a great deal from experimental studies of initial reactions to non-traditional media representations, and this has been the primary approach of psychologists in this field so far.

One point which should be stressed before summarizing this work is that experimental evidence of effects due to counter-stereotyped media does not provide a mirror-image account of what happens when people use stereotyped media. The latter, as we have seen, are *integrated* with numerous other societal processes, whereas counter-stereotypes provide a quite different learning opportunity, with cognitive and affective salience that cannot be expected of ordinary media images and events which simply echo the familiar. Hence, it may be erroneous to assume (as many do) that detection of a change in subjects' beliefs or behaviour following exposure to counter-stereotyped media amounts to evidence that stereotyped media has made them what they were in the first place.

Nevertheless, evidence of the consequences of counter-stereotyped media is important because it points to a level at which psychologists, in collaboration with media producers, can contribute towards positive change in alleviating the dysfunctional constraints due to traditional sex roles. In fact there is considerable evidence that the media can play a part in encouraging people to reconsider certain aspects of their sex roles, though the contributions they can make are not boundless.

Most of the studies so far have been conducted with children. Several of these have found significant effects upon children's beliefs and attitudes following exposure to non-traditional stories (De Lisi & Johns 1984; Scott & Feldman-Summers 1979), films (Flerx, Fidler & Rogers 1976), and television programmes (Durkin & Akhtar, in prep.; Johnston & Ettema 1982). Studies with adults have been rarer, but Jennings (Walstedt), Geis and Brown (1980) and Geis *el al*. (1984) found that undergraduate women exposed to sex-role reversals in TV commercials showed more independence of judgement in conformity tests or measures of personal achievement orientation administered afterwards.

However, we should not assume that simply reversing roles in children's entertainment media or TV commercials will resolve gender in-equities throughout society. First, despite the several successes that have been reported in the experimental literature, there are good *a priori* reasons not to expect all interventions to be so effective. Having already stressed the diversity of the audience, it should be obvious again here that not all people are predisposed to respond to counter-stereotypes in identical ways. In fact, several studies have found evidence of resistance and individual differences in this respect. For example, Drabman *et al*. (1981) found that children presented with doctors and nurses in reverse sex roles sometimes failed even to recognize the switch, despite careful emphasis in the materials. Durkin and Hutchins (1984) found that young adolescents retained, and in some cases intensified traditional sex-role beliefs with respect to careers after viewing non-traditional careers pro-grammes (advocating female plumbers, male secretaries, female doctors, etc.). Durkin (1985c) found that an authentic change in broadcast televi-sion, namely the introduction of a woman to the hitherto all-male panel of weather forecasters on British national television, led to different evaluations by males and females. Men showed no difference in rating male and female weather forecasters; women evaluated the female more harshly. Clearly, the audience's pre-existing values and prejudices can influence the reception of a non-traditional message in a medium, leading either to stark opposition or to subtle scepticism. Other studies indicate that the sex-role orientation of the individual viewer influences how she or he processes non-traditional information in the media (Eisenstock 1984; List, Collins & Westby 1983), and that there are developmental differences in ability to interpret such information (Durkin, 1985b).

Second, the fact remains that society is more than its media. Experimental evidence on short-term effects, due to fleeting experiences with books or unusual programmes, is valuable because it illustrates the potential and the pitfalls of counter-stereotyping. But of course in the real world people have many independent sources of sex-role information and pressure. We cannot assume that incidental counter-stereotypes will combat a powerful social system in its entirety. Indeed, the strongest and most enduring effects of such interventions are found when the media are supported by corresponding influences from other quarters, such as teachers (cf. Johnston & Ettema 1982; Durkin 1985b, provides a more extensive review of this literature and a discussion of the practical, ethical and theoretical issues at stake in counter-stereotyping work).

These qualifications do not detract from the importance of work in this field but simply indicate the multiplicity of factors impinging upon it. This challenges rather than precludes research and it is to be hoped that attention will be increasingly devoted to this area (Durkin, 1985b, c). What we can conclude for the present is that the audience will play a central part in determining the fate of media interventions and that long-term success depends upon careful attention to the social and cognitive contexts in which the messages are transmitted and received.

Conclusions

Sex roles in the mass media is becoming a large and productive field of enquiry among psychologists. It is an important field because it bears directly upon the everyday lives of millions of people. In the early work in the area, much of the attention was directed at the deficiencies of media representations of human beings and human potential, and the media provide ample data for critical analyses at this level. Such research is important, and continuous monitoring of the media is essential if we are to understand the broader environment in which sex roles are constructed (Durkin 1985a).

Still more important is to discover how the media are *used* by the audience. I have suggested that this question has been relatively neglected because of limited theoretical conceptions of media effects, which assume that they operate unilaterally upon passive recipients (a view which has not received broad support in other areas of mass communications study (cf. Howitt 1982)). The limited research addressed to the issue of the effects of sex-stereotyped media suggests that the relationship is far more complex than early expectations indicated, and therefore makes the topic all the more demanding of future attention.

Finally, I have proposed that one of the most positive developments in this field, with exciting prospects for applied psychologists, is the recent growth of counter-stereotyping studies. These complement the actual commitments of some professionals *within* the media, and collaboration between psychologists and broadcasters or writers can lead beyond complaints about the state of the world, towards constructive attempts to change it.

References

Aronoff, C. E. (1974) Sex roles and aging on TV. Summary in *Journal of Communication*, 2, 127.

Baehr, H. (1980) The 'Liberated Woman' in television drama. *Women's Studies International Quarterly, 3*, 29–39.

Birk, J., Brooks, L., Juhasz, J., Barbanel, L., Herman, M., Seltzer, R. & Trangri, S. (1974) A content analysis of sexual bias in commonly used psychology textbooks. *JSAS Catalog of Selected Documents in Psychology*, 4, 107, cited in M. Butler & W. Paisley (eds) *Women and the mass media: sourcebook for research and action*. New York: Human Sciences Press.

Braman, O. (1977). Comics. *In* J. King & M. Stott (eds) *Is this your life?: images of women in the mass media*. London: Virago.

Butler, M. & Paisley, W. (1980) *Women and the mass media: sourcebook for research and action*. New York: Human Sciences Press.

Connor, J. M. & Serbin, L. A. (1978) Children's responses to stories with male and female characters. *Sex Roles, 4*, 637–645.

De Lisi, R. & Johns, M. L. (1984) The effects of books and gender constancy development on kindergarten children's sex-role attitudes. *Journal of Applied Developmental Psychology, 5*, 173–184.

Dominick, J. R. (1979) The portrayal of women in prime time, 1953–1977. *Sex Roles, 5*, 405–411.

Drabman, R. S., Robertson, S. J., Patterson, J. N., Jarvie, G. J., Hammer, D. & Cordua, G. (1981) Children's perception of media-portrayed sex roles. *Sex Roles, 7*, 379–389.

Durkin, K. (1984) Children's accounts of sex-role stereotypes in television. *Communication Research, 11,* 341–362.

Durkin, K. (1985a) Television and sex role acquisition 1: Content. *British Journal of Social Psychology 24,* 101–113.

Durkin, K. (1985b) *Television, sex roles and children: a developmental social psychological analysis.* Milton Keynes: Open University Press.

Durkin, K. (1985c) Sex roles and television roles: can a woman be seen to tell the weather as well as a man? *International Review of Applied Psychology, 34,* 191–201.

Durkin, K. (1985d) Television and sex role acquisition 2: Effects. To appear in *British Journal of Social Psychology 8, 24,* 191–210.

Durkin, K. (1985e) Television and sex role acquisition 3: Counterstereotyping. *British Journal of Social Psychology 88, 24,* 211–222.

Durkin, K. & Akhtar, P. (in preparation) Effects of a professionally produced counterstereotype programme on young children's sex-role beliefs. Manuscript in preparation, Social Psychology Research Unit, University of Kent at Canterbury.

Durkin, K. & Hutchins, G. (1984) Challenging traditional sex-role stereotypes via careers education broadcasts: the reactions of young secondary school pupils. *Journal of Educational Television, 10,* 25–33.

Eisenstock, B. (1984) Sex-role differences in children's identification with counterstereotypical televised portrayals. *Sex Roles, 10,* 417–430.

Flerx, V. C., Fidler, D. S. & Rogers, R. W. (1976) Sex role stereotypes: developmental aspects and early intervention. *Child Development, 47,* 998–1007.

Foreit, K. G., Agor, T., Byers, J., Larue, J., Lokey, H., Palazzini, M., Patterson, M. & Smith, L. (1980) Sex bias in the newspaper treatment of male-centered and female-centered news stories. *Sex Roles, 6,* 475–480.

Frueh, T. & McGhee, P. E. (1975)Traditional sex role development and amount of time spent watching television. *Developmental Psychology, 11,* 109.

Geis, F. L., Brown, V., Jennings (Walstedt) & Porter, N. (1984) TV commercials as achievement scripts for women. *Sex Roles, 10,* 513–525.

Gerbner, G. (1972) Violence in TV drama: trends and symbolic functions. *In* G. A. Comstock & E. A. Rubinstein (eds) *TV and social behavior,* vol.1. Washington, DC: US Government Printing Office.

Gunter, B. & Wober, M. (1982) Television viewing and perceptions of women's roles on television and in real life. *Current Psychological Research, 2,* 277–288.

Harris, A. J. & Feinberg, J. F. (1977) Television and aging. Is what you see what you get? *The Gerontologist, 17,* 464–468.

Harvey, S. E., Sprafkin, J. N. & Rubinstein, E. (1979) Prime time television: a profile of aggressive and prosocial behaviours. *Journal of Broadcasting, 23,* 179–189.

Hodges, K. K., Brandt, D. A. & Kline, J. (1981) Competence, guilt and victimization: sex differences in attribution of causality in television dramas. *Sex Roles, 7,* 537–546.

Howitt, D. (1982) *Mass media and social problems.* Oxford: Pergamon Press.

Jennings (Walstedt), Geis, F. L. & Brown, V. (1980) Influence of television commercials on women's self-confidence and independent judgement. *Journal of Personality and Social Psychology*, 2, 203–210.

Johnston, J. & Ettema, J. S. (1982) *Positive images: breaking stereotypes with children's television*. Beverly Hills and London: Sage.

Karpf, A. (1980) Women and radio. *Women's Studies International Quarterly*, 3, 41–54.

Lemon, J. (1977) Women and blacks on prime time television. *Journal of Communication*, 27, 70–79.

List, J. A., Collins, W. A. & Westby, S. D. (1983) Comprehension and inferences from traditional and non-traditional sex-role portrayals on television. *Child Development*, 54, 1579–1587.

Lull, J., Mulac, A. & Rosen, S. L. (1983) Feminism as a prediction of mass media use. *Sex Roles*, 9, 165–178.

McArthur, L. Z. & Resko, B. G. (1975) The portrayal of men and women in American television commercials. *Journal of Social Psychology*, 97, 209–220.

Manstead, A. S. R. & McCulloch, C. (1981) Sex-role stereotyping in British television advertisements. *British Journal of Social Psychology*, 20, 171–180.

Miller, S. (1975) The content of news photos: women's and men's roles. *Journalism Quarterly*, 52, 70–75.

Morgan, M. (1982) Television and adolescents' sex-role stereotypes: a longitudinal study. *Journal of Personality and Social Psychology*, 43, 947–955.

Ruble, D. N., Balaban, T. & Cooper, J. (1981) Gender constancy and the effects of sex-typed television toy commercials. *Child Development*, 52, 667–673.

Schwartz, L. A. & Markham, W. T. (1985) Sex stereotyping in children's toy advertisements. *Sex Roles*, 12, 157–170.

Scott, K. P. & Feldman-Summers, S. (1979) Children's reactions to textbook stories in which females are portrayed in traditionally male roles. *Journal of Educational Psychology*, 71, 396–402.

Sexton, D. & Haberman, P. (1974) Women in magazine advertisements. *Journal of Advertising Research*, 14, 41–46.

Slaby, R. G. & Frey, K. S. (1975) Development of gender constancy and selective attention to same-sex models. *Child Development*, 46, 849–856.

Welch, R. L., Huston-Stein, A., Wright, J. C. & Plehal, R. (1979) Subtle sex-role cues in children's commercials. *Journal of Communication*, 29, 202–209.

CHAPTER ELEVEN **Sex Roles and Work**
Oonagh Hartnett and
Jenny Bradley

Introduction

This chapter focuses upon aspects of the division of labour between men
and women including non-paid as well as paid work. There are three sections. The first describes the variation between male and female patterns
of work. The second attempts to use psychological perspectives to
account for these differences. The third briefly discusses a possible future
scenario for work in the context of the unemployment crisis in many
industrialized countries.

Male and female patterns of work

It is a truism that in many industrialized nations, including the UK, the
employment roles of the majority of men and women differ in obvious
ways. There is at least equal variation between the sexes in non-paid
work roles. However not all men and women differ in their employment
roles. At the present time employment patterns are changing considerably, particularly for women.

Men have, by and large, accepted and conformed to a role which
commits them to lifelong, full-time paid employment with all the advantages and disadvantages that this role entails. Now that the profession of
midwifery is open to men (previously males could only be gynaecologists
and paediatricians), they are to be found working across the full range
of professions and occupations. They are also to be found at the higher
levels of all of these occupations, even those in which women are more
numerous when the occupation is looked at as a whole. The corollary of
men accepting this commitment to full-time paid employment is that they
play a comparatively minor role in the unpaid work of managing the
household, furthering the development of their children, caring for other
dependents and maintaining social networks outside of the sphere of
employment.

In contrast, the majority of women are in precarious forms of employment, in jobs that are regarded as unskilled, and of low status, and which are part-time, temporary and comparatively poorly paid:

> The situation of women as regards employment is exacerbated by the effects of public expenditure cuts on social infra-structures such as creches and pre-primary education. Females account for almost half the registered unemployed even though they represent little more than a third of the communities' working population. Even on entry into the labour market, young women are more affected by unemployment than young men. In spite of the inroads made by certain women in non-traditional occupations, the overall concentration of women in a very limited range of occupations has hardly changed. (Commission of the European Communities 1982, p. 6).

In the European Community as a whole in 1983, 37 per cent of women were in part-time employment as compared with only 5 per cent of men. A total of 58 per cent of men were employed. The corresponding figure for women was 33 per cent (Commission of the European Communities 1984). In Britain in 1983, 11 million men were employed of whom 700,000 were part-time. For women the statistics were 8 million employed, nearly 4 million of whom were part-time (Equal Opportunities Commission 1984). On average, in this country, women are likely to be out of employment for a total of seven years while they are bringing up a family (Equal Opportunities Commission 1984). Men are not expected to carry this responsibility and so are free to continue in employment without interruption. It needs to be emphasized that these differences in work patterns between men and women must be set against a background which is changing over the longer term. In Britain in 1981, the once 'typical family' with husband in full-time employment and wife at home with dependent children, is now found to be the case in less than one-sixth of families (General Household Survey 1981). The proportion of married women in employment increased by some 400 per cent between the fourth and eighth decades of this century. Contrary to expectation perhaps, the majority of women are as satisfied, globally speaking, with their jobs and are as highly motivated in them as men even though the jobs which women fill might not appear, to an observer, to be as rewarding as the jobs men occupy (Commission of the European Communities 1979). Women's pay and promotion prospects continue overall to be lower than men's, despite recent improvements resulting from the Amended Equal Pay Act of 1984 and the efforts of the Equal Opportunities Commission.

Psychological perspectives on the differences between male and female work roles

The data presented in the previous section raise a number of questions. Why do women, even when committed to employment, tend to be restricted to a comparatively narrow range of occupations while men are not confined to the same extent? Why do men occupy the more prestigious and powerful positions even in occupations in which women are more numerous? Why do women, even when employed, carry out the overwhelming majority of the work associated with the management of the household and the development and care of dependents when there is no reason to believe that men, having gained experience, could not do practically all of it just as well? Why are women being given fewer promotions in their jobs than men? Why despite this are women apparently as satisfied with their jobs as men are with theirs? Finally, how did this division of labour become established in the first place, and why do the patterns appear to be undergoing some change at the present time?

Any attempted answers to the questions about the origins of the sex roles and the sources of change are much disputed. However, psychologists can help to throw some light on the other problems listed above. They can say that the variation between the sex roles is not explicable in terms of differences in ability between the sexes, as other chapters in this book have made clear. They can also help explain how it is that sex roles, once initiated, can come to be sustained and accentuated despite not being justified on the grounds of any relevant innate sex differences. Possible explanations seem to lie in psychological theories of the kind discussed in Chapters 2 and 3 which are concerned with such concepts and constructs as 'the self' and 'identity', 'internalization', and 'sex-role stereotyping'. In the following discussion we focus on the concept of 'conflict' and we discuss three types of conflict relevant to male and female occupational roles, namely intrapersonal, interpersonal and group, and role conflict.

Intrapersonal conflict

At this point it is useful to recall that sex stereotypes are applied to school subjects, to academic disciplines and to occupations as well as to people, men as well as women. There is considerable agreement (despite conceptual and methodological problems) as to the nature of these stereotypes. The positively valued masculine stereotype is associated with competence and dominance while the feminine one is associated with expressiveness and warmth. There is evidence that these stereotypes have changed very little, in so far as the measures are sufficiently sensitive to subtle change, since the research into this area was begun in the 1960s. The exception is the trait 'intellectual', which now appears to be seen as equally appropriate for women and men. Examples of sex-role stereotyping of occupations include supreme court judge, miner, high government official, company president, carpenter and electrician, which are rated as masculine, and nurse, receptionist, private secretary, physician's assistant and social worker, which are rated as feminine. Some readers may be consoled to know that the occupation of clinical psychologist was found not to be stereotyped as either masculine or feminine. School psychologist was not stereotyped either. Other forms of psychologist were not mentioned. Another important aspect of sex-role stereotyping is that the masculine stereotype is assigned a higher status than the feminine stereotype. These stereotypes are very powerful in that no area of life seems to be unaffected by them (even if a particular occupation is not stereotyped, paid employment in general is thought to be more appropriate for males). Additionally no person, irrespective of sex, social class, educational level or marital status escapes their influence, though a few people seem to be more independent of them than is generally the case. Furthermore, sanctions are applied when individuals deviate from what is considered to be the appropriate stereotype (e.g. Broverman *et al.* 1970, 1972; Di Sabatino 1976; Ruble & Ruble 1982; Shinar 1975; Weinreich-Haste 1979; Women's National Commission 1984).

As has been said, there is nothing in the current literature on sex differences which would account for such major differences in the work roles of men and women. However one explanation is in terms of the internalization of the sex role stereotypes and the consequent problems for the maintenance of identity and a sense of self-worth and congruence if an individual, whether man or woman, attempts to behave in a way which does not conform to these stereotypes.

Numbers of studies show that women still feel uncomfortable with the concept of female career orientation. Richardson (1975) found that among college women, many had decided that a career was not for them and that even those who did see themselves as 'career women' had conflicts about this and had not necessarily decided to act upon their aspiration. Both men and women reject an atypical career for similar reasons (e.g. Di Sabatino 1976; Women's National Commission 1984). In general it has been found that those women 'whose employment status is mis-matched with their personal sex role attitudes have higher levels of somatic anxiety' (Parry 1984, p. 22). These tendencies are reinforced by vocational counselling which is itself influenced by the stereotypes. Oliver (1975) and Thomas and Stewart (1971) found that counsellors of both sexes approved less of career goals which deviated from the stereotypes than they approved of conforming goals.

In the context of intrapersonal conflict, it is also necessary to consider Martina Horner's well-known and thought-provoking concept 'fear of success'. She defines the concept as 'an internal psychological represent-ative of the dominant social stereotype which views competence, independence, competition and intellectual endeavour as qualities basically inconsistent with femininity even though positively related to masculinity and mental health' (Horner 1972, p. 157). Controversy centres around the precise nature of 'fear of success'. Is it a realistic awareness of difficulties and possible social sanctions rather than, as Horner seems to suggest, more a case of intrapersonal conflict? Some studies based on projective tests have given contradictory results (Condry & Dyer 1976; Ward 1979). In any case Horner's work has undoubtedly focused attention on the fact that some women fear success rather then failure particularly in competition with males. Fear of success seems to first develop alongside the growth of interest in the opposite sex when girls reach puberty. Therefore it is likely to be at its height at an age when crucial decisions are being made about career development.

So far the focus has been on identity problems for women should they seek a successful career, particularly one which is male stereotyped and of high status. In the present context of high unemployment men are likely to suffer from similar problems if they lose their jobs or cannot find employment. An unemployed man undoubtedly does not conform to the masculine stereotype. Studies of the effects of unemployment on men do indeed show many adverse effects on physical and mental health, self-esteem, a sense of identity and general outlook on life (Jahoda 1982; Sinfield 1981; Warr 1983a, 1983b, 1984). Mitigating variables include financial security, marital support, age and class. (Those near retiring age seem to cope better, as do middle-class men). Relatively little research has been done into the effects of unemployment upon women perhaps because the stereotypes would lead one to believe that unemployment should not bother women. The research done on women indicates that the fewer their sources of domestic identity confirmation, then the more likely they are to suffer in a similar way to a man (Warr & Parry 1982). Most married women at least have some source of identity from their roles as home-makers which no doubt makes them better able to cope with unemployment problems than do men.

Given the identity problems already outlined, how can we explain exceptions? For there undoubtedly exists a small but significant percentage of women who do not conform to the prevailing general pattern of female employment. These women continue to put full-time work before other considerations. They pursue and fulfil career ambitions sometimes in non-stereotypic fields and against the odds they succeed in male-defined terms (Douvan 1976; Mednick, Tangri & Hoffman 1975).

It seems that one set of explanations can be found by looking into family background and the effects this may have had on identity formation. Hoffman (1972) and Lipman-Blumen (1972) concur in finding that psychological distancing between mother and daughter tends to be associated with career orientation in women. Oliver (1975) found that career-oriented women were significantly more father-identified than were women who were content with their traditional role. Lipman-Blumen (1972) and Arvey and Gross (1977) have both found that women's dissatisfaction with the 'housewife' role is related to whether their mothers were happy in that role and to whether or not the mothers worked outside the home.

Another explanation for exceptions emerges from recent studies of what is known as 'psychological androgyny'. The evidence indicates that for some people, men as well as women, the conventional sex stereotypes are not a crucial part of their sense of identity. A small proportion of these people identifies with the stereotype of the opposite sex. A greater number seem to be able to transcend both stereotypes and manage to integrate into their identity the desirable traits from both stereotypes. Research indicates that such individuals are more capable of being flexible in behaviour than sex-stereotyped individuals – that is they are more prepared and happier to carry out masculine or feminine stereotyped tasks as the situation requires irrespective of their sex. Also they have higher levels of self-esteem than individuals who identify with the feminine stereotype (Bem 1974, 1975; Bem & Lenney 1976; Spence, Helmreich & Stapp 1975).

Other research tends to support the implications of these findings. Women who want a career have been found to be higher in traits variously described as 'autonomy', and 'self determination'. For instance Tangri (1972) makes an association between autonomy and role innovation among women.

This evidence suggests that people who are more psychologically androgynous are unlikely to suffer from the same levels of debilitating conflict as most people, if they try to adopt work patterns which do not conform to the stereotypes. This does not mean that they will escape, any more than anyone else, from other forms of conflict such as interpersonal and group conflict; and it is to this topic we now turn.

Interpersonal and group conflict

In the last fifteen years there has been a number of studies that have explored the subject of group and social identity (Tajfel 1981; Turner 1975). The question of the association of interpersonal and intergroup behaviour is discussed by Tajfel. He says that individuals do not necessarily deal with each other as individuals *per se*:

> Quite often they behave primarily as members of well defined and clearly distinct social categories. When in conditions of racial discrimination people find it difficult to obtain accommodation or employment, it is not because they are ugly or handsome, short or tall, smiling or unsmiling, but because they are black. (Tajfel 1981, p. 228)

People tend to define themselves, as well as others, in terms of their location within social groupings. When such group membership is relevant to self-acceptance, self-esteem and evaluation, then there will be a distancing from and discrimination against the 'outgroup'. Such reasoning and evidence is surely as applicable to sex discrimination as it is to race discrimination.

There is an overwhelming amount of evidence that sex discrimination is a powerful factor influencing both sexes to remain in stereotyped work roles. Men are very much less likely to be given parental leave than women. Also in smaller ways men are discriminated against in this respect. The experience of many years in employment, anecdotal though it may be, leads us to believe that men are regarded with disapproval if they wish, for instance, to leave a late-running meeting for the purpose of carrying out some family task, even when it is well known that they regularly undertake that particular responsibility and are depended upon to do so. Women on the other hand are more discriminated against in the area of paid employment. In 1983, 57 per cent of men in the European Community thought that their sex had been an advantage to them in their job. The corresponding figure for women was 27 per cent. This difference tended to increase with the age of the respondents and was most marked at medium education levels (Commission of the European Communities 1984). Both men and women are influenced by the norms of the groups with which they identify; furthermore the group identity can transcend interpersonal relationships *per se* and monetary rewards (Turner 1975). The findings of the Commission of the European Communities (1984) conform to this view. Even in low income groups, where presumably there is financial need, 59 per cent of women wish to be in paid employment of some kind but only 28 per cent of husbands are prepared to support them in this wish. Also a majority of women, as well as men, were in agreement strongly or mildly with the idea that in times of high unemployment men have greater right to a job than do women. Education tends to modify the view of both sexes. The higher their level of education the more in favour of female access to paid employment people are.

Men and women are both sometimes discriminated against in selection for jobs, women more so than men, because the number of stereotypically feminine jobs is smaller and these are assigned lower status than stereotypically masculine jobs (Cohen & Bunker 1975). The qualities believed to be necessary for high status occupations are qualities considered to be the prerogative of the male group. It is not surprising, therefore, that those women who do reach the top suffer an increasing sense of alienation. In the United States this phenomenon is referred to as being 'cored out'. What this means is that the characteristics perceived to be at the core of a group's identity are considered to be quite different from the characteristics of the core identity of an individual who is required to work in that group environment. This construct appears to be a nice marriage between concepts of alienation and group identity. This should be put into proportion. Men also suffer stress at work. However the label more likely to be applied to the symptoms of stress in men is 'burn-out'. Work stressors include rigid and meaningless demands and expectations, role ambiguity, feeling unappreciated, thwarted career development, too difficult or too much work, conflicting demands and expectations, too much responsibility, constant change, and so on (e.g. Farmer, Monohan & Hekeler 1984; McLean 1979; Paine 1982). The differential labelling of what may be the same symptoms in men and women could of course serve to maintain distinctions between groups.

As mentioned earlier, discrimination and prejudice are likely to begin long before any selection interview. In addition to career counsellors being stereotyped, the available careers information can be biased, as can vocational interest measures (Prediger & Cole 1975). During and after the interview, discrimination continues in the areas of access to training and promotion. Training opportunities are more limited for females (Women's National Commission 1984) as are promotion opportunities.

In the case of unemployment, predictions made with group identity theory in mind would suggest that men would be less well able to cope with unemployment than women, and that the proportion of girls and women who are unemployed, even though available for employment, would be greater then for men and boys. The evidence indicates that both of these predictions are being fulfilled.

Another problem now arises. Why is it, as indicated earlier, that women express as much global satisfaction with their jobs as men despite, on average, the lower status and levels of financial reward associated with the work women do?

A caveat is necessary here. The personal and environmental features identified by Warr as relevant to work motivation and job satisfaction are not easy to disentangle. Further, the complexity of the theories and the shortcomings of job satisfaction measures make both accurate prediction and practical data gathering very difficult (Warr 1978). The sources of satisfaction and dissatisfaction from work appear to differ for the sexes despite the similarity in global measures. Men tend to place more value on features such as 'security' and 'prospects' while women rank 'interesting work' and 'companionship' as more important (Martin & Roberts 1984). Women tend to express less satisfaction than men with items such as job status and promotion prospects (Commission of the European Communities 1979). Given all these differences it is difficult to sustain the idea that 'job satisfaction' has the same meaning for both sexes. Therefore direct comparisons are suspect. However let us suppose, for a moment, that there are no grounds for suspicion. Is there any reason for being surprised that women do not express less job satisfaction than men given the differences in the jobs men and women tend to do? One such reason might be that, because of 'occupational apartheid', women are more likely to choose their comparison others from among their own sex group rather than from among men, and therefore not feel as deprived as they otherwise might (Festinger 1968; Wheeler 1969). A further reason which leads one to believe some factor like this could be operating, is that there is not a substantial difference between measures of global satisfaction among men even though they may be in jobs which seem, to an observer, to differ greatly in possible rewards.

Finally it is instructive to remember that even if one were prepared to accept that women and men assigned the same meaning to job satisfaction, there is still more than one way of looking at the evidence. Probably the more obvious way is to be surprised that women express as much global job satisfaction as men. A less obvious question is why men do not express more satisfaction than women. Presumably the latter question has not been asked before because of the stereotypes which result in men's opinions being viewed as less problematical than those of women. However looking at the evidence in this apparently less obvious manner gives one an interesting perspective. It leads one to question whether men's expressions of satisfaction with their lot in life and with the division of labour and the work roles are any less surprising, any more reliable, or any more indicative of happiness than women's may be.

Role conflict

It now becomes important to underline the distinction between work, any work, and a career; between uninterrupted paid employment and intermittent employment combined with working in other areas.

Nearly all women and some men suffer from role confllict because the organization of employment makes it extremely difficult, and well-nigh impossible in many cases, to combine management of the household and family responsibilities with filling a job with high status and high levels of intrinsic and extrinsic reward. It also makes it impossible for men to compensate for the inadequate status and rewards associated with some of the jobs they fill by having an identity that is nourished by more varied, interesting and rewarding work in the home such as furthering the development of their children, cooking interesting meals and having more responsibility for and control over the structuring of their own time and activities.

Not surprisingly, married women workers experience more role conflict than either single women or full-time housewives (Nevill & Damico 1974), and this is also associated with psychological distress (Parry 1984). Martin and Roberts (1984) analyse, in some detail, the ways in which child-rearing affects the employment experience of women in Britain. The evidence indicates a downward occupational move to be typical between the last job women occupied before giving birth to their first child and the job currently held. The choice made by many married women is of a gradual return to employment in a succession of part-time jobs, perhaps working more hours as their children get older but taking work of lower status and with fewer prospects than their original occupation. The object is to work the hours and at the locations which fit in with their children's needs. This is a compromise evolved in an attempt to reduce role strain and conflict (Hudis 1976).

As the wife's job decreases in status, the husband's job is likely to increase relatively in importance. This explains why the husband's job, its location, the hours he works and the employment pressures he experiences also play a significant part in determining women's employment choices (Mortimer, Hall & Hill 1978).

Little research has been done on role conflict among men in this context (though plenty of work has been done on the effects of role conflict and ambiguity on men inside the employment situation, showing it to have deleterious effects – see reference to work stressors earlier in this chapter). This paucity of research has its counterpart in the comparatively little work that has been done on the effects of unemployment upon women. Researchers are not immune from the effects of sex-role stereotyping. It influences the questions they ask and the explanations they are inclined to give, just as it influences the general population in its expectations and behaviour. However a few researchers have managed, at least partially, to break this particular set. Holahan and Gilbert (1978) made a study of dual career marriages in which men had a less traditional ideology. They found highly similar patterns of conflict for male and female subjects in the areas of 'Professional vs Self', 'Spouse vs Parent', and 'Parent vs Self'.

In times of high unemployment men are likely to have other problems because of the role divisions. In addition to the provision of income, employment has many 'latent benefits' such as confirmation of identity; giving of status, independence and purpose; relief from feelings of isolation; and the provision of structure (Jahoda 1979). When people become unemployed they obviously lose these latent benefits, and the male's concentration upon the employment role results in his perceiving himself as having no other source from which to secure such benefits. Becoming involved in the management of the household conflicts with the role set he considers to be appropriate. As has been said, women's dual role appears to give them an advantage when unemployment is high. Indeed many women, who are not in paid work, refused to label themselves as 'unemployed' (Martin & Roberts 1984).

To sum up, the evidence indicates that the present stereotypic structuring of the work roles is disadvantageous, in one way or another, to both sexes. Women have less opportunity for securing the status, monetary rewards and other benefits associated with paid employment. Men have much less opportunity for participating in the management of the household and furthering the development of their children. They also have no alternative source of identity should they become unemployed or not achieve the enjoyment and success in paid employment for which they hope. One can only wonder what disadvantages the children may be suffering with mothers whose careers have had to be scrapped, and with fathers who are anxious about security and who are more characterized by their absence than by their presence. The question now arises as to what, if anything, can be done to improve the situation. Methods of combating unfair sex discrimination at work by psychologists and others have been delineated elsewhere (Hartnett 1976, 1978, 1984; Hartnett & Novarra 1980) and will not be further discussed here. In this chapter it is more apposite to consider a future scenario in which, to the benefit of both sexes, the employment roles of men are considered to be as problematic and as open to change as those of women have been considered to be in the relatively near past.

A possible scenario for the future

When attempting to think about the future it is sensible to reflect upon the past and to consider what light the present may throw upon each in the context of the other.

As has already been indicated, the traditional sex roles and stereotypes seem to be in a greater state of flux or change than has been the case for some time. Which psychological theory, if any, might give some insight into what might be happening? That which seems most helpful is known as sociotechnical systems theory. It was first evolved by Trist and Bamforth (1951) when they were studying work groups in an industry with changing technology. These researchers came to the conclusion that the social and technical systems are interdependent. Changes in one are associated with changes in the other. This is not to argue that the technical aspects of the system drive the social or vice versa. It is simply to say that they are in dynamic interaction. They have enabling effects on one another. One feeds the other. Thus questions about goodness of fit arise, the fit between the social and technical aspects and the fit between the resulting sociotechnical system and the needs of the people involved (Burns & Stalker 1961; Emery & Trist 1965; Katz & Kahn 1978; Trist & Bamforth 1951; Trist, Higgin & Pollock 1963). In this second half of the twentieth century one would deny that we are undergoing a surge of technological change. This is in terms of 'software', for example the knowledge and skill bases, and in terms of 'hardware', for example the sources of energy or lack of them, the sources of destruction, the equipment, machinery, drugs and medicines available to us. One would expect such changes to be associated with a corresponding surge of change in the social system. It can surely be no accident that a change in the role of women is associated with increased knowledge of the biochemistry of human reproduction and the evolution of effective means of contraception. For the first time women are able to direct their own fertility. Once this was achieved possibly the greatest barrier to participation, for practical purposes, in any other area of endeavour they chose had been removed. Again, a caveat, this is not to say that the change caused women to be more involved in other areas, it is merely to say that it allowed them to do something which apparently they want to do for whatever reason. Such change can also enable men to participate in the upbringing of their children. They now know that they too need not think in terms of a dozen children at unknown intervals. They can anticipate having an average of two children, who importantly are likely to survive into adulthood. Over a lifetime this allows them plenty of time for other activities.

Another change in the technological system is the development of automated control and therefore a corresponding wane in the demand for muscularity. This means that many jobs denied to women on the grounds of lack of physical strength are now obviously open to them. This includes even military activities. Again this is not to say that the change causes women to go into these jobs or men to go into others. Rather, it enables them to do so if they choose.

Yet another important aspect of technological change, which has been in process for a number of centuries, is the development of equipment, materials and food which makes the management of the household less time-consuming. Alongside this is the transfer of the manufacture of materials and food, and the provision of services such as education and care of the sick from the private domain of the household to the public domain of employing organizations. The management of the household in medieval times must have been more challenging and interesting, and demanding of a greater variety of skills than it is today. Therefore it is perhaps not too much to suggest that some women are seeking to recover this challenge and interest by tracking it into the public domain.

When all of these and other changes are taken in conjunction, the

Women's Movement can be seen as part of a move to achieve goodness of fit between the social and technical systems, and between the socio-technical systems and human characteristics.

Now seems to be the time to focus equally on men. More recently, technological change is resulting in long-term, structural unemployment which appears to be causing many men a great deal of suffering. The remedy would seem to reside in adjustments which improve the types of goodness of fit already mentioned. Such adjustments could include job sharing; shorter working hours; greater provision for sabbaticals and for retraining (likely to be needed, in any case, to keep up with technological innovation); involvement of men in the management of the household, which will provide another source of identity; and proper provision of parental leave for men as well as women.

There is already a trend towards some of these adjustments. The Commission of the European Communities has produced a new draft directive requiring improved parental leave for both men and women which is not interchangeable between them. Sweden is in advance of the Community in this respect. Many members of the European Parliament are endeavouring to secure a reduction in working hours. Efforts are being made to improve the status of part-time work so that terms, benefits and conditions are at least *pro rata* to those of full-time employment. New working arrangements such as these may have many problems which require careful thinking through. However they undoubtedly have many advantages. The various forms of employment available can be more equitably distributed. The stresses associated with work and the various forms of conflict already discussed are likely to be reduced.

Now it happens that women have spearheaded these new forms of employment, but there is no reason why men should not take a similar initiative and there are a good many reasons why they are likely to find it to their advantage to do so. A small survey of job sharers was carried out in Britain by the Equal Opportunities Commission (1981). It is relevant to quote one respondent who saw job sharing as 'an opportunity to attempt total equality in marriage...a kind of life without sex defined roles at home or at work' (p. 19).

To conclude, whatever one's view may be about the origins of the stereotypes, it is clear that there is a dearth of research evolved from a perspective capable of considering the masculine stereotype, the male role and men's expression of belief and opinion to be as problematical as the feminine stereotypes the female role and women's expression of belief and opinion. Future research needs to pay much more attention to this area; to question what stresses and strains the stereotypes may impose upon males; to consider the extent to which men's behaviour and expression of attitude may be distorted by pressures of social desirability, fear of rejection and loss of status; and to develop programmes which will permit men to adopt more flexible roles, should they so wish, without fear of losing face.

References

Arvey, R. D. & Gross, R. H. (1977) Satisfaction levels and correlations of satisfaction in the homemaker job. *Journal of Vocational Behaviour, 10,* 25–34.

Bem, S. L. (1974) The measurement of psychological androgyny. *Journal of Consulting and Clinical Psychology, 42,* 155–162.

Bem, S. L. (1975) Sex role adaptability: one consequence of psychological androgyny. *Journal of Personality and Social Psychology, 31,* 634–643.

Bem, S. L. & Lenney, E. (1976) Sex typing and the avoidance of cross-sex behaviour. *Journal of Personality and Social Psychology, 33,* 48–54.

Broverman, I. K., Broverman, D. M., Clarkson, F. E., Rosencrantz, P. S. & Vogel, S. R. (1970) Sex role stereotypes and clinical judgements of mental health. *Journal of Consulting Psychology, 34,* 1–7.

Broverman, I. K., Vogel, S. R., Broverman, D. M., Clarkson, F. E. & Rosencrantz, P. S. (1972) Sex-role stereotypes: a current appraisal. *Journal of Social Issues, 28,* 59–79.

Burns, T. & Stalker, A. M. (1961) *The management of innovation.* London, Tavistock.

Cohen, S. L. & Bunker, K. A. (1975) Subtle effects of sex-role stereotypes on recruiters' hiring decisions. *Journal of Applied Psychology, 60,* 1–14.

Commission of the European Communities (1979) *European men and women in 1978: a comparative study of socio-political attitudes in the European Community.* Brussels: Commission of the European Communities.

Commission of the European Communities (1982) A new community action programme on the promotion of equal opportunities for women. *Bulletin of the European Communities, Supplement 1/82.* Brussels: Commission of the European Communities.

Commission of the European Communities (1984) Women and men of Europe in 1983. *Supplement No. 16 to Women of Europe.* Brussels: Commission of the European Communities.

Condry, J. & Dyer, S. (1976) Attribution of cause to the victim. *Journal of Social Issues, 32,* 63–83.

Di Sabatino, M. (1976) Psychological factors inhibiting women's occupational aspirations and vocational choices: implications for counseling. *Vocational Guidance Quarterly, 25,* 43–49.

Douvan, E. (1976) The role of models in women's professional development. *Psychology of Women Quarterly, 1,* 5–20.

Emery, F. E. & Trist E. L. (1965) The causal texture of organizational environments. *Human Relations, 18,* 21–32.

Equal Opportunities Commission (1981) *Job-sharing: improving the quality and availability of part-time work. Alternative working arrangement 1.* Manchester: Equal Opportunities Commission.

Equal Opportunities Commission Statistics Unit (1984) *The fact about women is* ... Manchester: Equal Opportunities Commission.

Farmer, R. E., Monohan, L. H., Hekeler R. W. (1984) *Stress management for the human services.* London: Sage.

Festinger, L. A. (1968) A theory of social comparison processess. *In* H. Hyman, & E. Singer (eds) *Readings in group theory and research.* New York: Free Press.

General Household Survey (1981) London: HMSO.

Hartnett, O. M. (1976) Affirmative action programmes. *Women Speaking, 5(2),* 12–13.

Hartnett, O. M. (1978) Sex role stereotyping at work. *In* J. Chetwynd, & O. M. Hartnett (eds) *The sex role system.* London: Routledge & Kegan Paul.

Hartnett, O. M. (1984) Sex discrimination in psychology. *In* D. J. Muller, D. E. Blackman, A. J. Chapman (eds) *Psychology and law.* London: John Wiley.

Hartnett, O. M. & Novarra, V. (1980) Single sex management training. *Personnel Management, 12,* 32–35.

Hoffman, L. W. (1972) Early childhood experiences and women's achievement motives. *Journal of Social Issues, 28,* 129–156.

Holahan, C. K. & Gilbert, L. A. (1978) Interrole conflict for dual career couples. The effects of gender and parenthood. Paper presented at the annual meeting of the American Psychological Association, Toronto, Canada.

Horner, M. S. (1972) Towards an understanding of achievement-related conflicts in women. *Journal of Social Issues, 28,* 157–175.

Hudis, P. (1976) Commitment to work and to family: marital status differences in women's earnings. *Journal of Marriage and the Family, 38,* 265–278.

Jahoda, M. (1979) The impact of unemployment in the 1930's and 1970's. *Bulletin of the British Psychological Society, 30,* 309–314.

Jahoda, M. (1982) *Employment and unemployment. A social-psychogical analysis.* Cambridge: Cambridge University Press.

Katz, D. & Kahn, R. L. (1978) *The social psychology of organisations,* 2nd edn. New York: John Wiley.

Lipman-Blumen, J. (1972) How ideology shapes women's lives. *Scientific American, 226(1),* 34–42.

McLean, A. A. (1979) *Work stress.* London: Addison-Wesley.

Martin, J. & Roberts, C. (1984) *Women and employment: a lifetime perspective.* The report of the 1980 DE/OPCS Women and Employment Survey, London: HMSO.

Mednick, M. T., Tangri, S. & Hoffman, L. W. (1975) *Women and achievement.* New York: Halstead Press, John Wiley.

Mortimer, J., Hall, R. & Hill, R. (1978) Husbands occupational attributes as constraints on wives' employment. *Sociology of Work and Occupations, 5,* 185–313.

Nevill, D. & Damico, S. (1974) Role conflict in women as a function of marital status. *Human Relations, 28,* 487–498.

Oliver, L. (1975) The relationship of parental attitudes and parent identification to career and homemaking orientation in college women. *Journal of Vocational Bahaviour, 7,* 1–12.

Paine, W. S. (1982) (ed.) *Job stress and burnout.* London: Sage.

Parry, G. (1984) The mental health of employed and unemployed mothers: beyond the global comparison. SAPU Memo 576, MRC/SSRC Social and Applied Psychology Unit, University of Sheffield.

Prediger, D. J. & Cole, N. S. (1975) Sex-role socialization and employment realities: implications for vocational interest measures, ACT Research Report No. 68. Research and Development Division, American College Testing Program, PO Box 168, Iowa City, Iowa 52240.

Richardson, M. S. (1975) Self-concepts and role-concepts in the career orientation of college women. *Journal of Counseling Psychology, 22,* 122–126.

Ruble, D. N. & Ruble, T. L. (1982) Sex stereotypes. In A. G. Miller (ed.) *In the eye of the beholder.* New York: Praeger.

Shinar, E. H. (1975) Sexual stereotypes of occupations. *Journal of Vocational Behaviour, 7,* 99–111.

Sinfield, A. (1981) *What unemployment means.* London: Martin Robertson.

Spence, J. T., Helmreich, R. & Stapp, J. (1975) Ratings of self and peers on sex role attributes and their relation to self esteem and conception of masculinity and femininity. *Journal of Personality and Social Psychology, 32,* 29–39.

Tajfel, H. (1981) *Human groups and social categories,* Cambridge: Cambridge University Press.

Tangri, S. S. (1972) Determinants of occupational innovation among college women. *Journal of Social Issues, 28,* 177–199.

Thomas, A. H. & Stewart, N. R. (1971) Counselor response to female clients with deviate and conforming career goals. *Journal of Counseling Psychology, 18,* 352–357.

Trist, E. L. & Bamforth, K. W. (1951) Some social and psychological consequences of the long-wall method of coal getting. *Human Relations, 4,* 3–38.

Trist, E. L., Higgin, G. W., Murray, H. & Pollock, A. B. (1963) *Organizational choice.* London: Tavistock.

Turner, J. C. (1975) Social comparison and social identity: some prospects for intergroup behaviour. *European Journal of Social Psychology, 5,* 5–34.

Ward, C. (1979) Is there a motive in women to avoid success? In O. Hartnett, G. Boden & M. Fuller (eds) *Sex-role stereotyping.* London: Tavistock.

Warr, P. (1978) Attitudes, action and motives. In P. Warr (ed.) *Psychology at work.* Harmondsworth: Penguin.

Warr, P. (1983a) Work, jobs and unemployment. *Bulletin of the British Psychological Society, 36,* 305–311.

Warr, P. (1983b) Job loss, unemployment and psychological well-being. In E. Van de Vliert & V. Allen (eds) *Role transitions.* New York: Plenum Press.

Warr, P. (1984) Economic recession and mental health: a review of research. SAPU Memo 609, MRC/SSRC, Social and Applied Psychology Unit, University of Sheffield.

Warr, P. & Parry, G. (1982) Paid employment and women's psychological well-being. *Psychological Bulletin, 91,* 498–516.

Weinreich-Haste, H. (1979) What sex is science? In O. Hartnett, G. Boden, M. Fuller (eds) *Sex-role stereotyping.* London: Tavistock.

Wheeler, L. (1969) Factors determining the choice of a comparison other. *Journal of Experimental Social Psychology*, 5, 219–232.

Women's National Commission (1984) *The other half of our future*. London, SW1: Cabinet Office.

CHAPTER TWELVE

Sex Roles in Leisure and Sport
Ann Colley

Introduction

This chapter examines the determining influence of adult sex roles on participation in leisure activities and on sport in particular. Sex-role socialization, which continues throughout infancy and childhood, establishes norms for the attitudes, behaviour, and hence the life styles of males and females. In Chapters 3 and 4 of this book, the reciprocal nature of sex-role socialization is discussed. As part of this complex process, parents and other significant adults behave differently towards male and female children. Exploration and independence are encouraged in males, while dependence is encouraged in females by a more protective approach to exploration (e.g. Lewis 1972). Tolerance of styles of play differs for the two sexes. Physical play is encouraged for boys but discouraged for girls, while the reverse is true for nurturant play (e.g. Fagot 1978).

Since the sex-stereotyping of play is an integral part of sex-role socialization, it is not surprising that adult 'play' in the form of participation in leisure activities is also to some extent sex-stereotyped. The encouragement of physical play in boys is a natural precursor to sport participation (Greendorfer 1983), which is predominantly a male pastime.

The first part of this chapter will discuss the constraints on leisure which result from adult sex roles, and the different attitudes to leisure of males and females. The second part of the chapter will focus on sport, and will discuss findings from empirical studies of sport socialization, sex-stereotyping of sports and the role conflict experienced by female athletes.

Sex roles in leisure

Leisure participation by males and females

Demographic studies which have looked at leisure (e.g. General Household Survey 1977) have found that men and women differ in both their patterns and rates of leisure participation. The most marked sex difference found in the General Household Survey (GHS) of 1977 was in sport participation, where women participated less than men in both outdoor and indoor sport. When active sport participation declined for older respondents and participation as a spectator increased, again there was greater participation from men. Sport will be discussed in some detail in the next part of this chapter. Other activities in which men took part more than women were social drinking, gardening, betting and 'do-it-yourself'. As might be expected, few if any men spent their time in traditionally female pastimes such as needlework and knitting. Both sexes watched television, listened to records and tapes, went to the theatre and cinema and went sightseeing. More women than men went to bingo. The results of this survey were very much as might be expected, in that some leisure activities both within and outside the home were sex-typed, and these are easy to predict. Rates of participation were also examined in the GHS of 1977, and women were found generally to have lower rates of participation in most activities than men. This is some indication that women may have less leisure time available.

Apart from the sex of the individual, perhaps the other most important determinants of leisure patterns are marital status and presence of children. Marriage has been found to result in a reduction in sport participation for both sexes (Boothby *et al.* 1981). Sillitoe (1969) found that parenthood reduced sport participation for men. Instead of occupying more leisure time than other activities, sport fell into second place behind watching television. Marriage and parenthood then, may reduce and change leisure for men. Neulinger and Breit (1971) examined perceptions of leisure time and found that married men perceived themselves as having less leisure than single men. However in a 'traditional household' the woman, whether in full-time employment or not, typically takes more responsibility for running the home and for child care, so that family commitments would be expected to have a particularly marked effect on women's leisure. Deem (1982) investigated the leisure behaviour of a sample of women in Milton Keynes, UK, who were active in some form of leisure activity outside the home. Many of the participants in this study felt that they did not have enough time for leisure, and this applied particularly to married women with children under twelve and women in full-time work with children under seventeen. From the questionnaires and interviews used in the study, constraints which applied to leisure within and outside the home could be identified. For leisure outside the home, these were the husband or partner's attitude to going out alone or with friends, his working hours and work-related social commitments, baby-sitting arrangements for children, the difficulty of releasing time from housework, the necessity to transport children to their leisure activities, lack of access to a car, absence of a companion, lack of money and tiredness. As far as leisure activities within the home were concerned, constraints cited were interruptions from the demands of other family members, and lack of space. How far some or all of these constraints apply to men is not clear, since only women took part in Deem's study, but it is unlikely that the majority of men would be restricted by their families in the same way or to the same extent.

Sex-role stereotypes and attitudes to leisure

One important determinant of the type of leisure engaged in by the women in Deem's sample was the attitude of the partner or husband towards going out. Negative attitudes were expressed towards activities which involved social contact with the opposite sex such as drinking in pubs or attending dances. Attendance at more formal or female-dominated activities such as women's organizations, bingo or evening classes was considered more acceptable. Women's leisure then may be constrained by the attitudes and expectations of those around them. Witt and Goodale (1981) looked at restrictions on leisure in relation to family stages and found that women felt increasingly limited by the expectations of others, with age. For males these expectations were less important and more constant. However, this finding may in part be due to the gradual liberalizing of attitudes towards the role of women in society which has taken place in recent years. The older female respondents presumably experienced more traditional expectations from their peers than the younger women in the sample.

Attitudes toward the suitability of particular leisure activities for males and females may be based on sex-role stereotypes from either or both of two sources. First, as indicated by the studies cited so far, they may be based on views of what is appropriate for the roles men and women enact at work and in the home. Second, attitudes may reflect stereotypes of male and female physical and psychological attributes. The latter explanation is particularly relevant to differences in male and female sport participation, and this issue will be further explored in the next section.

Sex-stereotyping of leisure activities is apparently very pervasive. As part of a more general study of leisure behaviour, we (Colley, Round &

Wheatley, cited in Colley 1984) asked a sample of male and female undergraduates to indicate which of a list of leisure activities were suitable for males only, females only and both sexes. We expected little sex-stereotyping to occur in this sample due to a general consciousness of sexual equality. We were, however, wrong. Over 40 percent of respondents scored carpentry, mending cars, darts, fishing and football as suitable for males only. Over 60 percent of the sample scored needlework and knitting as suitable for females only. Unfortunately the reasons for this stereotyping were not explored. Empirical work examining the foundations for such stereotypes would be a valuable addition to research in this area.

Definitions of leisure

Talbot (1979) has suggested that many women may find difficulty in defining what is leisure and what is leisure time. Most employed men and single employed women have a clearly-defined working day, so the distinction between work and leisure time is a relatively clear one. For women with heavy domestic commitments, this distinction is not as clear-cut since housework and child care do not occupy set hours. 'Time-off' may come in short and sometimes unpredictable periods throughout the day. Also, it may be difficult to decide whether a particular activity is 'leisure' or not. Is time spent playing with children a necessary part of child care and hence not leisure, or is it relaxing and enjoyable in the same way as more clearly defined social leisure activities? Similarly, shopping may be necessary but may also have a recreational element. This same dilemma arises when the leisure time of men with families is examined, although in a traditional household with a working man and home-based woman, time spent in this way may be rather less for the man. This issue has in the main been avoided by leisure researchers but has implications for the interpretation of the results of studies which have found lower participation rates in leisure activities by women.

The greater difficulty of defining leisure for women than for men may have led to the adoption of different criteria. Iso-Ahola (1979), using hypothetical leisure situations, investigated three dimensions which might affect definitions of leisure in males and females. These were relation to work, freedom of choice to participate and source of motivation (intrinsic-extrinsic). Respondents were asked to rate situations within which these dimensions were represented on a ten-point scale which ran from 'not leisure at all' to 'leisure at its best'. A sex difference emerged in the findings such that lack of relation to work increased rating for females regardless of freedom. Iso-Ahola suggested that this could be because women, particularly if working and running a home, tend to work harder than men, so they appreciate leisure more and are more open to leisure. A second possibility is that difficulty of defining leisure results in women emphasizing a criterion which overcomes this problem – leisure occurs away from their other commitments. A third possibility is that since women are constrained in their leisure by many aspects of their sex role, freedom to choose is a less relevant dimension for them.

Needs fulfilled by leisure

One possible way of resolving the dilemma of defining leisure, particularly if investigating whether or not women are disadvantaged by constraints on their activities and leisure time, is to try to identify needs which are fulfilled by leisure participation. If these needs are fulfilled by activities other than those strictly classified as leisure, then a low rate of participation in leisure may not mean that a given individual is disadvantaged or deprived.

If it is assumed that leisure choice is determined by the psychological needs of the individual, then it must closely relate to the life-style and sex role of the individual, which will determine the situations which precede leisure. Various theories have proposed needs which are fulfilled in leisure, and these have been summarized under five headings by Witt and Bishop (1970). These are surplus energy theory (e.g. Lore 1968) which proposes that leisure activities use up energy not already used elsewhere; relaxation theory (e.g. Sapora & Mitchell 1961) which proposes that leisure is relaxation from tiring activities or diversion from tedious ones; catharsis theory (e.g. Axline 1947) which sees leisure as a means of purging tension and anxiety; compensation theory (e.g. Mitchell & Mason 1934) which suggests that leisure activities may allow goals to be realized which are blocked elsewhere, and task generalization theory (Hagedorn & Labovitz 1968) which suggests that activities may be chosen for leisure which resemble situations in other areas of life which are rewarding. Witt and Bishop (1970) looked at the usefulness of each of these theories in explaining leisure choice. They asked respondents to rate how much they felt like taking part in each of a list of leisure activities after various hypothetical situations which were chosen to

represent the needs suggested in the theories. They found that differences
in the choice of leisure activities did emerge when the antecedent situation was varied, and that the surplus energy, catharsis and compensation
theories were useful in predicting them. If situational antecedents determine choice of leisure activity, then these may contribute to sex
differences in participation. For example, a male in a sedentary occupation may have surplus energy to use in physical recreation whereas a
working mother may not. Lack of mental stimulation in the daily routine
of a home-based female may cause her to compensate for this in leisure,
whereas her working husband may gain sufficient mental stimulation
from his job.

   Related to this question of needs, males and females may derive
different satisfactions from the same leisure activities. Sillitoe (1969)
asked male and female participants in sport and games to rank five
possible incentives to participate. These were keeping fit, the pleasure of
competition, a chance to mix with other people, taking your mind off
things and being in the open air. The chief incentive for women was the
social one, while the pleasure of competition had the least appeal. Men
did not relate the social incentive as highly as women. Younger men
favoured a competitive incentive, but older men favoured the incentive
of being in the open air. Boothby *et al.* (1981) presented male and female
respondents who were or had been active in sport with eight statements
describing positive attributes which they had to rate on a five-point scale
running from 'strongly disagree' to 'strongly agree'. More females than
males agreed with the statements 'Sport helps you to meet other people'
and 'Sport is just a bit of fun', and slightly more females than males
agreed with the statement 'Sport is just a way of passing time'. Slightly
more males than females agreed with the statements 'You get satisfaction
from winning' and 'Sport helps you to keep fit'. This is further evidence
that males and females may participate in the same leisure activities for
different reasons. For sport the major incentive for women seems to be
social and for men seems to be competitive. This clearly reflects sex-role
socialization and also relates to the lower participation rates for women.
There are other leisure activities which provide as much, if not more
opportunity to socialize than sport.

Sex-role identity and leisure

One possiblility which has recently been investigated is that individuals
who are not rigidly sex-typed may show different patterns of leisure from
those who are. The self-report inventories of Bem (1974) and Spence,

Helmreich and Stapp (1974) allow individuals to be classified as sex-typed (masculine and feminine) or balanced (androgynous or undifferentiated). Both Bem's BSRl (Bem Sex Role Inventory) and Spence *et al.*'s PAQ (Personal Attributes Questionnaire) contain items belonging to masculine and feminine scales. The items were selected to be stereotypically characteristic of males and females respectively. Sex-typed individuals obtain a high score on the scale which contains items for their own sex and a low score on the other scale. Androgynous individuals obtain high scores on both scales; undifferentiated individuals obtain low scores on both scales. It is possible that balanced individuals may be less constrained by the expectations of those around them, and participate in a broader range of leisure activities than others of their sex.

Gentry and Doering (1979) looked at leisure participation in college students and found sex to be a better predictor of leisure then sex-role identity. However, the findings indicated that androgynous individuals were more active recreationally than sex-typed individuals and that they participated in a broader range of activities, from traditionally feminine activities to traditionally masculine ones. College students have fewer constraints on their leisure than other adult groups, so it would be interesting to see if the findings of this study apply to the adult population in general.

Sex roles in sport

Sport socialization

As discussed previously in this chapter, more males than females participate in sport. The most obvious explanation for this is that sport socialization for males is continuous with and part of sex-role socialization. The behavioural traits encouraged in males, for example independence, competitiveness, leadership, are also encouraged in most sports. Skills obtained through physical play in infancy and childhood, and confidence in expressing these skills, lead naturally to enjoyment of sport and competence in sporting performance. Sport socialization for females is, however, at odds with sex-role socialization since the traits emphasized in sport and physical styles of play are discouraged in females (see Greendorfer (1983) for a discussion of this).

Lewko and Greendorfer (1978) reviewed the literature on sport socialization for both males and females and drew the following conclusions. First, the family rather than the school or peer group is the most influential agent for children's sport socialization. Within the family the parents are more influential than siblings, and the father is the most influential figure of all. The school has a more influential role for boys than girls, possibly because ridicule from teachers and peers can have an aversive effect on less able boys (as discussed later in this section). Second, perception of sex-appropriateness influences active participation and this affects females in particular in a negative way. Third, boys have more rigid perceptions of the sex-appropriateness of sporting activities than girls; and finally, boys value sport more highly than girls.

Since the family exerts a strong influence on sport socialization, it would seem reasonable to predict that females who participate in sport should have a supportive family background. This could moderate the effects of sex-role socialization. This prediction is supported by empirical findings. Snyder and Spreitzer (1976) found a background of positive family support for female adolescent sport participants. Further confirmation comes from Lewko and Ewing (1980) who classified a sample of 9–11-year-old children as having high or low active sport involvement. Using a questionnaire which included statements about family influence on sport participation, they found that father's influence could discriminate high- from low-involved boys. However, the influences of father, mother, sister and brother *all* discriminated between high- and low-involved girls. Greendorfer (1974, 1979) found that many female intercollegiate athletes came from families where both parents were sport participants and had played sports and games with them during childhood. This type of family background not only gives positive support, but also provides role models which do not sex-type sport. Greendorfer's findings has been extended by Gregson and Colley (in press) to a sample of varying sporting ability. In this latter study, data was collected on the participation patterns and sporting achievements of the family members of 15–16-year-old males and females. For the females, paternal and maternal sport participation, and maternal achievement in sport correlated significantly with the number of hours per week spent playing sport outside of compulsory sessions at school. No such relationship was found for males.

Most studies in this area are heterogeneous with respect to the type of sport played by the subjects. The importance of the influence of 'significant others' may vary with type of sport. Weiss and Knoppers (1982) examined socializing agents for female volleyball players in the 1979 Big Ten volleyball championships. They found that, in a comparison of the influence of immediate family members on sport involvement, only brothers had a significant influence. This was true both during childhood and during college years. Weiss and Knoppers do not attempt to discuss why brother's influence might be important to volleyball players. One possible explanation is that volleyball is a team sport and that teams are a more typical feature of male sports and games than of female sports and games. Interaction and play with brothers may be important for female attraction to team sports.

Finally, since sport socialization can be viewed as an integral part of male sex-role socialization, the socializing experiences of males who do not participate in sport are worthy of investigation. Snyder and Spreitzer (1978) have discussed aversive socializing experiences and their role in producing a negative attitude to sport. Coaches, teachers or peers may ridicule the less able and as a result some boys may avoid situations where their ability is under scrutiny. Snyder and Spreitzer present anecdotal evidence in support of this, although there may be other contributory factors, for example personality variables, lack of rigid sex-role socialization from family members, which warrant investigation.

Role conflict and sport participation by women

Since many aspects of sport participation are apparently incompatible with the female sex role, researchers have looked for evidence of role conflict in sportswomen. Sage and Loudermilk (1979) administered a questionnaire containing items on perceived and experienced role conflict to 268 female collegiate athletes. Roughly a quarter of their sample felt role conflict to a great or very great extent, but this varied according to sport. Participants in sports such as tennis, swimming and gymnastics which are considered fairly acceptable for women felt less role conflict than participants in less acceptable sports such as softball, basketball and field hockey. A difference emerged between the role conflict perceived by these women, that is which they themselves felt, and that which they had actually experienced through the behaviour of others towards them. They perceived greater role conflict than they had experienced (this was also found in a similar study by Anthrop and Allison, 1983).

One question which arises from this finding is whether role conflict is a form of paranoia on the part of female athletes or whether female sport participation is regarded negatively and as a contradiction of roles. Griffin (1973) found that undergraduates felt that female athletes and college professors were farthest from their image of the 'ideal' woman, while 'mother' and 'girlfriend' were closest. Fisher *et al.* (1978) presented slides of Canadian sportswomen in action, to male and female athletes and non-athletes. They asked these respondents to rate each slide on a ten-point scale to indicate how close the sportswoman pictured was to the 'ideal' woman. They found that ratings varied with sex and with sport participation. Males and non-athletes gave generally lower ratings than females and athletes. Other studies have confirmed that males have a more negative attitude to female sport participation than females (Colley *et al.* 1985; Nixon, Maresca & Silverman 1979; Selby & Lewko 1976). There is, therefore, evidence to suggest that 'athlete' and 'woman' are not seen as entirely compatible roles, but perceptions of compatibility vary.

To try to reduce the dissonance resulting from the contradictory roles of 'woman' and 'athlete', it has been suggested (e.g. Felshin 1974) that female athletes exhibit 'apologetic' behaviours. That is, they emphasize their femininity in the way they dress and also by espousing traditional sex-role attitudes. Empirical investigations of 'apologetic' attitudes among female athletes have produced inconsistent findings. Snyder and Kivlin (1977) gave a large sample of late adolescent female athletes and non-athletes a questionnaire in which items describing aspects of the female sex role had to be endorsed. They found that the athletes expressed more traditional attitudes than the non-athletes. However, Uguccioni and Ballantyne (1980) found no difference between the sex-role attitudes of female athletes and non-athletes using the Attitudes Toward Women Scale (AWS; Spence & Helmreich 1972). These discrepant findings are probably due to differences in sex-role attitudes which have been found *among* female athletes. Colker and Widom (1980) found that highly committed female athletes had more pro-feminist sex-role attitudes (as measured by the AWS) than female athletes with low commitment. Female athletes who wish to succeed at a high level in sport may adopt attitudes which question traditional sex-role norms and allow them to resist pressures to conform. Del Rey (1977) investigated the possibility that female participants in less acceptably feminine sports would show more traditional sex-role attitudes than those who participate in acceptable sports. Her assumption was that greater role conflict would be experienced by female athletes in less acceptable sports, resulting in a greater desire to adhere to traditional norms. She administered the AWS to female participants in basketball, softball, swimming and tennis. Since swimming and tennis are more acceptable than softball and basketball, she predicted that the tennis players and swimmers would have more liberal attitudes. This was borne out in part in her results. Tennis players had more liberal attitudes than swimmers and softball and basketball players.

Sex-typing of sports

Metheny (1965) described the characteristics of sports which are acceptable and unacceptable for female participation. Acceptable sports (e.g. tennis, fencing, golf, gymnastics, figure-skating, skiing) are aesthetically pleasing to watch, demand accuracy but not undue strength and may be competitive but do not involve bodily contact. In summary, the participants look 'feminine' and are not too rough.

Unacceptable sports (e.g. wrestling, boxing, weightlifting, rugby and other team sports) often require strength, face-to-face opposition and bodily contact. They, therefore, are rough and often overtly aggressive. Colley *et al.* (1985) investigated sex-typing of fifty sports/physical activities and obtained findings which supported Metheny's descriptions of twenty years before. More sports were sex-typed for males than for females. These included traditional male team sports (e.g. rugby, baseball), combat sports (e.g. boxing, wrestling), high-risk sports (e.g. mountaineering, potholing) and water sports requiring risk-taking and/or obvious use of strength (e.g. surfing, canoeing). Sports sex-typed for females included the traditionally female team sports (e.g. netball, rounders) and noncompetitive activities (e.g. yoga, popmobility).

In 'acceptable' sports, a traditionally 'feminine' appearance may be maintained which, as indicated in the study by Sage and Loudermilk (1979) described in the previous section, may result in less role conflict for the female participants. Snyder and Kivlin (1977) asked their sample of female athletes if they felt there was a stigma attached to their sport and 56 per cent of basketball players responded positively in comparison with 31 per cent of gymnasts. Snyder and Spreitzer (1976) looked at self-perceptions of femininity in female gymnasts and basketball players. In this study 70 per cent of gymnasts felt themselves to be very feminine as against only 44 per cent of basketball players.

The general acceptability of only certain sports for women reflects sex-stereotyping of both physical and psychological attributes. In other words, the stereotype of female as the 'weaker' sex is reflected in expectations of their sport participation and performance. Psychological characteristics such as aggressiveness, competitiveness and willingness to take risks are stereotyped as masculine (e.g. Bem 1974). Sports in which the display of such characteristics is most apparent are the least acceptable for female participation.

Physically, women are expected to be weaker and slower than men. Although physical differences between the sexes exist, Dyer (1982) argues that the effect of these on sporting performance is exaggerated by social and cultural factors. The potential level of performance of women in many physical activities is difficult to evaluate since they have restricted access to training facilities and to competition. Dyer presents evidence which demonstrates that in the speed sports (e.g. field events, swimming), women are catching up with men in participation and performance. He argues that physical sex differences ought to confer some advantages as well as disadvantages to female sporting performance. In long distance running, for example, women have the advantages of greater energy reserves, better mechanisms for temperature regulation and more efficient aerobic energy systems. However, the stereotype of the 'weak' woman is so well-established that such physical advantages have been largely ignored. As Dyer points out, 'In the whole history of track athletics it is just those events at which women are biologically most suited from which they have been banned or discouraged from participating' (p. 159). Dyer also discusses and dismisses 'myths' about potential damage to the female reproductive system from vigorous exercise and the masculinizing of women's bodies through training.

Sport is of course only one of many areas of human behaviour in which sex-stereotyping occurs. It is perhaps not surprising then, that Colley *et al.* (1985) found that general sex-role attitudes (measured using the AWS) significantly predicted the number of sports sex-typed for males and for females. The traditional view of female sport is reinforced by much media coverage of sport (see discussion in Dyer (1982) and Boutilier & SanGiovanni (1983)). Where coverage is given to female sports participants, their achievements may be trivialized, with greater attention being directed to their appearance than to their skill. Dyer (1982) includes a quote from a Sydney newspaper which had published an article on Jan Stevenson, the Australian golfer:

> Australia's Jan Stevenson was nominated today as the sexiest swinger in golf. Her sinuous body movements remind us of Marilyn Monroe ... the sexy kid from Sydney is a 23 year old suntanned blond with an enticing smile and 110 pounds laid out just right on a 5 foot 5 inches frame. (p. 107)

Any dissonance in integrating femininity with sporting ability can be resolved by the media in instances such as that above, by emphasizing the femininity of the participant rather than those qualities which may conflict with traditional sex-role expectations. This is less easy to do in those sports in which it is difficult to maintain a 'feminine' appearance.

Sex-role identity and sport participation

The traits demanded by competitive sport participation, for instance competitiveness, aggression and dominance, are those which are stereotyped as masculine. A reasonable prediction would therefore be that competitive sports participants, both male and female, would produce high scores on the masculinity scales of sex role inventories such as the BSRI or PAQ. Individuals of both sexes with high masculinity scores have been found to have both a higher achievement motivation and a greater interest in competitive interaction styles than those with low masculinity scores (Baxter & Shepherd 1978; Spence & Helmreich 1978). This prediction has been confirmed (Duquin 1978; Myers & Lips 1978; Uguccioni & Ballantyne 1980). A high proportion of masculine and androgynous individuals are found in sports participant groups. Many female participants are androgynous, that is they have high masculinity and femininity scores. The high femininity score is clearly attributable to the fact that they are female, but may also relate to the expressive, aesthetic component of sports which are acceptable for them and in which they participate. A comparison of the sex-role identity of participants in Metheny's 'acceptable' and 'unacceptable' sports would be of interest here since the 'unacceptable' sports do not have a clear expressive component.

A problem arises in the interpretation of the relationship between sex-role identity and sport participation. Individuals who score high on masculinity may be attracted to sport because it is an instrumental activity. A second possibility, however, is that sports participants become more aware of their masculine-stereotyped qualities through participation and hence give themselves higher ratings on these attributes than non-participants. Thirdly, sports participation may increase masculine attributes and therefore result in higher masculinity scores.

Non-participation in sports by males may relate to sex-role identity. Lower scores on masculinity are found in male non-participants (e.g. Colley, Roberts & Chipps 1985). Problems in interpretation arise again here, however. Males low on masculinity may choose not to participate in sports, or males who perceive themselves to be low on ability in sport may deny their instrumental attributes in order to find a more acceptable reason for their non-participation.

Summary and conclusions

This chapter has discussed the implications of psychological and sociological aspects of sex roles and sex-role socialization for participation in leisure activities in general and in sport in particular. Inevitably much of the discussion has focused on the constraints which apply to women. Women have more limited leisure lives than men according to the criteria used to collect data on leisure participation, and they participate in sport far less than men.

In general leisure, many differences in male and female patterns and rates of participation can be attributed to differing life-styles and home responsibilities. The domestic commitments for which sex-role socialization prepares women have a restrictive effect on leisure time in particular. Accompanying attitudes toward the sex-appropriateness of different leisure activities have an additional constraining effect. It is interesting to note that in this area of investigation into sex differences, as in others, there is an underlying orientation in the literature which emphasizes the injustices suffered by women by having fewer and more limited opportunities than men. 'The factors contributing to women's overall subordinate position in society thus contribute to their scant leisure' (Deem 1982, p. 29). It is certainly clear that women are severely constrained in their leisure behaviour. However, Gregory (1982) has suggested that this approach does not do justice to the way in which women have coped with and integrated the varying demands of their role. As Gregory points out, changing patterns of employment may fundamentally change the lives of men. They may start to share the problems of women in having a less clear-cut work/leisure distinction and a greater involvement in the domestic side of their lives. Knowledge of the way in which women integrate their commitments with leisure may be of considerable importance here. Traditional attitudes towards styles of female and male leisure, if they perpetuate, may result in poor adjustment to a less structured life-style for many men.

Sport is an area of leisure which, through sex-role socialization, becomes the clear province of the male. The domestic constraints which apply to women in general leisure apply to sport, but more important are the psychological constraints imposed by the incompatibility of sport with the female sex role. Many female participants in sport perceive their feminine and athletic roles to be in conflict. The sports considered acceptable for women, and in which the majority of women participate, are those in which masculine attributes are least apparent. They have an expressive as well as an instrumental component. Again in considering the constraints on female participation in sport, there is a tendency to emphasize the desirability of male traits. Birrell (1983), Duquin (1978) and Oglesby (1978) have all argued for a reconceptualization of sport such that female traits are also valued.

> Sport need not be narrowly viewed only as an arena for the display of power and dominance behaviours; it could also serve as a showcase for other valuable traits associated more with females than males. For example, nurturance and sensitivity are valued attributes which should be welcomed in sport. Furthermore, studies ... suggest the ethic of fair play is more frequently endorsed by females than males; it is not inconceivable that females can contribute a renewed emphasis on fairness and integrity to sporting activity. (Birrell 1983, p. 67)

References

Anthrop, J. & Allison, M. T. (1983) Role conflict and the high school female athlete. *Research Quarterly for Exercise and Sport, 54*, 104–111.

Axline, V. M. (1947) *Play therapy*. Boston: Houghton Mifflin.

Baxter, L. A. & Shepherd, T. L. (1978) Sex-role identity, sex of other, and affective relationship as determinants of interpersonal conflict–management styles. *Sex Roles, 4*, 813–825.

Bem, S. L. (1974) The measurement of psychological androgyny. *Journal of Consulting and Clinical Psychology, 42*, 155–162.

Birrell, S. (1983) The psychological dimensions of female athletic participation. *In* M. A. Boutilier and L. SanGiovanni (eds) *The sporting woman*. Champaign: Human Kinetics Publishers.

Boothby, J., Tungatt, M., Townsend, A. R. & Collins, M. F. (1981) *A sporting chance*? London: Sports Council.

Boutilier, M. A. & SanGiovanni, L. (1983) *The sporting woman*. Champaign: Human Kinetics Publishers.

Colker, R. & Widom, C. S. (1980) Correlates of female athletic participation: masculinity, femininity, self-esteem, and attitudes toward women. *Sex Roles, 6*, 47–58.

Colley, A. (1984) Sex roles and explanations of leisure behaviour. *Leisure Studies, 3*, 335–341.

Colley, A., Nash, J., O'Donnell, L. & Restorick, L. (1985) Attitudes to the female sex role and sex-typing of physical activities. Manuscript submitted for publication.

Colley, A., Roberts, N. & Chipps, A. (1985) Sex-role identity, personality and participation in team and individual sports by males and females. *International Journal of Sport Psychology, 16*, 103–112.

Deem, R. (1982) Women, leisure and inequality. *Leisure Studies, 1,* 29–46.

Del Rey, P. (1977) In support of apologetics for women in sport. *In* D. M. Landers and R. W. Christina (eds) *Psychology of motor behaviour and sport – 1976.* Champaign: Human Kinetics Publishers.

Duquin, M. E. (1978) The androgynous advantage. *In* C. A. Oglesby (ed.) *Women and sport: from myth to reality.* Philadelphia: Lea & Febiger.

Dyer, K. (1982) *Catching up the men.* St Lucia: University of Queensland Press.

Fagot, B. I. (1978) The influence of sex of child on parental reactions to toddler children. *Child Development, 49,* 459–465.

Felshin, J. (1974) The triple option ... for women in sport. *Quest, 21,* 36–40.

Fisher, A. C., Genovese, P. P., Morris, K. J. & Morris, H. H. (1978) Perceptions of women in sport. *In* D. M. Landers & R. W. Christina (eds) *Psychology of motor behaviour and sport – 1977.* Champaign: Human Kinetics Publishers.

General Household Survey (1977) London: HMSO.

Gentry, J. W. & Doering, M. (1979) Sex role orientation and leisure. *Journal of Leisure Research, 11,* 102–111.

Greendorfer, S. L. (1974) The nature of female socialization into sport: a study of selected college women's sport participation. Unpublished doctoral dissertation, University of Wisconsin.

Greendorfer, S. L. (1977) Role of socializing agents in female sport involvement. *Research Quarterly, 48,* 304–310.

Greendorfer, S. L. (1979) Childhood sport socialization influences of male and female track athletes. *Arena Review, 3,* 39–53.

Greendorfer, S. (1983) Shaping the female athlete. The impact of the family. *In* M. A. Boutilier & L. SanGiovanni (eds) *The sporting woman.* Champaign: Human Kinetics Publishers.

Gregory, S. (1982) Women among others: another view. *Leisure Studies, 1,* 47–52.

Gregson, J. & Colley, A. (in press) Concomitants of sport participation in male and female adolescents. *International Journal of Sport Psychology.*

Griffin, P. S. (1973) What's a nice girl like you doing in a profession like this? *Quest, 19,* 96–101.

Hagedorn, R. & Labovitz, S. (1968) Participation in community associations by occupations: a test of three theories. *American Sociological Review, 33,* 272–283.

Iso-Ahola, S. E. (1979) Basic dimensions of definitions of leisure. *Journal of Leisure Research, 11,* 28–39.

Lewis, M. (1972) State as an infant-environment interaction: an analysis of mother-infant behaviour as a function of sex. *Merrill-Palmer Quarterly, 18,* 95–121.

Lewko, J. H. & Ewing, M. E. (1980) Sex differences and parental influence in sport involvement of children. *Journal of Sport Psychology, 2,* 62–68.

Lewko, J. H. & Greendorfer, S. L. (1978) Family influence and sex differences in children's socialisation into sport: a review. *In* D. M. Landers & R. W. Christina (eds) *Psychology of motor behaviour and sport – 1977.* Champaign: Human Kinetics Publishers.

Lore, R. K. (1968) Activity drive hypothesis: effect of activity restriction. *Psychological Bulletin, 70,* 566–574.

Metheny, E. (1965) *Connotations of movement in sport and dance*. Dubuque: William C. Brown.

Mitchell, E. D. & Mason, B. S. (1934) *The theory of play*. New York: Barnes.

Myers, A. M. & Lips, H. (1978) Participation in competitive amateur sports as a function of psychological androgyny. *Sex Roles*, *4*, 571–578.

Neulinger, J. & Breit, M. (1971) Attitude dimensions of leisure: a replication study. *Journal of Leisure Research*, *3*, 108–115.

Nixon, H. L., Maresca, P. J. & Silverman, M. A. (1979) Sex differences in college students' acceptance of females in sport. *Adolescence*, *14*, 755–764.

Oglesby, C. A. (1978) The masculinity/femininity game: called on account of . . . In C. A. Oglesby (ed.) *Women and sport: from myth to reality*. Philadelphia: Lea & Febiger.

Rheingold, H. L. and Cook, K. V. (1975) The contents of boys' and girls' rooms as an index of parents' behaviour. *Child Development*, *46*, 459–463.

Sage, G. H. and Loudermilk, S. (1979) The female athlete and role conflict. *Research Quarterly*, *50*, 88–96.

Sapora, A. V. and Mitchell, E. D. (1961) *The theory of play and recreation*. New York: Plenum Press.

Selby, R. & Lewko, J. H. (1976) Children's attitudes towards females in sports: their relationship with sex, grade and sports participation. *Research Quarterly*, *47*, 453–463.

Sillitoe, K. K. (1969) *Planning for leisure*. London: HMSO.

Snyder, E. E. & Kivlin, J. E. (1977) Perceptions of the sex-role among female athletes and non-athletes. *Adolescence*, *45*, 23–29.

Snyder, E. E. & Spreitzer, E. (1976) Correlates of sport participation among adolescent girls. *Research Quarterly*, *47*, 804–809.

Snyder, E. E. and Spreitzer, E. (1978) *Social aspects of sport*. Englewood Cliffs, NJ: Prentice-Hall.

Spence, J. T. & Helmreich, R. (1972) *The attitudes toward women scale*. Washington, DC: American Psychological Association.

Spence, J. T. & Helmreich, R. L. (1978) *Masculinity and femininity: their psychological dimensions, correlates and antecedents*. Austin: University of Texas Press.

Spence, J. T., Helmreich, R. & Stapp, J. (1974) The Personal Attributes Questionnaire: a measure of sex-role stereotypes and masculinity-femininity. *JSAS Catalog of Selected Documents in Psychology*, *4*, 43. (Ms. no. 617).

Talbot, M. (1979) *Women and leisure*. A review for the Sports Council/SSRC Joint Panel on Leisure and Recreation Research.

Uguccioni, S. M. & Ballantyne, R. H. (1980) Comparison of attitudes and sex roles for female athletic participants and non-participants. *International Journal of Sport Psychology*, *11*, 42–48.

Weiss, M. R. & Knoppers, A. (1982) The influence of socializing agents on female collegiate volleyball players. *Journal of Sport Psychology*, *4*, 267–279.

Witt, P. A. & Bishop, D. W. (1970) Situational antecedents to leisure behaviour. *Journal of Leisure Research*, *2*, 64–77.

Witt, P. A. & Goodale, T. L. (1981) The relationship between barriers to leisure enjoyment and family stages. *Leisure Sciences*, *4*, 29–49.

CHAPTER THIRTEEN   Sex Roles and Mental Health
Suzanne Skevington

'Mr Woodhouse: 'Young ladies should take care of themselves. Young ladies are delicate plants. They should take good care of their health and complexion. My dear, did you change your stockings?' (Jane Austen, *Emma*, 1816)

As the quotation suggests, the notion of health is inextricably bound up with sex roles. The relationships between mental and physical health and sex roles will be explored in this chapter. The chapter starts with a discussion of some of the mental health statistics, which is followed by a consideration of the effects of work and marriage on well-being. Questions are asked about how the professionals view their patients and whether this affects the way the statistics are recorded. The decision-making processes whereby people become patients are discussed, and individual differences which affect the reporting of illness are included. Life expectancy and constitutional factors are considered, followed by a brief examination of the arguments surrounding sex differences in reproductive biology with special reference to menstruation and the menopause. The measurement of stress is tackled in the debate about how far the sexes respond differently to stressors. How sex roles affect the perception of and coping with stress is also discussed. Comments on social support and the hardy personality precede a final section on helplessness, depression and uncontrollability, and the chapter concludes with ideas about ways of taking greater control over events.

While it is impossible to ignore political, economic and sociological factors within these discussions the debates in this chapter follow process-oriented sociocognitive lines, rather than the more medically oriented labelling approach of the disease model of mental health.

Health psychologists today are bound to take an interactionist and multifactorial perspective of the complex processes which affect mind and body. Physical illnesses such as coronary heart disease, rheumatism and breast cancer not only have psychological consequences but may also be triggered, sustained and inhibited by psychological factors. This is the subject of matter of the new field of behavioural medicine and must be included in a discussion of mental health and sex roles where diseases are sex-related. More familiar to the psychologist is the converse example of psychological disturbance which is accompanied by physical symptoms, as instanced by the dizziness and palpitations of the person with an anxiety state (Lader & Marks 1971). In some disorders physical and psychological symptoms may be of similar magnitudes. Fordyce (1976) comments on the considerable numbers of patients who experience intense pain with profound depression. For the psychologist interested in admission rates and decisions to seek and persist with treatment, these findings raise questions about why some people will be treated in psychiatric outpatients, while others with similar symptoms will be referred to a pain clinic run by anaesthetists and neurologists (Skevington 1983).

The 'facts'

Using the 1975 DHSS statistics, Reid and Wormald (1982) reviewed mental health admissions in Britain. They found that male admissions were higher for alcoholism and alcoholic psychosis; that the sexes were similar in their admissions for schizophrenia, drug dependency and personality disorder, but that female admissions were higher for depression, other psychoses, senile and presenile dementia and the psychoneuroses. Other studies of sex differences in Britain, the United States and elsewhere tend to confirm the higher incidence of certain types of mental disorder among women.

A famous paper by Gove and Tudor (1973) reviewed nineteen studies done in the United States and found a higher percentage of mentally ill women than men. More recently, Goldman and Ravid (1980) compared eighteen studies where sixteen confirmed the finding of Gove and Tudor, and the other two showed no significant differences. Like other writers they note that studies before 1950 consistently show higher rates of mental illness in men, so indicating a social rather than biological explanation for the current sex differences. None of the studies they reviewed (published between 1952 and 1970) included the diagnostic category of personality disorder, and Gove and Tudor excluded this category from their review. As men are known to have higher levels of personality disorder in the United States such category omissions would bias the statistics by omitting particular groups of men from the survey. The type of study performed, and diagnostic criteria used should be scrutinized in any evaluation of this area.

The impact of work and marriage

Sociodemographic analysis of health and well-being shows that particular subgroups are susceptible or vulnerable to mental disorders so that generalizations become nonsensical. In a major review of well-being and employment, Warr and Parry (1982) concluded that psychological distress and self-report measures of happiness have rarely been found to be related to whether or not a woman has a job. However there is some slight association between psychiatric condition and having a job, in working-class groups. Warr and Parry (1982) could find no cases in which women with paid employment emerged as having significantly lower well-being than those without a job. Like men, single women without children have high occupational involvement, so unemployment in this subgroup is significantly related to low psychological well-being. This relationship is less marked for married women without children, and is negligible for married women with children at home. Employed and unemployed married women are no different from each other. It appears that there is a significant relationship between psychological distress and wanting to work, and that the *quality* of a woman's employment is very important. Reviewing studies on men's unemployment, Cochrane (1983) shows how work is especially important in maintaining men's psychological well-being. The human costs of an economic recession cannot be calculated.

These studies are particularly important at a time when increasing numbers of women are entering and re-entering employment. The proportion of economically active women increased by 45 percent between 1931 and 1970, and in the same period the number of married women increased fourfold. The proportion of men in the labour force remained stable during this time. By 1980 there were approximately 10.4 million women and 15.6 million men at work in Britain (Coote & Campbell 1982).

The relative importance of gender and social class on subjective well-being has been evaluated using *meta-analysis* by Haring, Stock and Okun (1984). Meta-analysis transforms results from individual studies to a common metric called effect size, then uses statistics to evaluate the results from a broad range of studies on a particular topic so that diverse findings can be assessed. Haring, Stock and Okun conclude that gender is significantly related to well-being, with men having slightly higher scores on measures of well-being than women. While the difference between the sexes remains when social class is entered into the analysis, the sex difference then accounts for less than 1 percent of the variance in subjective well-being. Regrettably the authors did not examine marital status.

While studies such as this are clearly major advances in the interpretation of the data, most studies of gender and social class are based solely on the social gradings of *male* occupations, because until Britten and Heath's paper in 1982, nobody had grasped the nettle of systematically evaluating the prestige of occupations held by women. Even the latter study has not come to terms with the problems of evaluating the social standing of different patterns of homemaking, unpaid voluntary work and part-time employment for women, although Britten and Heath make some interesting observations on cross-class marriages.

Marital status is yet another variable which needs consideration in this context. The statistics show that married men have better mental health than married women, although some recent research suggests that a mentally disturbed man is much more likely to be cared for at home than a similar woman. Reid and Wormald (1982) speculate whether current trends towards role reversal will alter mental hospital admission rates.

Gove and Tudor (1973) have suggested that marriage is less satisfying for women than for men. They argue that married men have satisfaction from their careers as well as being head of the household, so that if one fails the other may still provide satisfaction and well-being. With the growing numbers of women entering employment this may be less true today. Gove and Tudor identify several sources of distress in being a housewife. Housewives do not have opportunities for achievement and competence in the predominantly unskilled work of the home, which is low in prestige, is unstructured, 'invisible', and leaves ample time and opportunity to dwell on troubles. In entering employment but viewing their careers as secondary, not only do housewives take on a double load, but also they are more susceptible to discrimination when promotion is an issue. Finally they are continually adjusting to the needs of their husband and children, so having less control over events in their lives which will be shown later in the chapter to contribute to helplessness and depression. Regrettably there are too few good studies on black women and men to enable an adequate analysis of race and gender here. Most British researchers, for example, have not considered race a sufficiently important variable to warrant inclusion.

Views of the professionals

What exactly is meant by psychological health or well-being? The stereotypic views of men and women are particularly relevant to the mental health debate when we come to consider how health professionals view them and use them. Their training does not give them immunity from sex-role stereotyping, although hopefully in some cases it may give them a greater awareness of the problem. Despite the growing numbers of women entering the medical profession since the Sex Discrimination Act in 1975, most doctors are still men, and men form a large majority of consultants. Chesler (1972) reported that in the United States 90 percent of psychiatrists and 85 percent of clinical psychologists were men. This has implications for the judgement and interpretation of symptoms upon which the national statistics on health and illness are based. In a detailed historical analysis Ehrenreich and English (1979) trace the rise in male medical and psychomedical experts back to the purging of wise women in the sixteenth century. At that time wisdom about health and healing was passed on between women. It is interesting that social psychology in the 1970s has brought a renewed interest in, and re-established the importance of naive theories and common-sense approaches in the development of attributional and accountability theories and their relevance for health (e.g King 1983).

A particularly interesting study by Broverman *et al.* (1970) sought to investigate the role of sex-role stereotypes in clinical diagnosis. Seventy-nine medical clinicians (doctors, psychologists and social workers) completed the Rosencrantz Sex Role Questionnaire. One group were asked to rate a 'healthy, mature, socially competent adult person', and the other two groups were asked to rate a similarly described man or woman. They also made ratings of the person's health. No difference was found between the ratings of male and female clinicians, but socially desirable characteristics were seen as healthier for men than for women. Healthy women are seen as more excitable in minor crises, more easily influenced, less competitive, less aggressive and less objective, for example, than healthy males. Beliefs about what constituted a healthy adult were much closer to the view of the healthy man than to that of the healthy woman, reflecting a powerfully negative view of women. A disturbing implication of this study is that women may be more readily diagnosed as psychologically disordered and unstable because they differ so much more from the view of the ideal healthy adult even when healthy.

Other factors also affect the reporting of mental health statistics. For example, fashions in diagnosis change. A diagnosis of alcoholism was most uncommon for women thirty years ago (Litman 1978) because doctors were unwilling to stigmatize the fairer sex with this label, preferring to label them as depressed. The figures for the incidence of cirrhosis of the liver reflect more accurately the *actual* rates of drinking at this time. So the apparent dramatic rise in the incidence of alcoholism in women during the 1960s and 1970s, which has been blamed on the social change in women's lives brought about by the women's movement (Royal College of Physicians 1979) to some extent at least, reflects changes in the readiness to apply the diagnostic label as the stigma has diminished.

There are also cultural differences in diagnosis which could account for discrepancies in the frequency of particular disorders, despite attempts to standardize diagnosis. Psychiatrists trained in different schools in Britain, and between Britain and the United States show quite low levels of agreement about diagnosis (Vernon 1969). American psychiatrists tend to have a broader definition of schizophrenia, for example, and apply it in a much less conservative way than those in Britain, although this is changing with the common use of International Classification of Diseases and DSM III.

Decision-making by patients

Another factor which is of relevance here is the propensity to seek help, or action taken to report symptoms. The person in the street assumes that when people are ill they go to see a doctor, and most surveys of health and illness are compiled on the basis of this assumption. However, epidemiological studies of communities show that there is a large 'subclinical' population who, for a variety of reasons, do not visit their doctor and therefore are never included in the statistics.

In a large and detailed study in Wisconsin, Greenley and Mechanic (1976) amply demonstrate the breadth of sources consulted by distressed students. In addition to medical and psychiatric services, students consulted counsellors, clergymen, psychologists, social workers, T groups, 'Samaritan' type organizations, VD clinics, family courts, drug information centres, community law offices, Veteran's Administration hospitals, and university lecturers and administrators. They found three factors which were generally related to help seeking, namely being female, having a propensity to seek help for psychological problems and being oriented towards introspective others. In no case were women students under-users of any service in this study, so it is not just that they seek more help from doctors than men, but they seek more help from *all* available resources more frequently.

Sanders (1982) comments that there are considerable costs in relying on expert information, namely time and effort, ease of disclosure, pain and discomfort, bad news, recrimination, commitment, individuality and money. He describes the individual differences which could influence decisions to seek lay consultation. These are self-disclosure, self-esteem, extraversion, trust and dominant − submissive relationships. These features would seem to be linked to traditional sex roles. There are sex differences in the expression of feelings and complaints even at an early age, according to Mechanic (1964).

Ingham and Miller (1976) report that once individuals come to places such as psychiatric clinics for treatment, doctors are unwilling to admit that treatment is not required. In other words, they tend to diagnose and prescribe for those seeking help. This raises questions about why women report their symptoms more frequently. Pennebaker (1982) in a series of studies shows that women are much more attentive to their internal bodily state than men, and seek medical attention based on the perception of their symptoms. Why this is so is not entirely clear. The findings do give answers to questions about why, across cultures and ages, women report more symptoms, take more prescribed and non-prescribed medication and visit physicians more often than men. Pennebaker's work also implies that the well-established finding of greater longevity in women could be in part to do with being more 'tuned in' to their bodies, which leads them to take greater care of their health. This may be coupled with a greater inclination to take action to correct discomforts whenever necessary. The lower levels of internal attentiveness in men might account for the higher diagnosed rates of chronic hypertension, ulcers and cancer. This might also account for the shorter longevity of men, particularly if they disregard the signs of a heart attack and angina. This results in a delay in taking action, frequently at great cost! The argument goes that if men went to the doctor earlier with symptoms they might live longer. In a chapter on the symptom-reporting personality Pennebaker (1982) describes high symptom reporters as self-conscious, anxious, with low-self esteem and aspiring to (but not necessarily able to) control aspects of their environment. These are to some extent, aspects of the stereotypic female personality.

Longevity

The findings about longevity are interesting and relevant to sex roles and well-being. Researchers have been puzzled by why women seem to be more ill, but live longer. While longevity has been increasing in most countries of the Western world this century due to better public health and diet, the gap between men and women has widened noticeably. In 1900 in the United States, on average men survived 46.3 years and women 48.3 years; but by 1976 men were living for 68.7 years and women 76.5 years (Harrison 1978) so women have more years in which to consult a doctor. Recent increases in alcohol consumption and smoking in women may affect their longevity in the future (Reid & Wormald 1982).

Women are likely to consult more often because of the apparent greater complexity of their reproductive systems. Women menstruate between 300 to 400 times in their lives. They are likely to consult their doctors more often than men for advice on contraception from the age of menarche, which statistically is declining yearly in Britain. They are likely to see doctors more often when pregnant, and regularly when the children are ill (Bristol Women's Studies Group 1979). They may also seek advice at the menopause. It seems possible that these periodic visits for matters concerned with the reproductive cycle and child care may facilitate the reporting of other symptoms, given the greater opportunities for developing closer interpersonal relations with the doctor.

We would also expect women to feature more often in the statistics because they are a majority in the population. This is not so at conception where it is estimated that between 108 and 120 males are fertilized for every 100 females. More boys are aborted, so that the figures decline to 105 boys at birth for each 100 girls. More boys than girls die of childhood diseases and abnormalities so that 51.2 percent of the adult population are women (Harrison 1978)

The reasons for this can be explained in genetic terms, and for a fuller account a text on genetics should be consulted (e.g. Sinnott, Dunn & Dobzhansky 1958). A closer examination of the genes on the sex chromosomes accounts for the greater vulnerability of males. In brief, each of the forty-six chromosomes in human cells are made up of genes, which transmit information about the individual's characteristics, for example hair colour, personality traits, etc. Two of these chromosomes determine the person's sex and sex-related characteristics, and are called X and Y. At conception two X chromosomes are paired for a female, and an X with a Y for a male. Ova only contain X chromosomes, but sperm can carry an X or Y. When paired, some of the genes on each chromosome will match each other while others remain unmatched.

A feature of unmatched genes is that the characteristic they carry will be exhibited or expressed in the new human being. As the X chromosome is longer than the Y, when they pair a 'tail' of genes on the X remains unmatched and are therefore expressed in the male. Genes for sex-linked disorders are thought to exist largely in this 'tail', but not all have been identified. Baldness, for example, is expressed for genetic reasons in men but is carried through the female line of the family unexpressed. However this 'tail' may contain a variety of genes responsible for sex-linked mental and physical abnormalities, and is thought to be responsible for the vulnerability of males and the high levels of perinatal mortality in boys.

Here biology challenges the notion of men as the stronger sex, but this has not been true in sociobiology where there is a long tradition of using animal studies to demonstrate the physical weaknesses of women and hence their incapacity for education and work (Sayers 1982). Despite the explosion of psychological literature on the socialization of sex roles, with its emphasis on the importance of the environment and learning in the past twenty years, Wilson (1978) has recently pronounced on the costs of circumventing 'innate predispositions' in the advancement of sexual equality, even though much of his academic career has been devoted to the investigation of insect rather than human societies. In this field anthropomorphism is rife.

Studies of baboon societies by Lorenz (1969) and Tiger and Fox (1974) show how primate and human societies have social hierarchies which are determined by innate aggression. This is then used to argue for the biological determinants of human sex roles, citing the effects of hormones such as testosterone on behaviour. Many modern ethologists such as Gould (1977) are not prepared to make such definitive statements about the parallels between human and non-human behaviour. They study animals in their own right, rather than with the purpose of extrapolating up the evolutionary scale and refer to the propositions on which such arguments are based as 'crude biological determinism'. Similarly sexual inequality has been defended through the investigation of sex differences in the brain. Sayers points out how, couched in biological terms, these arguments appear to offer a legitimate scientific basis for opposition to equal education and work. Around the turn of the century it was argued that work would impair the monthly rhythm and the capacity and fitness of women to reproduce and have healthy children. Also it was believed that women were less well developed physically and mentally than men because their energy had to be reserved for reproduction. Similar and more subtle forms of these arguments are still in use today.

Reproductive cycle and mental health

What is the evidence that a woman's reproductive cycle affects her emotions and hence her mental health? Dalton (1969) believes that the premenstrual syndrome (PMS) is the result of changes in the mineral salts of the body. Her studies claim that schoolgirls perform less well on tests, teachers hand out more punishments, there are more accidents, suicides and crimes such as shoplifting, and that more women are admitted to psychiatric hospital during the premenstrual period. However there are lots of methodological problems in the investigation of a woman's reproductive cycle. It is impossible to separate completely the effects of physical from psychological symptoms in the cycle, because the physical ones are obvious and well learned. It is now believed that perceptual and social factors, as much as biological ones, affect mood change (Koeske & Koeske 1975). In addition, any awareness by subjects that their menstrual cycle is being monitored is likely to stimulate belief systems about the cycle, and knowledge about the cycle influences the reporting of symptoms (Slade 1984). Paige (1973) in common with other investigators, says that women with symptoms during menstruation also show the same types of symptoms at other times which suggests that a general trend to report may underlie results in this area. An interesting attributional study where male and female students were given thumbnail sketches about women which included a mention of the stage of their cycle, showed that knowledge about biology is important in explaining negative moods such as depression and irritability premenstrually, but not positive moods. In conclusion, the evidence linking mood and hormones is not as convincing as it appears (Archer & Lloyd 1982).

The menopause and so called 'empty nest syndrome' have also been a focus for research, and claims have been made for substantial psychological disturbance at this stage in the life cycle. In a large national health and nutrition survey, data was collected from 3,742 women and an analysis of age and well-being performed (Lennon 1982). The psychological consequences of menopause varied with the person's age. Most women *expect* the menopause in mid-life, but the greatest psychological distress is caused when the biological event is off-schedule with expectations. Young women (ages 24–43) were distressed, even though cessation of periods could well have been amenorrhea caused by poor diet, disease or stress. Depression was also high among the older age group (54–74). So the menopause *per se* does not seem to be psychologically stressful for most women.

The psychology of pregnancy is too broad to be covered here. Good reviews of the literature are to be found in Breen (1975), Fransella and Frost (1977) and Reading (1983). As a postscript to this section it is worth noting that remarkably few studies have been done on men to investigate the relationship between their emotions, mental health and the not inconsiderable fluctuations in testosterone (Archer & Lloyd 1982).

Stress, control and depression

To conclude this chapter the processes of stress and control will be reviewed in relation to depression in women, as depression is more often found in women than men. Klerman and Weissman (1980), reviewing the literature, conclude that of the population of women in Britain, America and Scandanavia, between 20 and 30 percent experience one or more depressive episodes at some point in their adult lives, which are often of moderate severity. Of these, only about a quarter with depressive symptoms will seek help from a physician. Evidence of depression comes not only from observations of patients coming to treatment, but also from studies of suicide and suicide attempters who are commonly very depressed, and from studies of grief and bereavement.

A variety of researchers have asked whether women are under more stress than men. This is a difficult question to answer. As Steptoe (1980) has pointed out, the use of the term *psychological stressor* fails to clarify ambiguities in the description of stress. In the area of stress reporting, the measurement of life events has been very influential, as exemplified by the development of scales such as the Schedule of Recent Events SRE (Holmes & Rahe 1967) and the extensive structured interviews used by Brown and Harris (1978). Makosky (1980) has suggested that life events scales were constructed (largely by men) with men in mind. They contain many questions about work, for example, about promotion and demotion, changes at work and interpersonal conflicts in the work environment. Only the respondent's stress level is assessed. Little attention is paid to the spouse's stress level, except where men are questioned about their wives' pregnancies, abortions, etc.

Makosky (1980) suggests that stress in one's spouse's life is probably more important for women than men, although research still needs to be done on the contagion of stress between wife and husband. Lists of life events systematically underestimate stress in women's lives. For example, the SRE uses the event of marriage as an anchor event and this was allocated an arbitrary value of fifty when the scale was designed. Other events were then compared to it. Makosky suggests that marriage probably causes more change in the lives of women than men.

Makoksy (1980) agrees with Klerman and Weissman (1980) that on the available evidence women neither report nor experience more stressful events, and there is no evidence to date to show that the sexes respond differently to comparable stress and stressors. So while the methodology seems to be suspect, so far there is no clear evidence to substantiate a sex difference in stress levels.

Relevant to this debate is the study of the 'hardy' personality. Kobasa (1982) identifies three components which comprise hardiness. Through prospective longitudinal studies she has shown, first, that hardy people tend to be *committed* to what they do in a variety of areas of life such as work, as opposed to feeling alienated. Secondly they believe that they have some degree of *control* over the causes of, and solutions to problems, rather than feeling helpless or powerless. Third they view demands for readjustment and change in life as opportunities and a *challenge*, not threats. She says hardiness accounts for the observation that some people who have high levels of stress do not automatically become ill. In Kobasa's study of 100 gynaecology outpatients, the 40 who had high stress and low illness had significantly more commitment to work, to family and to self, had greater personal control, and greater 'vigor of challenge' than the other 60 women with high stress and high psychiatric symptoms. Kobasa concludes that hardy people see stress more positively.

How people perceive and react to stress is also related to their sex roles. The concept of psychological androgyny (Bem 1974) is described in Chapter 2, and perhaps one of the most interesting discoveries to arise from its investigation is that under stressful conditions, psychologically androgynous women experience better health than those who are sex-typed (Williams 1979). This may be something to do with their more adaptable and flexible approach towards life. More recent research indicates that the masculine component in androgyny may be more important than the feminine contribution (Taylor & Hall 1982).

One of the most widely discussed studies of depression in the last decade was published by Brown and Harris (1978) in a book called *Social Origins of Depression*. They reported two community studies of women between eighteen and sixty-four years living in Camberwell in 1969–71 and 1974–5 and identified *vulnerability* factors, which they said were derived from the observation of a relationship between life events, chronic difficulties and the onset of depression. These vulnerability factors were not associated with depression unless the person had been exposed to adversity, or a chronic difficulty, such as loss of mother either through death or separation before age eleven, being unemployed, having three or more children under age fourteen or being without a husband or boyfriend in whom to confide. A replication of this study by Bebbington *et al.* (1984) confirms the finding that there are more depressed 'cases' among working-class women with children who have experienced stressful events, but failed to find any evidence in support of loss of mother. Investigation of the other two factors was inconclusive and only showed some significant associations in some conditions. Bebbington *et al* (1984) criticized the original study for its loose definition of 'cases', and for the overrepresentation of married women in the sample.

Reviewing the effects of social support, interpersonal relations and health, Suls (1982) concludes that despite a large body of evidence which suggests that social support is good for mental health, not all groups, social networks and significant others are necessarily helpful to those who need help. He points to research on helping behaviour which shows how people can mistrust others who give help without asking for rewards. Such relationships may well develop in families where chronic illness is present. The negative effects of social support are demonstrated in the lowering of self-esteem. This could account for the inconsistent results found by Bebbington *et al.* (1984) who found the influence of some husbands/boyfriends to be supportive, while others contribute to the woman's distress.

Finally, the incidence of depression in women has been explained through the application of the attributional learned helplessness hypothesis (Abramson, Seligman & Teasdale 1978) by writers such as Litman (1978) and Dweck and Licht (1980). Dweck and Licht show compellingly how girls learn to be more helpless than boys in achievement situations, and how this perception of incompetence generalizes to failure in a wide variety of situations. Repeated failure and loss of control is deemed to be the basis of this attributional interpretation of depression. Radloff (1980) takes the line that competent behaviour is rewarded by praise in our culture, and that this behaviour is more often attributed to men. In contrast women get fewer rewards, have less control over their rewards and more often see rewards as accompanied by punishment, producing conflicts that interfere with learning. Low self-esteem accompanies perceptions of uncontrollability and is said by Abramson *et al.* (1978) to be an integral part of depression and helplessness. Although women as a whole do not have lower self-esteem than men (Fransella & Frost 1977) in some situations, and with some subgroups, it is higher than in others. For example, women tend to be more socially skilled than men, and are thought to gain their self-esteem more from success in social situations than from career achievements (Fransella & Frost 1977). Recent moves to develop and teach assertiveness training have arisen from discussion within the women's movement about the importance of taking control of situations and thereby maintaining self-esteem and reducing feelings of perceived helplessness (e.g. Dickson 1982). The differences between real and illusory control in many contexts are now being explored by researchers, notably Langer (1983), and may well prove to be another important key to the understanding of sex differences in the mental health of women and men.

Conclusion

In this chapter we have examined the notion of women as the sicker and weaker sex from a variety of viewpoints. Interpretation of relevant statistics is by no means straightforward because they are confounded by a host of psychological factors which differentially affect the sexes. The epidemiological studies suggest that we are only looking at the tip of an iceberg of symptoms which seem to reflect a greater propensity in women to seek help. Women also seem much more sensitive to the detection of internal sensations which may prove to be a life-extending advantage, despite the greater costs to the health service in the provision of help.

The concept of control is a theme which runs through this chapter and may prove to be one of the most interesting frontiers for current research. Women are socialized into giving, caring, nurturing and responding to the demands of their families. It has been suggested that the stress in women's lives has been substantially underestimated, given the biases of measures such as the Schedule of Recent Events. The idea of a male breadwinner is now a myth (Land 1975), and today there is increasing economic necessity for both adults in a household to do paid work. Where women take on the double role of running a home and going out to work this does affect their well-being. Many feel intimidated by the Shirley Conran 'Superwoman' approach which entreats women in this position to take on everything uncomplainingly and never ask for help (Conran 1977) but they are often unaware of the alternatives.

The new skills of assertiveness training are helping women to ask for help both in the home and to satisfy their emotional needs in a non-aggressive way that defuses the anger and frustrations which arise in stressful situations. This way they are more in control of their lives rather than being subject to uncontrollable demands they may feel unable to meet and which can generate a loss of self-esteem, helplessness and the depression so commonly found in married women. There is a gathering body of evidence that expressing anger may also give some psychological immunity against diseases such as breast cancer.

The mental and physical health of men might also be helped through assertiveness training to cope with situations where traditional aggression normally occurs. Aggression, hostility, competition and impatience are part of the Type A syndrome which is a major predictor of the incidence of coronary heart disease, particularly in men, who have been much more widely researched than women, presumably because men figure more prominently in the statistics.

The so-called feminine characteristic of caring can also be considered in this context. In caring for and nurturing others, women sometimes cannot find enough time to care for themselves physically or emotionally. A change in consciousness has occurred during the 1970s with the rise of a women's health movement which has increased confidence about self-help, and which has stimulated community action to provide needed facilities such as pregnancy testing. This has caused a re-evaluation of the power of the helping professionals. The complex psychology of anorexia and obesity is too broad to be discussed here, but seems to be linked with sex roles and has profound consequences for mental as well as physical health. However, allowing the individual to take the right degree of control is crucial to the successful treatment of such disorders, with or without professional help (e.g Orbach 1978).

For men, learning to take care of others could well have beneficial effects in enriching their emotional lives and creating more fulfilling and closer relationships with their children. At a time when unemployment is returning an increasingly large number of men to the home, those who feel able to participate in the organization of the home and raising of children may well turn out to be in better mental and physical health than those who persist with their traditional sex-role behaviour, in terms of fending off helplessness and depression.

To do all this, researchers like Bem (1981) would argue that we have to reduce the importance of the gender dichotomy, with the aim of creating an aschematic society, and thereby improving mental health.

References

Abramson, L. Y., Seligman, M. E. D. & Teasdale, J. (1978) Learned helplessness in humans: critique and reformulation. *Journal of Abnormal Psychology, 87*, 49–74.

Archer, J. & Lloyd, B. (1982) *Sex and gender*. Harmondsworth: Penguin.

Bebbington, P. E., Sturt, E., Tennant, C. & Hurry, J. (1984) Misfortune and resilience – a community study of women. *Psychosomatic Medicine, 14*, 347–363.

Bem, S. L (1974) The measurement of psychological androgyny. *Journal of Consulting and Clinical Psychology, 42*, 155–162.

Bem, S. L. (1981) Gender schema theory: a cognitive account of sex typing. *Psychological Review, 8*, 354–364.

Breen, D. (1975) *The birth of a first child: towards an understanding of femininity*. London: Tavistock.

Bristol Women's Studies Group (1979) *Half the sky: an introduction to women's studies*. London: Virago.

Britten, N. & Heath, A. F. (1982) Women, men and families: proposals for a new social class classfication. Paper presented to the British Sociological Association conference on 'Gender and Society', Manchester.

Broverman, I. K., Broverman, D. M., Clarkson, F. E., Rosencrantz, P. S. & Vogel, S. R. (1970) Sex role stereotypes and clinical judgements of mental health. *Journal of Consulting and Clinical Psychology, 34*, 1–7.

Brown, G. W. & Harris T. (1978) *Social origins of depression: a study of psychiatric disorder in women*. London: Tavistock.

Chesler, P. (1972) *Women and madness*. New York: Doubleday.

Cochrane, R. (1983) *The social creation of mental illness. Applied Psychology*. London: Longman.

Conran, S. (1977) *Superwoman*. Harmondsworth: Penguin.

Coote, R. & Campbell, B. (1982) *Sweet freedom: the struggle for women's liberation*. London: Picador.

Dalton, K. (1969) *The menstrual cycle*. Harmondsworth: Penguin.

Dickson, A. (1982) *A woman in your own right: assertiveness and you*. London: Quartet.

Dweck, G. S. & Licht, B. G. (1980) Learned helplessness and intellectual achievement. *In* J. Garber and M. E. P. Seligman (eds) *Human helplessness – theory and applications*. London: Academic Press.

Ehrenreich, B. & English, D. (1979) *For her own good: 150 years of the experts' advice to women*. London: Pluto Press.

Fordyce, W. E. (1976) Learning processes in pain. *In* R. A. Sternbach (ed) *The psychology of pain*. New York: Raven Press.

Fransella, F. & Frost, K. (1977) *On being a woman: a review of research on how women see themselves*. London: Tavistock.

Goldman, N. & Ravid R. (1980) Community surveys and sex differences in mental illness. *In* M. Guttentag, S. Salasin & D. Belle (eds) *The mental health of women*. London: Academic Press.

Gould, S. J. (1977) *Ever since Darwin: reflections in natural history*. New York: Norton.

Gove, W. R. & Tudor, J. F. (1973) Adult sex roles and mental illness. *American Sociological Review*, *44*, 59–80.

Greenley, J. R. & Mechanic, D. (1976) Social selection in seeking help for psychological problems. *Journal of Health and Social Behaviour*, *17*, 249–262.

Haring M. J. Stock, W. A. & Okun, M. A. (1984) A research synthesis of gender and social class as correlates of subjective well being. *Human Relations*, *37*, 654–657.

Harrison, J. (1978) Warning: the male sex role may be dangerous to your health. *Journal of Social Issues*, *34*, 65–86.

Holmes, T. H. & Rahe, R. H. (1967) The social readjustment rating scale. *Journal of Psychosomatic Research*, *11*, 213–218.

Ingham, J. G. & Miller, P. Mc.C. (1976) The concept of prevalence applied to psychiatric disorders and symptoms. *Psychological Medicine*, *6*, 217–225.

King, J. (1983) Attribution theory and the health belief model. *In* M. Hewstone (ed.) *Attribution theory – social and functional extensions*. Oxford: Basil Blackwell.

Klerman, G. L. & Weissman, M. W. (1980) Depressions among women – their nature and causes. *In* M. Guttentag, S. Salasin & D. Belle (eds) *The mental health of women*. London: Academic Press.

Kobasa, S. C. (1982) The hardy personality – towards a social psychology of stress and health. *In* G. S. Sanders and J. Suls (eds) *Social psychology of health and illness*. New York: Erlbaum.

Koeske, R. K. & Koeske, G. F. (1975) An attributional approach to moods and the menstrual cycle. *Journal of Personality and Social Psychology*, *31*, 473–478.

Lader, M. & Marks I. (1971) *Clinical anxiety*. London: Heinemann.

Land, H. (1975) The myth of the male breadwinner. *New Society*, 9 October.

Langer, E. (1983) *The psychology of control*. London: Sage.

Lennon, M. C. (1982) The psychological consequences of the menopause – the importance of timing of a life stage event. *Journal of Health and Social Behaviour*, *23*, 253–366.

Litman, G. K. (1978) Clinical aspects of sex role stereotyping. *In* J. Chetwynd & O. Hartnett (eds) *The sex role system – psychological and sociological perspectives*. London: Routledge & Kegan Paul.

Lorenz, K. (1969) *On aggression*. New York: Bantam.

Makosky, V. P. (1980) Stress and the mental health of women – a discussion of research and issues. *In* M. Guttentag, S. Salesin & D. Belle (eds) *The mental health of women*. London: Academic Press.

Mechanic, D. (1964) The influence of mothers on their children's health attitudes and behaviour. *Paediatrics, 33,* 444–453.

Orbach, S. (1978) *Fat is a feminist issue – how to lose weight permanently – without dieting.* Feltham: Hamlyn.

Paige, K. E. (1973) Women learn to sing the menstrual blues. *Psychology Today, 7,* 41–46.

Pennebaker, J. W. (1982) *The psychology of physical symptoms.* New York: Springer.

Radloff, L. S. (1980) Risk factors for depression: what do we learn from them? *In* M. Guttentag, S. Salasin & D. Belle (eds) *The mental health of women.* London: Academic Press.

Reading, A. (1983) *The psychology of pregnancy.* London: Longman.

Reid, I. & Wormald, E. (1982) *Sex differences in Britain.* London: Grant McIntyre.

Royal College of Physicians (1979) *Alcohol and alcoholism: a report of a special committee of the Royal College of Physicians.* London: Tavistock.

Sanders, G. S. (1982) Social comparison, perceptions of health and illness. *In* G. S. Sanders & J. Suls (eds) *Social psychology of health and illness.* New York: Erlbaum.

Sayers, J. (1982) *Biological politics: femininist and anti-feminist perspective.* London: Tavistock.

Sinnott, E. W., Dunn, L. C. & Dobzhansky, T. (1958) *Principles of genetics,* 5th edn. Tokyo: McGraw-Hill.

Skevington, S. M. (1983) Chronic pain and depression: universal or personal helplessness? *Pain, 15,* 308–317.

Slade, P. (1984) Premenstrual emotional changes in normal women – factor or fiction? *Journal of Psychosomatic Research, 28,* 1–7.

Steptoe, A. (1980) Stress and medical disorders. *In* S. Rachman (ed.) *Contributions to medical psychology,* vol. 2. Oxford: Pergamon.

Suls, J. (1982) Social support interpersonal relations and health – benefits and liabilities. In G. A. Sanders and J. Suls (ed.) *Social psychology of health and illness.* New York: Erlbaum.

Taylor, M. C. & Hall, J. A. (1982) Psychological androgyny – theories methods, and conclusions. *Psychological Bulletin, 92,* 347–366.

Tiger, L. & Fox, R. (1974) *The imperial animal.* New York: Dell.

Vernon, P. E. (1969) *Personality assessment: a critical survey.* London: Tavistock.

Warr, P. & Parry, G. (1982) Paid employment and women's psychological well-being. *Psychological Bulletin, 91,* 498–516.

Williams, J. A (1979) Psychological androgyny and mental health. *In* O. Hartnett, J. Boden & M. Fuller (eds) *Sex role stereotyping.* London: Tavistock.

Wilson, E. O. (1978) *On human nature.* Harvard: Harvard University Press.

CHAPTER FOURTEEN

**Sex Roles and Sexual
Behaviour**
Kevin Howells

Introduction

Human sexual behaviour and its variations have been the subject of
scientific inquiry and theoretical analysis throughout most of this
century. In spite of the public and professional opposition which such
work has encountered, some progress has been made in unravelling the
myriad biological, social and psychological influences which interact to
determine adult sexual functioning (Bancroft 1983). The construct of *sex
roles* has been implicit in many attempts to describe the aetiology of
various patterns of sexual behaviour, though often conceptions of sex
roles have been unsophisticated, largely because they predated, or
developed in isolation from, contemporary theoretical formulations of
sex typing (Bem 1981; Feather 1984; Taylor & Hall 1982).

In recent work, more elaborate concepts of sex roles have been
adduced to describe and explain a wide range of sexual and sex-related
behaviours, including physique preferences (Maier & Lavrakas 1984),
choice of dating partner or potential spouse (Orlofsky 1982), patterns of
sexual arousal in response to erotica (Fisher 1983), homosexuality
(Whitam & Zent 1984), transsexualism (Barlow *et al.* 1980), rape (Check
& Malamuth 1983) and sexual dysfunction (Radlove 1983).

In the field of sex research it is important to clearly distinguish *sex role*
from other terms with which confusion is possible. *Gender identity*
refers, typically, to the subjective sense of being male or female and is
often assumed to be established in early childhood. *Sexual orientation*
refers to a preference for a particular class of sexual partner or sex
object. *Sex role* (sometimes *gender role* is used synonymously in the
literature) is best defined, in the way it is done throughout the present
volume, as referring to those behaviours understood or expected to
characterize males and females within a society. The importance of these
distinctions can be illustrated by considering a sexual variation such as
homosexuality (discussed in more detail below). Homosexual behaviour
is not generally the product of a gender identity disturbance. Individuals
with a gender identity disturbance (transsexuals) may show a sexual orientation consonant with their self-ascribed rather than their biological sex

and thus be behaviourally, though not subjectively, homosexual. People of this sort, however, account for only a tiny proportion of those who engage in homosexual behaviour. Whether homosexuality is sometimes a product of variation in sex role behaviour (sex-role inversion) is more controversial (see below), but it is clear that a homosexual orientation *can* develop without the individual being significantly deviant in relation to sex role (Storms 1981). Gender identity, sexual orientation and sex role, then, are capable of a marked desynchrony.

Cultural conceptions of male and female sexuality

There are indications within the human sexuality literature that beliefs and prescriptions derived from general sex-role expectations affect sexual behaviour itself. The content of sex-role stereotypes in the area of sexuality includes notions that males are, and should be, sexually dominant and females sexually passive. Zellman and Goodchilds (1983) have studied the developing sexual attitudes of American adolescents and report that it is generally expected that the male partner will initiate and control a sexual interaction. Males tend to be perceived as separating sex and love. Females, on the other hand, are expected to be sexually passive and to see sex as an expression of romantic love. These workers found that a general agreement exists that males have a higher level of sex drive than females, being more arousable sexually, and that this provides a rationale and partial justification for male sexual aggression. The role of the female is typically construed as being to set limits for male sexual advances. Zellman and Goodchilds's general conclusion is that gender-based sexual scripts are still powerful in determining sexual expression and that 'the gender roles assigned for sexual activity accord exceedingly well with the traditional gender-role differentiations for behaviours in general: the woman is the passive recipient and the man is the active, aggressive initiator' (1983, p. 63).

Some of these cultural assumptions about sex differences in sexual behaviour can, and have been tested empirically. The assumption which has generated most research is that men have a higher 'sex drive' than women. There are many conceptual problems with the construct of sex drive but it is useful to distinguish the *arousability* component (capacity to respond to a sexual stimulus with arousal) and the *appetitive* component (the tendency to seek out sexual stimuli) (Bancroft 1983). The evidence suggests that sex differences are generally small in relation to sexual arousability but are larger in relation to appetitive sexual behaviour (Fisher 1983). Fisher's thorough review indicates that men and women show broadly similar arousability to erotic photographs, fantasy, films and other material, in terms of both behavioural and physiological measures, and that Schmidt's (1975) conclusion is valid:

> In sum, the pattern and intensity of reactions to explicit sexual stimuli are in general the same for men and women. When significant differences between the sexes are found, they represent merely minor shifts in the total pattern. These variations should not divert attention from the fact that women can react to the same extent and in the same direction as men. (p. 335) [Quoted by Fisher, 1983]

Women, on the other hand, may be less appetitive than men, in the sense that they are less likely to seek out sexual material such as published erotica. Fisher's interpretation (1983) is that women do not use erotica because they have not been socialized to enjoy it, because quality erotica is not available for women and because the use of erotica by women is construed as socially undesirable. The degree of sex-role identification affects behaviours of this sort. The significant difference between men and women in rates of volunteering to see an erotic film, for example, is increased if sex-typed males are compared with sex-typed females, but disappears if androgynous males are compared with androgynous females (Kenrick *et al.* 1980). It appears, therefore, that sex-role socialization may have a significant impact on appetitive sexual behaviour of this sort.

Sexual maladjustment

The evidence, reviewed above, that sexuality is an area of experience subject to sex-role stereotyping effects, raises the questions of whether sex-role stereotyping promotes sexual problems and maladjustment and whether individual differences in degree of sex-role socialization predict the likelihood of sexual difficulties arising.

Females

Assertions that such relationships do exist for sexual difficulties in females have a strong face validity, in the sense that there is an apparent overlap between the content of stereotyped sex-role beliefs and the topography of clinical female sexual dysfunctions. Stock (1984) points to women's socialization as sexually restrained, passive and uninterested ('good girls do not participate in and enjoy sex'), and argues that 'the internalization of these expectations about female sexuality surely has an effect on female sexual satisfaction' (p. 257). Klein (1983) similarly argues that 'optimal sexual satisfaction for a woman and her partner involves a degree of self-assertion and initiative not prescribed by the traditional female script' (p. 81). Both female socialization and female sexual dysfunctions would seem to share the feature of *acquired sexual inhibition*. Female sexual socialization involves learning to inhibit sexual behaviour, at least to a greater degree than for men. The common female sexual dysfunctions, particularly problems of low arousability and inability to reach orgasm (Jehu 1979, 1984), are similarly products of inhibitory conditioning. Jehu (1984) comments, in relation to the aetiology of sexual maladjustment: 'the long association of fear, guilt and disgust with sexuality may not be easily reversible on marriage; instead it may persist and overgeneralize so that what should be an enjoyable and socially valued sexual relationship is impaired by some form of dysfunction' (p. 143). Extreme sex typing is one plausible source of such associative learning.

Such evidence is largely indirect. Direct empirical tests of the sex role hypothesis are rare. Derogatis and Meyer (1979) found that 'normal' females had significantly higher levels of both masculinity and femininity than a dysfunctional group. Walfish and Myerson (1980) compared the sexual attitudes of androgynous and feminine females and found that the former were significantly more 'comfortable' in their attitudes towards sexuality, though the measure used did not properly assess clinical levels of sexual dysfunction. More recently, Radlove (1984) has described a study showing that androgynous women tended to achieve orgasm more frequently than feminine women, the former being more likely to perceive active sexual behaviour (clitoral stimulation, coital thrusting and being on top of the partner) as appropriate behaviours for women.

Sexual adjustment is closely related to general marital and relationship problems, so that studies relating marital satisfaction to sex-role measures are also indirectly relevant to the present discussion. Baucom and Aiken (1984) have argued that both masculinity and femininity are important to a successful marital (or other intimate) relationship, the partners in such a relationship needing to be both instrumental/goal-orientated and sensitive/emotionally attuned. These authors provide some support for this theory. In their 1984 study androgyny was more common in their maritally satisfied group than in dissatisfied comparisons.

Males

There is much less of a consensus within the literature as to whether a relationship exists between male sex typing and male sexual problems. Klein (1983) has suggested that it is central to male sex-role identity to be sexually aggressive, powerful and in control. Such a sex-role identification is, perhaps, likely to make males performance and achievement-oriented in sexual contexts and to undermine 'feminine' interpersonal sensitivity. For Radlove (1984) a traditional sex-role identification is less damaging (sexually) for men than for women, the major causes of male sexual problems, such as erectile failure, being in other areas. It is feasible, however, that overly rigid sex-role typing could make males susceptible to the classic 'fear of failure' phenomenon. Occasional erectile failure, for example, is a normal event (Jehu 1979) but may pose such a threat to a strongly sex-typed male as to made subsequent failure more likely. In this sense, sex-typed males would be prone to a fear of failure in sexual encounters whereas sex-typed females would be prone to fear of success.

Zilbergeld (1978) has described other facets of masculinity in relation to sexuality and their attendant pressures, many of which are encapsulated in Stock's (1984) summary of the male sexual script as dictating that 'males control and orchestrate the sexual encounter, always be ready to perform, always have an erection, be free of emotional needs during sex, and always desire intercourse. The control and performance orientation of this script, if followed, limits sex to a physical act that is accomplished under great pressure' (p. 260).

Plausible though these suggestions are, empirical evidence is sparse. In Derogatis and Meyer's (1979) study, dysfunctional males had significantly *lower* masculinity scores than normal controls, disconfirming the hypothesis. The problem here, of course, is of disentangling causes and effects. The effect of sexual failure may be to *diminish* sex-role confidence. In Walfish and Myerson's study (1980) androgynous males tended to be more 'comfortable' in their sexual attitudes than their masculine counterparts, though this effect was only marginally significant statistically.

In summary, sex roles have high face validity as being important for sexual adjustment and there is indirect evidence to support the sex typing hypothesis. Research, as yet, however, has barely begun. Proper evaluation of this hypothesis awaits detailed empirical studies, using a range of validated sex-role and sexual functioning measures with both clinical and non-clinical groups.

Homosexual behaviour

Homosexuality and heterosexuality are likely to have a very distinctive and special status in gender-based schematic processing (Bem 1981). Heterosexuality, as Bem suggests, facilitates the generalization that the two sexes are, and ought to be, different. In addition, exclusive heterosexuality is often perceived as a necessary condition for adequate masculinity or femininity. Bem (1981) points out that 'regardless of how closely an individual's attributes and behaviour match the male or female prototypes stored within the gender schema, violation of the prescription to be exclusively heterosexual is sufficient by itself to call into question the individual's adequacy as a man or woman' (p. 361). To develop a homosexual interest or to engage in homosexual behaviour, may require a significant shift in the self-concept and sex-role identification. Changed sex-role behaviour is a likely *consequence*, therefore, of homosexuality. The question has also be asked whether sex-role variables are *causal* in relation to homosexual preference, and it is this question which will be addressed, in the main, for the rest of this section.

Sex-role identification theories of homosexuality have many competitors. Attempts have been made to explain this preference in terms of genetic influences, prenatal hormones, unusual parental relationships, aversive heterosexual experiences, erotic fantasy orientation and a range of other variables (Feldman 1984). Few theories pay more than lip-service to the likely heterogeneity of homosexuals, and attempts are made to provide explanations for *all* homosexual people.

The case for sex roles as important

It appears to be a common cultural stereotype that homosexuals differ from heterosexuals not only in their choice of sexual partner but also in terms of sex-role behaviours. Male homosexuals may be thought to be effeminate and limp-wristed while female homosexuals are masculine or 'butch' (Stokes, Kilmann & Wanlass 1983). The notion that homosexuality is related to sex-role inversion has a long history too in classical sexual and psychodynamic theory (Storms 1980). A number of empirical studies have been conducted to test this theory. Whitam and Zent (1984) have reviewed the evidence from such studies and point to the apparent consistency with which homosexuals do indeed show sex-role inversion. Follow-up studies of boys known to be effeminate suggest that they are more likely to become homosexual (Green 1979; Zuger 1978), though the children used in these studies are likely to be atypical of effeminate boys in general.

Retrospective studies in which homosexuals are asked about their childhood behaviour have also produced evidence consistent with inversion (Saghir & Robins 1973: Whitam 1977). Grellert, Newcomb and Bentler (1982) looked at the differences between homosexuals (male and female) and heterosexuals in reported childhood play and sport behaviour. In this carefully executed study, on all eight of the scales used there was a significant effect for sexual orientation. All differences between homosexuals and heterosexuals were in the direction of homosexuals being similar to the opposite sex heterosexual group. In a similar vein, Blanchard *et al.* (1983) investigated reported boyhood aggressiveness (defined as a generalized disposition to engage in physically combative or competitive interactions with male peers) in a number of groups, including male homosexuals. The latter obtained lower scores than heterosexuals, though not as low as the scores of transsexual homosexuals.

Two major, large-scale studies of non-clinical samples of homosexuals also support the general picture of childhood sex-role inversion. Bell, Weinberg & Hammersmith (1981) have reported the results of lengthy interviews with 979 homosexual and 477 heterosexual men and women in the San Francisco Bay area. Their results reveal a significant link between self-reported gender non-conformity in childhood and the development of homosexuality. As Bell *et al.* (1981) are careful to point out, not all homosexuals showed sex-role inversion and many heterosexuals showed cross-sex behaviour in childhood. In this sense, sex-role inversion is neither a necessary nor a sufficient condition for the development of homosexuality, but it does, nevertheless, increase the probability of its occurrence.

Detailed inspection of items in this survey reveals that male homosexuals were less likely to report enjoyment of 'boys' activities (baseball and football). More homosexual men, though still a minority, reported pretending to be a female or dressing in girls' clothes. Male homosexuals were also more likely to describe themselves as passive and submissive in childhood. A broadly similar (though reversed) pattern was found for female homosexuals. Fewer female homosexuals (than heterosexuals) enjoyed typical girls' activities (playing house, hopscotch) and they were more likely to enjoy baseball and football. More homosexual women also reported having worn boys' clothing and pretending to be a boy.

Van Wyk and Geist (1984), as part of a larger study of the development of homosexual orientation, also tested the hypothesis that a preponderance of opposite-sex playmates at age ten would be positively associated with a homosexual preference in adulthood. In a multiple regression analysis, sex-role inversion did predict adult homosexuality, though it was a stronger influence for males than for females, and it was a less powerful influence than sexual experience and subjective arousal. These authors interpret the sex-role association in terms of the 'familiarity breeds contempt' hypothesis. Cross-sex identification, interest in the activities of the opposite sex and absence of same-sex companions may sometimes induce a boy to become 'one of the girls' and a girl 'one of the boys', this effect subsequently inhibiting heterosexual attraction and encouraging attraction to the same sex, which is now viewed as 'different' and, perhaps, exotic.

A major problem with research of this sort is that sex roles are often conceptualized dichotomously. Masculinity and femininity are unlikely to be mutually exclusive (Bem 1974) and need to be independently assessed. Oldhams, Farnhill and Ball (1982) did use a bidimensional measure (the Bem Sex Role Inventory) to compare lesbians and heterosexual women and found that the former had higher masculinity scores but did not differ on femininity. Homosexual women were able to combine both masculine and feminine attributes.

Whether sex-role inversion and homosexual relationships are culture-specific has been investigated by Whitam and Zent (1984), who assessed groups in the United States, Guatemala, Brazil and the Philippines. With considerable consistency across the cultures, male homosexuals were more likely than heterosexuals to report childhood interest in female patterns of play and female clothing and to prefer the company of girls and adult females.

The case against sex roles as important

The thesis that sex roles are of aetiological significance for homosexuality has not gone unchallenged. Counter-arguments have typically been that some empirical evidence is inconsistent with the hypothesis, that there are methodological problems with the research methods used, or that other variables rather than sex roles have the major causal influence in the development of homosexuality (Ross 1980; Stokes, Kilmann & Wanlass 1983; Storms 1980, 1981).

Storms (1980) compared heterosexual, bisexual and homosexual men and women on the Personal Attributes Questionnaire (PAQ), which provides a masculinity scale, a femininity scale and a bipolar masculinity-femininity scale. Although there was an inconsistent trend in the direction suggested by the sex-role inversion hypothesis, the group differences were not significant statistically. Stokes, Kilmann and Wanlass (1983) studied similar groups (though recruited from a different part of the United States) using a different, though related measure, the Bem Sex Role Inventory (BSRI). No particular sex role was found to be significantly associated with any sexual orientation group and the authors concluded, albeit cautiously, that 'these results do not support the popular conception of homosexuals as deviant from conventional sex roles' (p. 431).

The apparent inconsistency between these two studies and the previous ones described may be attributable to their different methodologies. Studies such as those of Bell, Weinberg and Hammersmith (1981) and Whitam and Zent (1984) focus on *recall* of childhood behaviour and attitudes, while those of Storms (1980) and Stokes, Kilmann and Wanlass (1983) focus on *current* sex-role identification. It is possible that sex-role inversion may contribute to homosexual development in childhood without such an effect persisting into adulthood. There is some, albeit inconsistent, evidence that the sex-role identification of homosexuals *changes* from childhood to adulthood and through the different phases of adulthood (Harry 1983; Robinson, Skeen & Flake-Hobson 1982; Whitam 1977). Harry's (1983) study demonstrated that approximately two-thirds of homosexual males who were sex-role inverted in childhood had 'defeminized' in adulthood, becoming virtually indistinguishable from heterosexual males. Thus the majority of homosexual men, as Harry points out, may appear visibly gender-conventional while having been unconventional as children. Few homosexual men acquire cross-gender behaviour in adulthood without also having shown cross-gender behaviour in childhood, though visible and exaggerated effeminacy may sometimes be used as a symbolic 'coming out' behaviour in adolescence or early adulthood. Why defeminization should occur is not entirely clear though it is likely that cross-sex behaviour is strongly socially censured and 'punished' (Hayes & Leonard 1983), perhaps increasingly so in adolescence and adulthood.

Methodological problems

Studies of sex-role behaviour in homosexuals have been largely, though not exclusively, reliant on the retrospective method. The problems with this method are obvious and have been much discussed (Ross 1980). A homosexual, asked in a research study, to recall his/her childhood experience is engaged in a very different task from his/her heterosexual equivalent. Questions of causality do not arise spontaneously for heterosexuality, which may be seen as 'natural' and not requiring attribution or explanation. The development of homosexual interest or behaviour, however, often requires the person to find an attribution for this non-normative state of affairs. Thus homosexual people are much more likely to have already pondered why they are as they are and to have scanned childhood experiences, familial relationships and other areas which our lay psychological culture suggests are plausible causes of differences in sexual orientation. Homosexuals may also internalize stereotyped cultural theories of homosexuality (Ross 1980). How such processes may distort data and consequent conclusions in retrospective studies is not, as yet, clear. Problems of bias can be alleviated, to some degree, by using homosexuals as their own controls. Feldman (1984) has suggested, for example, that two major subclasses of homosexuality exist – primary and secondary. Primary homosexuals have never experienced heterosexual arousal at any stage, while secondary homosexuals have experienced significant heterosexual arousal. Neither of these groups is, at least intuitively, more likely than the other to give biased retrospective accounts of childhood experience. Studies, therefore, should subdivide homosexual groups. This would acknowledge the likely heterogeneity of the homosexual population and also allow more clear-cut interpretation of childhood differences found in a particular homosexual group.

A remaining methodological and conceptual problem is the elucidation of the precise causal status of sex-role inversion. Does sex-role inversion cause homosexual behaviour? Or is it that other precursors of homosexuality (early homosexual interest) cause sex-role inversion? Or may both forms of behaviour be caused by some third variable, such as parental behaviour? Current research is increasingly of an interactional and developmental nature, plotting the temporal and causal relationships between sex roles and other childhood variables such as early sexual experience, familial and other social relationships (Bell, Winberg & Hammersmith 1981, Van Wyk & Geist 1984). Bell, Weinberg and Hammersmith in particular, using path analysis, have shown the complex and varied causal chains involved in arriving at the endpoint of adult homo- or heterosexuality.

In summary, empirical work increasingly suggests that there is some relationship between sex-role inversion and homosexuality, though problems of interpretation persist. Many, though not all, homosexuals have shown cross-sex behaviour in childhood. The fact that not all homosexuals show this pattern confirms that there are other routes to the same destination (cf. Feldman 1984). Equally, sex-role-inverted boys and girls will often grow up to acquire conventional heterosexual orientations. Understanding how sex-role behaviour interacts sequentially with other biological, social and cognitive processes is a major task for the future.

Aggressive sexual behaviour

The psychological study of aggressive forms of sexual behaviour such as rape is relatively less advanced than the study of sexual orientation.

Feminist analyses of rape (e.g. Brownmiller 1975; Russell 1975, 1982), although sociocultural rather than psychological in form, have done much to broaden the perspective of clinicians and of experimentally orientated psychologists, who, in turn, have provided clinical and experimental support for many of the hypotheses generated by feminist analyses. Two broad theoretical approaches to rape are discernible within the literature. The first might be labelled as 'clinical' or 'typological' (Koss & Oros 1982). A large number of studies have assessed for example, the psychology and psychopathology of rapists as a discrete, abnormal, psychiatric/criminological group (Cohen *et al.* 1971; Groth 1979; Rada 1978; West, Roy & Nichols 1978). The second might be labelled as 'cultural' or 'dimensional' (Koss & Oros 1982). Within this approach, the emphasis is on criminal rape as the end point of a continuum of male sexual aggression rather than on individual pathology (Burt 1980; Sanday 1981). For this latter approach, the sex-role system is an important mediator of the cultural forces that create and maintain rape behaviour. Sex-role variables also feature, however, in clinical accounts, suggesting that a culture/individual pathology dichotomy is not an entirely useful one.

Culture and rape

Cultures and subcultures vary markedly in the prevalence of aggressive sexuality. In this sense, behaviour such as rape requires analysis at the cultural level as much as at the level of individual psychology. Particular cultures have been identified in which rape is rare (Mead 1935) or alternatively, endemic (Levine 1977). In the culture studied by Levine (the Gusii in Kenya), rape appears to be a product of sex-role socialization in that males are expected to behave, generally, in a coercive and antagonistic manner in sexual situations. Whether there is a *general* relationship between rape rates and configurations of cultural (including sex-role) attitudes, is the question addressed by Sanday (1981), who was able to demonstrate that rape-prone cultures differed significantly from rape-free cultures in their expectations for male and female behaviour. Rape-prone cultures promoted male–female antagonism, used rape to enhance male dominance, and regarded women as the economic property of men. Rape-free societies promoted sexual equality, valued female attributes and generally discouraged violence. In a correlational analysis, three cultural variables significantly related to rape probability. the general degree of interpersonal violence ($r = 0.47$); having a cultural ideology of male toughness ($r = 0.42$) and low female participation in decision-making ($r = 0.33$).

Attitudes to rape

It is possible to apply the sort of cultural analysis that Sanday (1981) has performed with non-Western societies to North American and European societies. The two important questions that might be asked, for the purposes of this chapter are, first, whether rape-promoting beliefs and expectations exist within a society and, second, whether there is any link between such beliefs, if they exist, and sex-role variables. Burt (1980) has conducted such a study in the United States and reports that America is a rape-supportive culture in the sense that 'rape myths' are prevalent. More than half of Burt's sample agreed, for example, that 'a woman who goes to the home or apartment of a man on the first date implies she is willing to have sex' (p. 229). More importantly, adherence to rape myths could be predicted from other, more general attitudes. Rape myth believers were more sex-role stereotyped, more adversarial and dominance-oriented in their conceptions of male–female relationships and more accepting of male–female violence. This work suggests, then, that strongly traditional sex-role socialization promotes rape-engendering beliefs, though, of course, such beliefs are not necessarily translated into sexually aggressive behaviour.

A number of other experimental studies have reported results consistent with those of Burt (Deitz, Littman & Bentley 1984; Feild 1978; Feild & Bienen 1980; Klemmack & Klemmack 1976; Krulewitz & Payne 1978; Schwarz & Brand 1983; Thornton, Ryckman & Robbins 1982). There are indications that such effects hold also for rape within marriage. Jeffords (1984) reports that traditional sex-role attitudes were negatively associated with norms against forced marital intercourse in a mail survey of Texas residents. Sex-role effects are not specific to North America. Broadly similar results were reported in a British sample by Howells *et al.* (1984) in a study of social perceptions of simulated newspaper accounts of rape. In this study males with traditional sex-role expectations blamed rape victims more and perceived them as less damaged psychologically by the rape than did males with non-traditional sex-role expectations.

Rape behaviour and rape proclivity

The demonstrated link between sex-role measures and rape attitudes does not prove that rape behaviour itself has a relationship to sex roles. There are two ways in which such a relationship might be assessed. Known rapists themselves could be studied to ascertain whether they differ from non-rapists in sex-role behaviour. Such studies are rare in the published literature, though frequent anecdotal observations have implicated sex roles as important. The second method would be to study 'normal' males with a 'rape proclivity' (Malamuth 1981) and to compare them with males without such a proclivity. The very existence, of course, of 'normal' males with a rape proclivity would tend to confirm the hypothesis that rape should be regarded as a continuum rather than as a discrete pathology found only in a few.

Clinical studies

There has been a large number of studies of convicted rapists, but the main emphasis of published work has been on assessing sexual arousal rather than sex-role variables (Howells 1984). Clinical accounts, however, do suggest extremes of sex-role identification. West, Roy and Nichols (1978) clinical description of rapists in therapy draws attention to impaired masculinity in this group as does Groth's description of the 'power' rapist (Groth 1979). Groth's account stresses that the rapist's behaviour is instigated by the need to control, capture and conquer the victim, rather than by a desire for sexual gratification. Groth suggests: 'Such offenders feel insecure about their masculinity or conflicted about their identity ... rape then becomes a way of putting such fears to rest, of asserting one's heterosexuality, of preserving one's sense of manhood' (p. 28). It is of interest that Groth highlights strong fears of homo-sexuality in this group (cf. previous section). Rape, for the 'power' rapist, then, is a form of masculinity validation. Groth's suggestions clearly need to be tested in terms of empirical comparisons, on sex-role measures, between rapists and controls.

Such clinical observations raise the possibility of a complex relation-ship between sex-role identification and aggressive sexuality. A male may be sexually aggressive because his behaviour conforms to an extreme degree to masculine stereotypes, or because he aspires to such a masculine ideal but *fails* to match his actual behaviour with his gender schema. As Bem (1981) suggests, the gender schema is a *prescriptive standard* in terms of which behaviour is regulated. Failure to meet this intended standard creates problems of self-esteem and instigates, perhaps, neurotic, ill-judged attempts at self-esteem repair. It may be that this neurotic type of sex-role problem is more frequent in psychiatric than in general population samples of rapists.

Proclivity studies

Studies of rape proclivity in the general population also implicate sex-role stereotyping as an important variable. Males may have a high rape proclivity in two senses: (1) they may report a high subjective likelihood of raping in particular situations or, (2) they may be sexually aroused by depictions of rape behaviour. These two sorts of proclivity are unlikely to be independent and both appear to have some relationship to sex-role behaviour.

Malamuth and other workers have investigated the psychological cor-relates of rape proclivity, defined as having a high self-rated likelihood of raping 'if you could be assured of not being caught and punished' (Briere & Malamuth 1983; Malamuth 1981; Malamuth, Haber & Feshbach 1980; Tieger 1981). Roughly 35 percent of Malamuth's subjects report some likelihood of raping on this measure, and those with high scores differ from those with low scores on measures of sex-role identification (Tieger 1981). Briere and Malamuth (1983) compared sexuality and cultural/attitudinal variables as predictors of likelihood of raping or using sexual force and found that the latter were more powerful. These were precisely the sorts of attitude shown by Burt (1980) to be related to stereotyped sex-role beliefs.

Check and Malamuth (1983) tested the relevance of sex roles more directly by assessing the relationship between a sex-role stereotyping measure and self-reported arousal to rape descriptions. High sex-role stereotyped individuals were shown to report high levels of sexual arousal to acquaintance rape depictions and to be similar in this respect to actual rapist samples. Sex-role stereotyped men were also more likely to report that they themselves might rape.

Taken together, such studies of rape attitudes and behaviour suggest the utility of including sex-role variables within explanatory theories of rape. The work suggests, in a preliminary fashion, that beliefs about rape, the proclivity to rape and, perhaps, even rape behaviour itself are correlated with extreme forms of traditional sex typing in males. This research clearly needs to be developed and elaborated, particularly in the area of study of known rapists, who would provide a better test of sex-role theory than is provided by studies of those with rape-creating beliefs of self-reported propensities for such behaviour.

Conclusions

This chapter provides only a brief introduction to psychological work which has used the construct of sex roles in attempts to explain particular patterns of sexual behaviour itself. In all three of the areas surveyed (sexual dysfunction, homosexuality and aggressive sexuality), sex-role concepts have been implicit in aetiological formulations for some time. For all three forms of behaviour, however, it is only in very recent years that sex-role concepts have been made sufficiently precise and operationalized in a sufficiently valid form for proper empirical work to be carried out. Even now, applications in this area lag behind advances in general sex role and gender schema theory (Bem 1981; Feather 1984;

Taylor & Hall 1982). Work has rarely, for example, taken sufficient account of the fact that masculinity and femininity may be independent dimensions and that they may interact in a complex fashion (Taylor & Hall 1982). Some substantial progress seems to have been made in the understanding of homosexuality from a set role perspective and an encouraging first step seems to have been made in unravelling the forces producing sexual aggression. For sexual dysfunction, perhaps, much of the work remains to be done. Further advances in all three areas depend, ultimately, on progress being made in core sex-role theory and measurement.

References

Bancroft, J. (1983) *Human sexuality and its problems*. Edinburgh: Churchill Livingstone.

Barlow, D. H., Mills, J. R., Agras, W. S. & Steinman, D. L. (1980) Comparison of sex-typed motor behaviour in male-to-female transexuals and women. *Archives of Sexual Behaviour, 9*, 245–253.

Baucom, D. H. & Aiken, P. A. (1984) Sex role identity, marital satisfaction, and response to behavioral marital therapy. *Journal of Consulting and Clinical Psychology, 52*, 438–444.

Bell, A. P., Weinberg, M. S. & Hammersmith, S. K. (1981) *Sexual preference*. Bloomington: Indiana University Press.

Bem, S. L. (1974) The measurement of psychological androgyny. *Journal of Consulting and Clinical Psychology, 42*, 155–162.

Bem, S. L. (1981) Gender schema theory: a cognitive account of sex-typing. *Psychological Review, 88*, 354–364.

Blanchard, R., McConkey, J. G., Roper, V. & Steiner, B. W. (1983) Measuring physical aggressiveness in heterosexual, homosexual and transsexual males. *Archives of Sexual Behaviour, 12*, 511–524.

Briere, J. & Malamuth, N. M. (1983) Self-reported likelihood of sexually aggressive behavior: attitudinal versus sexual explanations. *Journal of Research in Personality, 17*, 315–323.

Brownmiller, S. (1975). *Against our will: rape, women and men*. London: Secker & Warburg.

Burt, M. R. (1980) Cultural myths and supports for rape. *Journal of Personality and Social Psychology, 38*, 217–230.

Check, J. V. T. & Malamuth, N. M. (1983) Sex role stereotyping and reactions to depictions of stranger versus acquaintance rape. *Journal of Personality and Social Psychology, 45*, 344–356.

Cohen, M. L., Garofalo, R., Boucher, R. & Seghorn, T. (1971) The psychology of rapists. *Seminars in Psychiatry, 3*.

Deitz, S. R., Littman, M. & Bentley, B. J. (1984) Attribution of responsibility for rape: the influence of observer empathy, victim resistance and victim attractiveness. *Sex Roles, 10*, 261–280.

Derogatis, L. R. & Meyer, J. K. (1979) A psychological profile of the sexual dysfunctions. *Archives of Sexual Behavior*, *8*, 201–223.

Feather, N. T. (1984) Masculinity, femininity, psychological androgyny, and the structure of values. *Journal of Personality and Social Psychology*, *47*, 604–620.

Feild, H. S. (1978) Attitudes toward rape: a comparative analysis of police, rapists, crisis counsellors and citizens. *Journal of Personality and Social Psychology*, *36*, 156–179.

Feild, H. S. & Bienen, L. B. (1980) *Jurors and rape*. London: Lexington Books.

Feldman, P. (1984) The homosexual preference. In K. Howells (ed.) *The psychology of sexual diversity*. Oxford: Blackwell.

Fisher, W. A. (1983) Gender, gender-role identification, and response to erotica. *In* F. R. Algeier & N. B. McCormick (eds) *Changing boundaries*: *gender roles and sexual behaviour*. Palo Alto: Mayfield.

Green, R. (1979) Childhood cross-gender behaviour and subsequent sexual preference. *American Journal of Psychiatry*, *136*, 106–108.

Grellert, E. A., Newcomb, M. D. & Bentler, P. M. (1982) Childhood play activities of male and female homosexuals and heterosexuals. *Archives of Sexual Behavior*, *11*, 451–478.

Groth, A. N. (1979) *Men who rape*. New York: Plenum.

Harry, J. (1983) Defeminization and adult psychological well-being among male homosexuals. *Archives of Sexual Behaviour*, *12*, 1–19.

Hayes, S. C. & Leonard, S. R. (1983) Sex-related motor behaviour: effects on social impressions and social cooperation. *Archives of Sexual Behaviour*, *12*, 415–426.

Howells, K. (1984) Coercive sexual behaviour. In K. Howells (ed.) *The psychology of sexual diversity*. Oxford: Blackwell.

Howells, K., Shaw, F., Greasley, M., Robertson, J., Gloster, D. & Metcalfe, N. (1984) Perceptions of rape in a British sample: effects of relationship, victim status, sex, and attitudes to women. *British Journal of Social Psychology*, *23*, 35–40.

Jeffords, C. R. (1984) The impact of sex-role and religious attitudes upon forced marital intercourse norms. *Sex Roles*, *11*, 543–552.

Jehu, D. (1979) *Sexual dysfunction*: *a behavioural approach to causation, assessment and treatment*. Chichester: John Wiley.

Jehu, D. (1984) Sexual inadequacy. *In* K. Howells (ed.) *The psychology of sexual diversity*. Oxford: Blackwell.

Kenrick, D. T., Stringfield, D. O., Wagenhals, W. L., Dahl, R. N. & Rausdell, H. J. (1980) Sex differences, androgyny, and approach responses to erotica: a new variation on an old volunteer problem. *Journal of Personality and Social Psychology*, *38*, 517–524.

Klein, R. (1983) Gender identity and sex-role stereotyping: clinical issues in human sexuality. *In* C. Nadelson & D. B. Marcotte (eds) *Treatment interventions in human sexuality*. New York: Plenum.

Klemmack, S. H. & Klemmack, D. L. (1976) The social definition of rape. *In* M. J. Walker & S. L. Brodsky (eds) *Sexual assault*: *the victim and the rapist*. London: Lexington Books.

Koss, M. P. & Oros, C. J. (1982) Sexual experiences survey: a research instrument investigating sexual aggression and victimization. *Journal of Consulting and Clinical Psychology*, *50*, 455–457.

Krulewitz, J. E. & Payne, E.J. (1978) Attributions about rape: effects of rapist force, observer sex and sex role attitudes. *Journal of Applied Social Psychology*, *8*, 291–305.

Levine, R. A. (1977) Gusii sex offences: a study in social control. *In* D. Chappell, R. Geis & G. Geis (eds) *Forcible rape: the crime, the victim and the offender*. New York: Columbia University Press.

Maier, R. A. & Lavrakas, P. J. (1984) Attitudes toward women, personality rigidity, and idealized physique preferences in males. *Sex Roles*, *11*, 425–433.

Malamuth, N. M. (1981) Rape proclivity among males. *Journal of Social Issues*, *39*, 138–157.

Malamuth, N. M., Haber, S. & Feshbach, S. (1980) Testing hypotheses regarding rape: exposure to sexual violence, sex differences and the 'normality' of rapists. *Journal of Research in Personality*, *14*, 121–137.

Mead, M. (1935) *Sex and temperament in three primitive societies*. New York: William Morrow.

Oldhams, S., Farnhill, D. & Ball, I. (1982) Sex role identity of female homosexuals. *Journal of Homosexuality*, *8*, 41–46.

Orlofsky, J. L. (1982) Psychological androgyny, sex-typing, and sex role ideology as predictors of male-female interpersonal attraction. *Sex Roles*, *8*, 1057–1073.

Rada, R. T. (ed.) (1978) *Clinical aspects of the rapist*. New York: Grune & Stratton.

Radlove, S. (1984) Sexual response and gender roles. *In* E. R. Allgeier & N. B. McCormick (eds) *Changing boundaries: gender roles and sexual behaviour*. Palo Alto: Mayfield.

Robinson, B. E., Skeen, P. & Flake-Hobson, C. (1982) Sex role endorsement among homosexual men across the life span. *Archives of Sexual Behavior*, *11*, 355–359.

Ross, M. W. (1980) Retrospective distortion in homosexual research. *Archives of Sexual Behavior*, *9*, 523–531.

Russell, D. E. H. (1975) *The politics of rape*. New York: Stein & Day.

Russell, D. E. H. (1982) *Rape in marriage*. New York: Macmillan.

Saghir, M. T. & Robins, E. (1973) *Male and female homosexuality*. Baltimore: Williams & Wilkins.

Sanday, P. R. (1981) The socio-cultural context of rape: a cross-cultural study. *Journal of Social Issues*, *37*, 5–27.

Schmidt, G. (1975) Male–female differences in sexual arousal and behavior during and after exposure to sexually explicit stimuli. *Archives of Sexual Behavior*, *4*, 353–365.

Schwarz, N. & Brand, J. F. (1983) Effects of salience of rape on sex role attitudes, trust, and self-esteem in non-raped women. *European Journal of Social Psychology*, *13*, 71–76.

Stock, W. E. (1984) Sex roles and sexual dysfunction. *In* C. S. Widom (ed.) *Sex roles and psychopathology*. New York: Plenum.

Stokes, K., Kilmann, P. R. & Wanlass, R. L. (1983) Sexual orientation and sex role conformity. *Archives of Sexual Behavior, 12*, 427–433.

Storms, M. D. (1980) Theories of sexual orientation. *Journal of Personality and Social Psychology, 38*, 783–792.

Storms, M. D. (1981) A theory of erotic orientation development. *Psychological Review, 88*, 340–353.

Taylor, M. C. & Hall, J. A. (1982) Psychological androgyny: theories, methods and conclusions. *Psychological Bulletin, 92*, 347–366.

Thornton, B., Ryckman, M. & Robbins, M. A. (1982) The relationships of observer characteristics to beliefs in the causal responsibility of victims of sexual assault. *Human Relations, 35*, 321–330.

Tieger, T. (1981) Self-rated likelihood of raping and the social perception of rape. *Journal of Research in Personality, 15*, 147–158.

Van Wyk, P. H. & Geist, C. S. (1984) Psychosocial development of heterosexual, bisexual and homosexual behavior. *Archives of Sexual Behavior, 13*, 505–544.

Walfish, S. & Myerson, M. (1980) Sex role identity and attitudes toward sexuality. *Archives of Sexual Behavior, 9*, 199–203.

West, D. J., Roy, C. & Nichols, F. L. (1978) *Understanding sexual attacks.* London: Heinemann.

Whitam, F. L. (1977) Childhood indicators of male homosexuality. *Archives of Sexual Behavior, 6*, 89–96.

Whitam, F. L. & Zent, M. (1984) A cross-cultural assessment of early cross-gender behavior and familial factors in male homosexuality. *Archives of Sexual Behavior, 13*, 427–439.

Zellman, G. L. & Goodchilds, J. D. (1983) Becoming sexual in adolescence. *In* E. R. Allgeier & N. B. McCormick (eds) *Changing boundaries: gender roles and sexual behavior.* Palo Alto: Mayfield.

Zilbergeld, B. (1978) *Male sexuality: a guide to sexual fulfilment.* New York: Bantam.

Zuger, B. (1978) Effeminate behaviour present in boys from childhood: ten additional years of follow-up. *Comprehensive Psychiatry, 19*, 363–369.

CHAPTER FIFTEEN Sex Roles and Ageing
Ann Taylor

Theories of sex-role development in later life

There is a certain consensus of opinion concerning the course of sex-role development in late adulthood, although writers may vary considerably in the detail and the emphasis of their argument. When it comes to substantiating or disproving such opinion there is rather little firm data, although it is clear both that sex typing shows some variation through the life cycle and that there are apparent sex differences in later life, in personality and in adaptation to life events.

The consensus view appears to be that sex-appropriate behaviour (whether or not it is preprogrammed by genetic differences) is largely defined, and overwhelmingly reinforced, by parents, schools, peers, social and occupational constraints, and above all by the demands of parenting. The 'traditional' definition of sex-appropriate behaviour – of the man as active, aggressive, competitive and dominant and the woman as passive, nurturant and submissive – reflects the 'traditional' division of labour in the family, and particularly the (assumed) central importance of work and breadwinning for the man and of homemaking and child care for the woman. Socially sanctioned sex typing is thus most strongly in evidence in the parenting years: husbands are masculine, agentic (Bakan 1966) and instrumental (Spence & Helmreich 1978) while wives are feminine, communal and expressive. Events of later life, notably the 'empty nest' or launching of the youngest child from the home, retirement and bereavement, are such as to blur the breadwinner–homemaker distinction of earlier years, and it is commonly assumed therefore that sex typing diminishes in later life, such diminution being variously described as increased androgyny, increased frequency of combined sex roles, sex-role blurring (Sinnott 1977), sex-role transcendence (Hefner, Rebecca & Oleshansky 1975), sex-role reversal, and 'the normal unisex of later life' (Gutmann 1975).

The different terms indicate differences, at least of emphasis, concerning the characteristics and perhaps the timing of diminished sex typing. Gutmann (1975, 1977) emphasized parenting, above all, as the central motivator and shaper of human roles and attitudes, and argued that

traditional sex typing would decline after the end of active parenting —
that is, in middle age; the change, he held, is most marked for women,
who become 'domineering, independent and unsentimental' while men
become more passive, dependent, nurturant and emotional. In short,
Gutmann (1975) argued, there is sex-role reversal in that 'each sex
becomes to some degree what the other used to be' (p. 181); on the other
hand, his other famous phrase 'the normal unisex of later life' suggests
rather that men and women become alike, exhibiting both so-called
masculine and so-called feminine characteristics. The latter interpretation is also that of Sinnott (1977), who argued that normal and well-
adjusted men and women in later life tend to exhibit combined sex roles
(or sex-role blurring, or androgyny) in which activity and autonomy are
reconciled with the expression of dependence, nurturance and emotion.
Hefner, Rebecca and Oleshansky (1975) hypothesized that development
beyond sex typing is towards sex-role transcendence, or decreased sex-
role salience, rather than androgyny, which implies maintained salience,
but combination, of masculine and feminine orientations. They stated
explicity that transcendence is a desirable and adaptive stage for younger
as well as older adults, but one which many of them will not achieve: it
is less clear whether Sinnott regards androgyny as typical of, or merely
desirable in, old age.

Although Sinnott, like Gutmann, stresses the cessation of active
parenting as a trigger for the depolarization of sex roles, other events,
notably retirement, also receive consideration, and the emphasis is on
development in old, rather than middle, age. Nash and Feldman (1981)
also concluded that androgyny was triggered in 'grandparenthood' by a
release both from work pressures and from the demands of parenting.
The impact of retirement upon later-life development has received considerable attention. It has tended to be assumed that retirement is a
crucial event for men but a much less significant one for women, since
it marks an end to the identification of men as breadwinners but does not
substantially alter the domestic status of women. Retirement reduces
men's claims to possession of agency and dominance and at the same
time liberates them to develop generally domestic and affiliative attitudes
and behaviours. Thus one could hypothesize that retirement is the
principal stimulus for sex-role blurring in men, as the 'empty nest' is for
women.

It will be immediately noticeable that these analyses of sex-role
development implicitly assume a marriage with a single (male) breadwinner, and dependent wife and children, which is terminated by the

death of a partner in comparatively old age, as the defining context within which sex roles are acted out in adulthood. They thus largely exclude consideration of individuals who have never married, as well as other deviants from the 'normal' pattern such as the childless and those who were divorced, separated or widowed in early or middle adulthood. It is unclear how limiting these exclusions are for the generality of the theories advanced. Gutmann argues that sex typing is a product of innate sex-linked potentials, further structured by socialization and finally stamped in by the experience of parenthood. One might hypothesize that genetic potential and socialization would be enough, even in the absence of personal parenthood, to produce attitude and behaviour constellations in the unmarried and childless which correspond to sex-role norms. On the other hand such writers as Emmerich (1973) and Nash and Feldman (1981) stress the functional significance of sex typing as its chief determinant in the parenting stage: parents behave in sex-typed ways because sex typing is an efficient way of coping. Gutmann himself emphasizes the actual experience of parenthood as 'the ultimate source of the sense of meaning. For most adults the question 'What does life mean?' is automatically answered once they have children; better yet, it is no longer asked' (1975, p. 170). Gutmann's plausible description of active parenting as a stage of 'chronic emergency' tempts one to suggest that questions as to the meaning of life are no longer asked after the arrival of children not because parenthood has supplied a satisfactory answer but because parents no longer have time or energy to ask metaphysical questions. Unfortunately, although there are hints that never-married people in old age may be qualitatively different in certain respects from the married and the bereaved elderly (Gubrium 1975), evidence on sex typing in single and childless old people appears virtually non-existent; indeed such individuals tend to be specifically excluded from samples or, if they are included, form too small a subgroup for separate analysis.

By some criteria at least the traditional picture of role division in marriage is of limited validity even for the conventionally married; large numbers of wives, for example, have always worked outside the home, or within it in home-based industries, and even when they have not it is a mistake to regard the conventional role of 'wife and mother' as one characterized simply by nurturance, submissiveness and communion, since its efficient organization and execution require considerable 'instrumentality'. Even if the picture has been accurate, at least for the urban middle-class families who tend to dominate sex-role study samples, it is in many ways out of date for contemporary Western society, in which parenting ceases earlier than in preceding generations and in which growing numbers of women, including wives and mothers, are in paid employment (Hoffman 1977; Spence & Helmreich 1978). Hoffman (1977) has also reviewed evidence that the husbands of working wives are more likely to share housework and child care than are those of non-working wives, at least when family size and ages of children are matched for the two groups. She argues that the effect of these trends should be to reduce the polarizing effect of the 'parental imperative' and of parentally mediated socialization. McGee and Wells (1982), however, conclude that the depolarizing effect of work upon mothers is more evident than that of increased domestic participation upon fathers. Even when both partners work, and even when husbands 'help' more, the lion's share of housework and child care, and overall responsibility for them, are still undertaken by the wife. There is also some evidence that the husband's job is often regarded as more important than the wife's (probably largely reflecting the fact that men typically earn more than women). The extent of domestic task sharing also depends upon the status of the wife's employment: job or career, and the money it brings in (Bird, Bird & Scruggs 1984; Maret & Finlay 1984). By some definitions, therefore, traditional sex typing in the family, if weakening, is far from defunct.

The adaptive significance of adult sex-role development

For some writers, notably Gutmann, the implication is clear that during early adult years, and particularly during active parenting, traditional sex typing is adaptive, but that it becomes less so, and androgyny more so, in older age. Emmerich (1973) and Nash and Feldman (1981) also argued that life-cycle fluctuations in sex typing are functional responses to differing demands at different life stages: thus sex typing is adaptive in the parental stage and androgyny more adaptive in postparental and, in particular, in postretirement stages. Sinnott (1977) claimed further that sex-role flexibility represents a general and enduring trait of flexibility which enables its possessor to adapt successfully to changing life circumstances; thus the flexible person will be appropriately sex-typed at some life stages and androgynous at others. Androgyny is particularly adaptive for the elderly because the work and family responsibilities which justify sex typing have been largely removed and also because integration of distinct and complementary aspects of the personality – for example, the agentic and the communal – is seen as a fundamental developmental task for mature persons (Sinnott 1982).

Others, notably Bem (1975), have argued that younger adults are pressured by socialization into constricting sex roles which are more adverse than favourable in their effects upon individual well-being. According to this view it is androgynous individuals at all ages who have a behavioural flexibility and an independence of belief and attitude which enable them to adopt socially desirable and individually rewarding behaviour patterns of either or both sexes. The implication for ageing is that androgynous individuals are better equipped to cope with the blurring of sex-role expectations, lessening of opportunity for certain sex-linked behaviours and increased opportunities for others, which are likely to result from the life events of later adulthood. While predictions concerning the adaptiveness of androgyny may thus differ for the two positions outlined, they agree on the desirability of androgyny in the elderly.

A third view is that traditional sex roles are, on the whole, advantageous for men but disadvantageous for women; as Hefner, Rebecca and Oleshansky (1975) put it, 'both men and women are trapped in the prison of gender ... but the situation is far from symmetrical: men are the oppressors and women are the oppressed' (p. 144). There is a considerable accumulation of evidence, summarized by Taylor and Hall (1982), that psychological well-being (measured in various studies by such factors as self-esteem, adjustment and relative absence of anxiety, depression and psychosomatic symptoms) is generally more strongly related to masculinity than to femininity on such measures as the Bem Sex Role Inventory (BSRI) and appears not to distinguish reliably between sex-typed and balanced, or androgynous, individuals.

In spite of often-reported social 'punishment' for cross-sex behaviour, masculinity seems to be as advantageous to women as it is to men. There seems little reason to predict that the virtues of masculinity would be less for elderly than for younger adults, except on two possible counts: role integration may be an important and fulfilling task in late life, as Sinnott suggests, even if it is not so at earlier ages, and the behavioural correlates of masculinity may be more difficult to achieve and therefore more problematic for older people. Apart from such reservations, the prediction for ageing would be that increased androgyny and diminished sex typing are adaptive for older women but irrelevant to well-being for older men, as long as androgyny is taken to mean relatively high scores on both masculinity and femininity measures rather than a balance of scores which might be high or low.

Sex differences in life satisfaction

The notion that 'it pays to be masculine' receives some support from studies of sex differences in life satisfaction. Elderly men have often been found to have higher morale and lower incidence of mental disorder than elderly women (e.g. Atchley 1976; Gove & Tudor 1973; Spreitzer & Snyder 1974), and it has been argued that these sex differences reflect particular problems of ageing for women. These include the greater likelihood of widowhood (since women are typically younger than their husbands, live longer than men, and are less likely to remarry) and of low income in late life, and also the prevalence of ageism which may well be exacerbated for women, not least because of the greater premium placed upon physical attractiveness in women than in men (Sontag 1972). The stereotype of the old woman is not an attractive one in our society: old women tend to be more denigrated than old men in everyday language, for example, in humour (Palmore 1971). There are few socially valued roles for older women which would serve to enhance their status and self-esteem (Bart 1969).

On the other hand, while women fare less well than men in old age by some criteria, by others they fare better. Their physical health may be better (although the evidence is complex (Verbrugge 1976)), longevity is greater, and adaptation to life events appears more satisfactory. For example, when baseline sex differences are controlled, widows appear to suffer less depression than widowers and are less likely to suffer physical illness and to die shortly after bereavement (Rowland 1977; Stroebe & Stroebe 1983). This has lent support to the argument that women may be better, rather than worse, equipped to cope with the 'crises' of late life. Kline (1975), for example, argued that the life cycle of women is characterized by 'role inconstancy' – fluctuations in the onset, cessation and relative priorities of the roles of worker, housewife and mother – and that the experience of inconstancy facilitates adjustment to old age. Heyman (1970) and Lopata (1966) similarly argued that retirement is less critical for women than for men because employment is less 'central' for them, because they have other, concurrent roles and because they have had more experience of change and, in a sense, of retirement from work on marriage or on having children, and from parenting when the children leave home.

However, Atchley (1976) and Gratton and Haug (1983) found no sex differences in adjustment to retirement (which is not necessarily a traumatic event for either sex), although there may be differences between the sexes in factors influencing the decision to retire when retirement is not mandatory (George, Fillenbaum & Palmore 1984; Gratton & Haug 1983). Troll and Turner (1979) concluded that men and women are more or less equally advantaged and disadvantaged in dealing with the problems of ageing although the nature of the advantage or disadvantage may differ; and Liang (1982) and Collette (1984) demonstrated that sex differences in life satisfaction are principally to be attributed to differences between the sexes in income, socioeconomic status, health and social integration. It is also worth noting that the lower morale and greater depression reported by women applies most clearly to married women compared to married men; single or divorced women have been found to be higher in morale and lower in mental illness rates than their male counterparts (Gove & Tudor 1973; Rubinstein 1971). The moral might be that for maximal mental health all men should marry, and stay married, while women should stay single; this conclusion is in line with the view that marriage is good for men but bad for women (Bernard 1973), but poses something of a problem for social engineering.

It seems probable that any overall sex differences in adaptation and development in later life are dwarfed by individual differences, for instance in self-definition and in the respective values placed by women upon paid employment, child care and housework within the home. In such individual differences, moreover, it is highly likely that generational differences and secular trends contribute substantially to any observed relationship. More specifically, sex typing, rather than biological sex *per se*, might be expected in principle to offer better predictions of degree and mode of adaptation in old age.

Empirical studies of sex typing in later life

Evidence concerning the incidence of sex typing and androgyny in older adults and their relation to measures of adaptation and well-being is scanty, diverse and sometimes conflicting. Its diversity reflects the fact that the definition of sex-role blurring or reversal is not self-evident. It may refer to indulgence in sex-appropriate or sex-inappropriate behaviour; to the nature of beliefs and attitudes about appropriate behaviour in others; to one's self-concept, or self-identification, as male or female; or to the possession of 'masculine' or 'feminine' personality traits. Different studies tap different aspects of sex typing, and may confound two or more of them; further, different aspects may not be reliably correlated. To some extent, therefore, different measures of sex typing have to be considered separately and findings based on the use of different measures compared only cautiously.

The first support for hypotheses of increased androgyny in late life came from studies, several of them cross-cultural, employing the Thematic Apperception Test (TAT), Rorschach and other projective test data, sometimes supplemented by interview material: for reviews, see, for example, Gutmann (1975), Neugarten (1964, 1968), and Sinnott (1982). The classic study in this area was that of Neugarten and Gutmann (1958), who obtained TAT protocols from men and women aged between forty and seventy for an adapted stimulus picture showing four protagonists – young man, young woman, old man, old woman – in what was almost universally interpreted as a family group. There were both sex and age differences in responses: in particular, with increasing age of respondents the old man and old woman tended to reverse roles with respect to authority in the family. For 40–54-year-olds the old man was usually seen as the authority figure and the old woman either as submissive or as aggressive but controlled by the old man; for 55–60-year-olds the old woman was authoritative (either benignly or with hostile self-assertion), and the old man passive. Neugarten and Gutmann (1958) related these age differences to personality modifications with age, women becoming more tolerant of their own aggression and egocentrism and men of their own nurturant and affiliative impulses. Additional evidence suggested that such sex-role convergence, or at least general characteristics of integration to which it was held to be related, were associated with normal health rather than senility (Ames *et al.* 1954), to 'successful' ageing in terms of life satisfaction and adaptation to retirement (Neugarten 1964; Reichard, Livson & Peterson 1962) and indeed to longevity (Jewett 1973). However, the validation and interpretation of projective test data are uncertain in this context, as in others (McGee & Wells 1982), and it is unwise to accept these conclusions without considering evidence from other, more objective (though not necessarily more valid) measures.

The BSRI is a popular measuring instrument for the study of androgyny and sex typing, but has not been frequently used with older adult age groups. Feldman and Nash (1979), in an investigation of age and sex differences in responsiveness to babies, reported that grandfathers of infants had higher femininity scores (but not lower masculinity scores) than younger 'empty nest' fathers – that is fathers whose children had left home; grandmothers had higher masculinity scores (but not lower femininity scores) than 'empty nest' mothers. Feldman, Biringen and Nash (1981) obtained BSRI scores from subjects in eight stages of life, ranging from adolescents to grandparents, and found that grandparents were more 'cross sex typed' than other groups, grandmothers appearing as more autonomous than younger women and grandfathers as more compassionate and tender than younger men; but sex-typed traits were also elevated, with grandmothers also rating themselves comparatively high on compassion and tenderness and grandfathers rating themselves high on self-ascribed masculinity and, to a less extent, on autonomy. However, in both studies the absolute age differences between grandparents and members of younger but adjacent groups – 'mature parents' and 'empty-nesters' – were not considerable. Feldman, Biringen and Nash (1981) were able to hold age constant while varying stage, by comparing fifty-year-olds in each of the three groups quoted, and found that differences between stages were analogous to those between age/stage groups overall. Thus they argue that, at least to some extent, age effects are stage-of-life effects.

Hyde and Phillis (1979) administered the BSRI to individuals aged between thirteen and eighty-five, while Sinnott (1982) tested a large sample of 60–90-year-olds, comparing their scores with those of younger subjects reported by Bem (1974) and by Hoffman and Fidell (1979). Both studies found some evidence of diminished sex typing in older men, who were more likely to be androgynous, less masculine and more feminine than younger men. Older women, however, were more sex-typed rather than less: more older women than younger women were feminine and fewer were masculine. Hyde and Phillis (1979) found that only 14 percent of older women were non-polarized (androgynous or undifferentiated) compared to 65 percent of older men; Sinnott found no sex difference in non-polarization (about 63 percent of her elderly sample), but when women were polarized they were more likely than men to be so along traditional lines. Sinnott also found that androgyny was generally associated with better physical and mental health (based chiefly on self-report) and undifferentiation and femininity with poor mental health and depression, but also with low income, which can be seen as a confounding factor. Masculine individuals were distinct from the rest chiefly on the basis of high income, but masculinity scale scores overall were associated with good mental health.

It would be unwise to take these findings as evidence of genuine asymmetry in the sex role development of men and women in later life. In any cross-sectional study – that is one in which individuals of different ages are compared at the same point in time – age differences are inevitably confounded with cohort differences: older and younger groups differ not only in age but also in the historical, social and cultural era into which they were born. The early socialization experiences of now elderly people were almost certainly more 'traditional' with respect to sex-appropriate behaviour and attitudes than those of later cohorts. Sinnott suggests that greater femininity in older women reflects principally cohort differences, and that longitudinal investigation, in which the same individuals are studied over time, might well reveal increased androgyny in women from a much more strongly polarized baseline in youth. Further, Hyde and Phillis (1979) argued that masculinity items on the BSRI are related to 'youthful' traits, such as ambition and athleticism, which it would be difficult for women to acquire as they grow older, whereas femininity items reflect activities and attitudes, such as gentleness and love for children, which can feasibly be adopted or strengthened by the elderly, whether men or women. The finding of Feldman, Biringen and Nash (1981) that grandfathers rated themselves higher in masculinity than did younger men, is not irreconcilable with this argument; their grandfathers were comparatively young (mean age fifty-eight) and were also a highly selected group since only about 50 percent of these approached, as opposed to 80–90 percent of other groups, agreed to complete the questionnaire. It is also important that the subjects used by Feldman and her associates were middle-class, white and 'intactly married' while those of Sinnott were roughly comparable with US census data for the national older adult population, and thus included black as well as white individuals, some of whom were single, separated, divorced or widowed and for many of whom income and education level were comparatively low (information is incomplete for the Hyde and Phillis sample). Inconsistency in the nature of sex-role blurring shown by these studies, particularly with respect to masculinity scores, may well be explained at least in part by such sampling considerations.

Additional evidence comes from studies examining age differences in sex-role stereotypes, often within the context of marital relations. For example, Markides and Vernon (1984) asked subjects from three-generation Mexican American families (with median ages for successive generation subjects of twenty-six, forty-five and seventy-four) to rate statements concerning male dominance and female submissiveness within marriage, and women's participation in community and political affairs; they also completed indices of life satisfaction and depression. Women were found to be less traditionally oriented than men, most markedly in middle and younger generations, and sex-role orientation was more traditional in the oldest than in younger groups. There was thus no evidence for increased flexibility in older age, but age and cohort were of course confounded. For the oldest women, but not for the rest, traditional orientation was positively related to depression; for the oldest men there was no relation between orientation and depression or life satisfaction when income, marital status and education were controlled, although for younger men traditional orientation was negatively associated with well-being.

The confounding of age with cohort was avoided by Holahan (1984), who obtained longitudinal data on marital attitudes, particularly with reference to sex equality within the family, by retesting men and women who had been tested forty years earlier, at the median age of thirty, as part of the Terman Study of the Gifted (Terman & Oden 1947). She also tested a contemporary group of married thirty-year-old graduates to provide evidence of cohort effects. Longitudinal comparison showed that members of the retested group were more egalitarian at age seventy than they had been at age thirty, and that the change was particularly marked for women, with the exception that men changed more in the direction of agreement that 'spouses should express their love for each other in words' (although to a level of agreement still below that of women). Cohort comparisons of thirty-year-olds in 1940 with thirty-year-olds in 1981 yielded similar evidence of increased liberalization of attitude between earlier and later cohorts; women were again more egalitarian than men, but more uniformly so in the earlier than in the later cohort.

From these findings one might conclude that women become more instrumental and assertive, and men more expressive, as they age, and so become less sex-typed. However, both longitudinal and cohort comparisons are affected by secular, or time-of-testing, changes; where longitudinal and cohort differences are more or less identical it is difficult to assert that individuals become less traditionally sex-typed with age, independently of changes in contemporary attitudes accompanying their ageing. Holahan found that in one or two cases longitudinal changes were greater than cohort differences, suggesting that there is age-related change over and above adaptation to historical trends. Longitudinal trends were generally equivalent to cohort differences in the case of women but smaller in the case of men, and Holahan (1984) concluded that women appear to be more responsive to social change. It is not clear how far the intellectually gifted nature of her samples should limit generalization of her findings; nor it it easy to predict what age changes would be likely to occur over periods characterized by secular change towards decreased, rather than increased, sexual egalitarianism. Would individuals tested over time become more sex-typed, rather than less, with age, and would the effect be greater, or smaller, for women?

Other work on sex-role stereotypes has compared descriptions of 'ideal females' and 'ideal males' (Urberg 1979) or rated comparisons of young, middle-aged and older generations with respect to masculinity and femininity (Cameron 1976). Urberg found no difference in degree of stereotyping of 'ideal' descriptions between adults aged 25–40 and those aged 50–65. Cameron asked young, middle-aged and old subjects (mean ages twenty-one, forty-eight and seventy years respectively) to state which of 'the three age groups (young, middle-aged and old)' was most, and which least, masculine and which was most, and which least, feminine in overall personality style, possession of masculine (or feminine) interests and skills, and social pressure to do masculine (or feminine) sorts of things. For all age groups, the middle-aged generation was rated most masculine and also most feminine, and the old were rated least masculine and least feminine, in all respects (the young were in most respects rated similarly to the middle-aged). These findings are not too readily interpreted, since it is not clear whether subjects would naturally interpret their ratings as applying equally to both sexes (so that, for example, middle-aged people, whatever their sex, are seen as both more masculine and more feminine than members of other generations) or whether in practice they judged masculinity with respect to men and femininity with respect to women. If, as Cameron (1976) assumed, the former is the case, then subjects of all ages believe the middle-aged to be androgynous and the old undifferentiated; if the latter, they believe the middle-aged to be traditionally sex-typed and the old less so (either undifferentiated or cross-sex typed). However, subjects of all ages and both sexes rated themselves as above average in possession of their own gender characteristics – personality style, interests and skills – and below average in opposite gender characteristics, as compared to all others of their own sex. Thus, while some measures may indicate age-related differences in sex-role stereotypes and attitudes, self-identification as masculine or as feminine may well be strong, and constant, across the adult life-span.

Studies of overt behaviour which may be related to sex-typing are rare with respect to the elderly; one such is a study of responsiveness to babies, already mentioned, by Feldman and Nash (1979). They found that grandmothers of infants were more responsive to babies in a waiting-room situation, and showed more preference for pictures of babies in a picture viewing task, than mothers of adolescents or empty-nest mothers; a similar trend was observed for grandfathers, although different aspects of responsiveness were enhanced for the two sexes. Grandmothers were more responsive than grandfathers, while no sex differences appeared at earlier stages. These findings tend to support the suggestion of increased androgyny for older men but increased sex typing for older women, but as already reported, Feldman and Nash (1979) found BSRI scores indicating greater androgyny for both grandfathers and grandmothers. In fact, for their grandmothers, though not for grandfathers, recent exposure to babies was a better predictor of en-hanced responsiveness than were BSRI scores.

Finally, a number of studies have investigated husbands' participation in household tasks, generally by comparing preretirement and postretire-ment behaviour in elderly couples of whom the husband, but not the wife, has been in full-time employment. Generally the comparison made is between reports of current activity and retrospective reports of preretirement behaviour, obtained from already postretirement families. Lipman (1962), for example, reported that in a sample of 100 retired couples over 80 percent of wives reported that their husbands helped with the housework; he also found that his subjects emphasized love, understanding, companionship and compatibility as the most important qualities of a husband, or wife, over sixty years of age, and were less likely to cite the instrumental qualities of the good provider (for husbands) or the good housewife (for wives). He concluded that 'role differentiation by sex is reduced with increased age and retirement' (p. 484), but reported no evidence concerning the extent to which sharing of household tasks had increased from the preretirement period. Fur-ther, domestic-task sharing was highly selective. More than 75 percent of wives reported that their husbands took over or helped with 'garbage and trash' management and with grocery shopping; 50 percent were said to clear the table, wipe the dishes and pick up and put away clothes, but fewer would wash dishes, make breakfast, lay the table, hang out the washing, clean or dust, and fewer than 25 percent would make the beds or do the laundry. Similar non-random participation was reported by Ballweg (1967), although he also reported that retirees did take over more tasks than non-retired husbands of similar age. However, Keating and Cole (1980) reported no significant increase in household task par-ticipation by husbands, or in role interchangeability between husbands and wives with respect to housework, following retirement. In fact housework increased for wives following their husbands' retirement, both because there was more to do and because wives felt less freedom to schedule the work to suit themselves and more responsibility to make time available for responsiveness and support for their husbands and their involvement in social activities. It is worth noting that wives expressed considerable satisfaction with the postretirement stage in spite of its extra burdens, but that the extra attentiveness to their husbands' needs which wives reported was not always observed, or appreciated, by the husbands themselves.

Conclusion

From the diverse studies reviewed here it is possible to conclude tentatively that there is diminished sex typing in old age. It emerges in projective-test data and in longitudinal studies of marital attitudes, though not when cross-sectional designs, confounding age with birth cohort and early socialization, are employed; cross-sectional studies using the BSRI find reduced typing in men, though not reliably in women. Decreased sex typing may also occur for men in responsiveness to babies and in housework sharing, though evidence for the latter is strictly limited. Older women appear more sex-typed than men when the BSRI is used (perhaps because of scale limitations and cohort effects) but more egalitarian when marital attitudes are examined, even in cross-sectional studies. What evidence there is, from cross-sectional studies of the BSRI, marital attitudes and projective tests, suggests that lessened sex typing is positively associated with good mental and physical health and morale, with the important exception that a non-traditional orientation in marital relations seems not to be serviceable for older men.

Sinnott's (1982) BSRI data further indicate that, as with younger adults (Taylor & Hall 1982), masculinity may contribute substantially to well-being in elderly men and women, and that there is little to choose between the advantages of masculinity and those of androgyny.

However, changes in sex typing are not always substantial, and appear to depend upon the age of the elderly population and to be associated with other characteristics, such as income, educational and occupational level, health and marital status, which have been shown to underlie sex differences in psychological well-being and which also tend to differentiate elderly from younger adult samples. The rather disparate patterns of development in men and women with respect to sex typing require further exploration, and might be related to more general studies of personality development which suggest that different typologies or life-cycle accounts are needed to describe men and women (e.g. Lowenthal, Thurnher & Chiriboga 1975; Maas & Kuypers 1974).

Age-related changes in traditionally sex-linked behaviour, marital attitudes and stereotypes of sex-appropriate behaviour in others do not necessarily indicate fundamental changes in underlying personality traits, and may be more likely to reflect changes in the climate of opinion of the society and in the life circumstances of the individual. Sinnott's (1977) description of fluctuations in sex typing in terms of an adaptive, and enduring, trait of flexibility is of course consistent with this view. Neugarten (1964, 1977) concluded that with the exception of a tendency to increased introversion there is no consistent evidence that personality changes with advancing age; rather, enduring personality traits become more overt and more salient, so that people become 'more like themselves'. Other studies too have found stability rather than change to characterize ageing populations when cohort and secular effects are controlled (e.g. Schaie & Parham 1976). Even such frequently reported tendencies as greater dominance in women and greater passivity in men can to some extent be accounted for not by a hypothesis of personality change but by the simpler observation that in elderly couples the wife is typically younger, and probably in better health, than the husband.

Little evidence exists on the relation between sex typing and specific adjustments to, say, retirement and bereavement, and there is an urgent need for longitudinal studies in conjunction with successive-cohort comparisons to supplement the evidence gained from methodologically problematic cross-sectional studies. Finally, both conceptual and empirical analyses are needed to clarify the likely impact of secular changes upon sex-role development in men and women. Although the women's liberation movement, for example, appears not to be concerned with older women (Lewis & Butler 1972) there is no reason to suppose that older women, and indeed older men, cannot or will not be influenced by its arguments. Will such demographic trends as early retirement, high unemployment, women's work involvement and proportionately increasing numbers of elderly people, and such ideological developments as greater acceptance of at least a compromise feminism and the devaluation of the 'work ethic', radically change the nature of lifespan sex-role development? Or will innate potentials and the parental imperative ensure consistent differences in 'masculinity' and 'femininity' between the sexes, and comparable life-cycle fluctuations in their extent and nature, over succeeding cohorts? The data which will enable us to answer these questions, for the most part, have still to be collected.

References

Ames, L. B., Learned, J., Metraux, R. & Walker, R. (1954) *Rorschach responses in old age.* New York: Hoeber.

Atchley, R. (1976) Selected social and psychological differences between men and women in later life. *Journal of Gerontology, 31*, 204–211.

Bakan, D. (1966) *The duality of human existence.* Chicago: Rand McNally.

Ballweg, J. A. (1967) Resolution of conjugal role adjustment after retirement. *Journal of Marriage and the Family, 29*, 277–281.

Bart, P. (1969) Why women's status changes in middle age: the turns of the social ferris wheel. *Sociology Symposium, 3*, 1–18.

Bem, S. L. (1974) Measurement of psychological androgyny. *Journal of Consulting and Clinical Psychology, 42*, 155–162.

Bem, S. L. (1975) Sex-role adaptability: one consequence of psychological androgyny. *Journal of Personality & Social Psychology, 31*, 634–643.

Bernard, J. (1973) *The future of marriage.* New York: World Press.

Bird, G. W., Bird, G. A. & Scruggs, M. (1984) Determinants of family task sharing: a study of husbands and wives. *Journal of Marriage and the Family, 46*, 345–355.

Cameron, P. (1976) Masculinity/femininity of the generations: as self-reported and as stereotypically appraised. *International Journal of Aging and Human Development, 7*, 143–151.

Collette, J. (1984) Sex differences in life satisfaction: Australian data. *Journal of Gerontology, 39*, 243–245.

Emmerich, W. (1973) Socialization and sex-role development. *In* P. Baltes & K. W. Schaie (eds) *Life-span developmental psychology: personality and socialization.* New York: Academic Press.

Feldman, S. S., Biringen, Z. C. & Nash, S. C. (1981) Fluctuations of sex-related self-attributions as a function of stage of family life-cycle. *Developmental Psychology, 17*, 24–35.

Feldman, S. S. & Nash, S. C. (1979) Sex differences in responsiveness to babies among mature adults. *Developmental Psychology, 15*, 430–436.

George, L. K., Fillenbaum, G. G. & Palmore, E. (1984) Sex differences in the antecedents and consequences of retirement. *Journal of Gerontology, 39*, 364–371.

Gove, W. R. & Tudor, J. (1973) Adult sex roles and mental illness. *American Journal of Sociology, 78*, 812–835.

Gratton, B. & Haug, M. R. (1983) Decision and adaptation: research on female retirement. *Research on Aging, 5*, 59–76.

Gubrium, J. F. (1975) Being single in old age. *International Journal of Aging and Human Development, 6*, 29–41.

Gutmann, D. (1975) Parenthood: key to the comparative psychology of the life cycle? *In* N. Datan & L. Ginsberg (eds) *Life span developmental psychology.* New York: Academic Press.

Gutmann, D. (1977) The cross-cultural perspective: notes toward a comparative psychology of aging. *In* J. E. Birren & K. W. Schaie (eds) *Handbook of the psychology of aging.* New York: Van Nostrand.

Hefner, R., Rebecca, M. & Oleshansky, B. (1975) Development of sex-role transcendence. *Human Development*, *18*, 143–158.

Heyman, D. K. (1970) Does a wife retire? *Gerontologist*, *10*, 54–56.

Hoffman, D. M. & Fidell, L. S. (1979) Characteristics of androgynous, undifferentiated, masculine, and feminine middle-class women. *Sex Roles*, *5*, 765–781.

Hoffman, L. W. (1977) Changes in family roles, socialization and sex differences. *American Psychologist*, *32*, 644–657.

Holahan, C. K. (1984) Marital attitudes over 40 years: a longitudinal and cohort analysis. *Journal of Gerontology*, *39*, 49–57.

Hyde, J. S. & Phillis, D. E. (1979) Androgyny across the life span. *Developmental Psychology*, *15*, 334–336.

Jewett, S. (1973) Longevity and the longevity syndrome. *Gerontologist*, *13*, 91–99.

Keating, N. C. & Cole, P. (1980) What do I do with him 24 hrs a day? Changes in the housewife role after retirement. *Gerontologist*, *20*, 84–89.

Kline, C. (1975) The socialization process of women. Implications for a theory of successful aging. *Gerontologist*, *15*, 486–492.

Lewis, M. I. & Butler, R. N. (1972) Why is women's lib ignoring old women? *Aging and Human Development*, *3*, 223–231.

Liang, J. (1982) Sex differences in life satisfaction among the elderly. *Journal of Gerontology*, *37*, 100–108.

Lipman, A. (1962) Role conceptions of couples in retirement. *In* C. Tibbitts & W. Donahue (eds) *Social and psychological aspects of aging*. New York: Columbia University Press.

Lopata, H. Z. (1966) The life cycle of the social role of housewife. *Sociology and Social Research*, *51*, 5–22.

Lowenthal, M. F., Thurnher, M. & Chiriboga, D. (1975) *Four stages of life: a comparative study of women and men facing transition*. San Francisco: Jossey-Bass.

Maas, H. S. & Kuypers, J. A. (1974) From thirty to seventy. San Francisco: Jossey-Bass.

McGee, J. & Wells, K. (1982) Gender typing and androgyny in later life: new directions for theory and research. *Human Development*, *25*, 116–139.

Maret, E. & Finlay, B. (1984) The distribution of household labor among women in dual-earner families. *Journal of Marriage and the Family*, *46*, 357–364.

Markides, K. S. & Vernon, S. W. (1984) Aging, sex-role orientation, and adjustment: a three-generations study of Mexican Americans. *Journal of Gerontology*, *39*, 586–591.

Nash, S. C. & Feldman, S. S. (1981) Sex-role and sex-related attributions: constancy and change across the family life cycle. *In* M. E. Lamb & A. L. Brown (eds) *Advances in developmental psychology*, vol. 1. Hillsdale, NJ: Erlbaum.

Neugarten, B. L. and associates (1964) *Personality in middle and late life*. New York: Atherton.

Neugarten, B. L. (1968) *Middle age and aging*. Chicago, IL: University of Chicago Press.

Neugarten, B. L. (1977) Personality and aging. *In* J. E. Birren & K. W. Schaie (eds) *Handbook of the psychology of aging*. New York: Van Nostrand.

Neugarten, B. L. & Gutmann, D. (1958) Age-sex roles and personality in middle age: a thematic apperception study. *Psychological Monographs*, 72 (17, whole no. 470).

Palmore, E. (1971) Attitudes toward aging as shown by humor. *Gerontologist*, *11*, 181–186.

Reichard, S., Livson, F. & Peterson, P. G. (1962) *Aging and personality*. New York: John Wiley.

Rowland, K. F. (1977) Environmental events predicting death for the elderly. *Psychological Bulletin*, *84*, 349–372.

Rubinstein, D. (1971) An examination of social participation found among a national sample of black and white elderly. *Aging and Human Development*, *2*, 172–188.

Schaie, K. W. & Parham, I. A. (1976) Stability of adult personality: fact or fable? *Journal of Personality and Social Psychology*, *34*, 146–158.

Sinnott, J. D. (1977) Sex role inconstancy, biology, and successful aging. A dialectical model. *Gerontologist*, *17*, 459–464.

Sinnott, J. D. (1982) Correlates of sex roles of older adults. *Journal of Gerontology*, *37*, 587–594.

Sontag, S. (1972) The double standard of aging. *Saturday Review*, *55*, 29–38.

Spence, J. T. & Helmreich, R. L. (1978) *Masculinity and femininity. Their psychological dimensions, correlates, and antecedents*. Austin, University of Texas Press.

Spreitzer, E. & Snyder, E. (1974) Correlates of life satisfaction among the aged. *Journal of Gerontology*, *29*, 454–458.

Stroebe, M. S. & Stroebe, W. (1983) Who suffers more? Sex differences in health risks of the widowed. *Psychological Bulletin*, *23*, 279–301.

Taylor, M. C. & Hall, J. A. (1982) Psychological androgyny: theories, methods and conclusions. *Psychological Bulletin*, *92*, 347–366.

Terman, L. M. & Oden, M. H. (1947) *The gifted child grows up. Genetic studies of genius*, vol. 4. Stanford, Stanford University Press.

Troll, L. E. & Turner, B. F. (1979) Sex differences in problems of aging. *In* E. S. Gomberg & V. Franks (eds) Gender and disordered behaviour: sex differences in psychopathology. New York: Brunner/Mazel.

Urberg, K. A. (1979) Sex role conceptualization in adolescents and adults. *Developmental Psychology*, *15*, 90–92.

Verbrugge, L. M. (1976) Females and illness: recent trends in sex differences in the United States. *Journal of Health and Social Behaviour*, *17*, 387–403.

Author Index

Subject Index